D1526798

Handbook of Experimental Pharmacology

Volume 183

Editor-in-Chief

K. Starke, Freiburg i. Br.

Stefan Bauer • Gunther Hartmann
Editors

Toll-Like Receptors (TLRs) and Innate Immunity

Contributors

S. Akira, A. Asea, W. Barchet, S. Bauer, C. Brikos, M. Gangloff, N.J. Gay, H.S. Goodridge, S. Hamm, G. Hartmann, H. Hochrein, V. Hornung, A. Krug, T. Müller, M. O'Keeffe, L.A.J. O'Neill, S. Pascolo, M. Schlee, D. Tormo, T. Tüting, S. Uematsu, D.M. Underhill, J. Wenzel

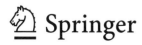 Springer

Prof. Dr. Stefan Bauer
Institut für Immunologie
BMFZ
Philipps-Universität Marburg
Hans-Meerwein-Str. 2
D-35043 Marburg, Germany
stefan.bauer@staff.uni-marburg.de

Prof. Dr. Gunther Hartmann
Abteilung für Klinische Pharmakologie
Universitätsklinikum Bonn
Sigmund-Freud-Str. 25
D-53105 Bonn, Germany
gunther.hartmann@ukb.uni-bonn.de

ISBN 978-3-540-72166-6   e-ISBN 978-3-540-72167-3

Handbook of Experimental Pharmacology ISSN 0171-2004

Library of Congress Control Number: 2007933837

Cover Design: WMXDesign GmbH, Heidelberg

Printed on acid-free paper

9 8 7 6 5 4 3 2 1

spinger.com

Preface

In the second half of the 20th century innate immune responses of cellular or humoral type were treated like stepchildren by many immunologists: that is, somewhat neglected. This disregard turned into an exciting research field over the past several years and led to the identification of receptor families involved in the recognition of microbes. This has resulted in a remarkable refinement of our understanding of innate immunity as it relates to host defense. Additionally, it has led to the appreciation of the role of the innate immunity in "guiding" the development of the adaptive immune system.

The Toll-like receptors represent an important family within the innate immune system. Originally identified in *Drosophila* as Toll receptors, various homologous Toll-like receptors (TLRs) have been identified in vertebrates. These receptors recognize chemically diverse ligands such as lipoproteins, proteins, lipopolysaccharides, nucleic acid, and nucleoside analogues and lead to the activation of immune cells. The mechanisms of TLR-driven cellular activation are quite well understood; however, information on the ligand-receptor interaction of the TLRs are scarce. A great body of evidence suggests that TLR ligands, especially nucleic acid and its analogues, have great pharmacological potential in the treatment of infectious diseases and cancer.

This book reviews and highlights our recent understanding on the function and ligands of TLRs, as well as their role in autoimmunity, dendritic cell activation and target structures for therapeutic intervention.

Overall, recent research on TLRs has led to tremendous increase in our understanding of early steps in pathogen recognition and will presumably lead to potent TLR-targeting therapeutics in the future.

Marburg, Germany
Bonn, Germany

Stefan Bauer
Gunther Hartmann

Contents

Contributors

Shizuo Akira
Department of Host Defense, Research Institute for Microbial Diseases,
Osaka University, 3-1 Yamada-oka, Suita Osaka 565-0851, Japan.
`sakira@biken.osaka-u.ac.jp`

Alexzander Asea
Division of Investigative Pathology, Scott & White Clinic and The Texas A&M
University System Health Science Center College of Medicine, 1901 South 1st
Street, Temple, TX 76508 USA. `aasea@swmail.sw.org`,
`asea@medicine.tamhsc.edu`

Winfried Barchet
Division of Clinical Pharmacology, University Hospital, University of Bonn, 53105
Bonn, Germany

Stefan Bauer
Institut für Immunology, Philipps-Universität Marburg, BMFZ, Hans-Meerweinstr.
2, 35043 Marburg. `stefan.bauer@staff.uni-marburg.de`

Constantinos Brikos
School of Biochemistry and Immunology, Trinity College Dublin, Dublin 2,
Ireland. `brikosc@tcd.ie`

Monique Gangloff
Department of Biochemistry, University of Cambridge, 80, Tennis Court Rd.,
Cambridge, CB2 1GA, UK. `mg308@mole.bio.cam.ac.uk`

Nicholas J. Gay
Department of Biochemistry, University of Cambridge, 80, Tennis Court Rd.,
Cambridge, CB2 1GA, UK. `njg11@mole.bio.cam.ac.uk`

Helen S. Goodridge
Immunobiology Research Institute, Cedars-Sinai Medical Center, 8700 Beverly
Blvd., Los Angeles, CA 90048, USA. helen.goodridge@cshs.org

Svetlana Hamm
4SC AG, Am Klopferspitz 19a, 82152 Martinsried, Germany

Gunther Hartmann
Division of Clinical Pharmacology, University Hospital, University of Bonn,
Sigmund-Freud-Str. 25, 53105 Bonn, Germany.
gunther.hartmann@ukb.uni-bonn.de

Hubertus Hochrein
Bavarian Nordic GmbH, Fraunhoferstrasse 13, D-82152 Martinsried, Germany.
hubertus.hochrein@bavarian-nordic.com

Veit Hornung
Division of Clinical Pharmacology, Department of Internal Medicine, University of
Munich, 80336 Munich, Germany

Anne Krug
II. Medizinische Klinik, Klinkum Rechts der Isar, Technische Universität München,
Trogersstraße 22, D-81675 München, Germany anne.krug@lrz.tum.de

Thomas Müller
Institut für Medizinische Mikrobiologie, Immunologie und Hygiene, Technische
Universität München, Trogerstrasse 30, 81675 München

Meredith O'Keeffe
Bavarian Nordic GmbH, Fraunhoferstrasse 13, D-82152 Martinsried, Germany.
meredith.okeeffe@bavarian-nordic.com

Luke A.J. O'Neill
School of Biochemistry and Immunology, Trinity College Dublin, Dublin 2,
Ireland. laoneill@tcd.ie

Steve Pascolo
Institut for Cell Biology, Department of Immunology, University
of Tuebingen, Auf der Morgenstelle 15, 72076 Tuebingen, Germany.
steve.pascolo@uni-tuebingen.de

Martin Schlee
Division of Clinical Pharmacology, University Hospital, University of Bonn, 53105
Bonn, Germany

Damia Tormo
Department of Dermatology, University of Bonn, Germany

Thomas Tüting
Department of Dermatology, University of Bonn, Sigmund-Freud-Strasse 25,
53105 Bonn, Germany. thomas.tueting@ukb.uni-bonn.de

Satoshi Uematsu
Department of Host Defense, Research Institute for Microbial Diseases,
Osaka University

David M. Underhill
Immunobiology Research Institute, Cedars-Sinai Medical Center, 8700 Beverly
Blvd., Los Angeles, CA 90048, USA. david.underhill@cshs.org

Joerg Wenzel
Department of Dermatology, University of Bonn, Germany

Toll-Like Receptors (TLRs) and Their Ligands

Satoshi Uematsu and Shizuo Akira(✉)

Abstract The innate immune system is an evolutionarily conserved host defense mechanism against pathogens. Innate immune responses are initiated by *pattern recognition receptors* (PRRs), which recognize microbial components that are essential for the survival of the microorganism. PRRs are germline-encoded, nonclonal, and expressed constitutively in the host. Different PRRs react with specific ligands and lead to distinct antipathogen responses. Among them, *Toll-like receptors* (TLRs) are capable of sensing organisms ranging from bacteria to fungi, protozoa, and viruses, and they play a major role in innate immunity. Here, we review the mechanism of pathogen recognition by TLRs.

1 Introduction

In mammals, host defenses sense pathogen invasion through PRRs. Toll-like receptors are evolutionarily conserved transmembrane proteins and play crucial roles as PRRs. Recent molecular biological studies have clarified the function of TLRs

Shizuo Akira
Department of Host Defense, Research Institute for Microbial Diseases, Osaka University, 3-1 Yamada-oka, Suita Osaka 565-0851, Japan
sakira@biken.osaka-u.ac.jp

S. Bauer, G. Hartmann (eds.), *Toll-Like Receptors (TLRs) and Innate Immunity.*
Handbook of Experimental Pharmacology 183.
© Springer-Verlag Berlin Heidelberg 2008

in microbial infection. TLRs recognize specific components of microorganisms, including fungi, protozoa, and viruses, and they induce innate immune responses. Here, we summarize the current knowledge regarding TLR family members and their ligands.

2 Innate Immunity

The mammalian immune system is divided into two types of immunity: *innate* and *adaptive*. Adaptive immunity is characterized by specificity and develops by clonal selection from a vast repertoire of lymphocytes bearing antigen-specific receptors that are generated by gene rearrangement. This mechanism allows the host to generate immunological memory. However, it takes time for specific clones to expand and differentiate into effector cells before they can serve for host defense. Therefore, the primary adaptive immune system cannot induce immediate responses to invasive pathogens. To induce immediate responses when it encounters a pathogen, a host is equipped with innate, nonadaptive defenses that form preemptive barriers against infectious diseases. Although the innate immune system was first described by Elie Metchnikoff over a century ago, it has long been ignored: viewed as merely a nonspecific response to simple phagocytose pathogens and as something that presents antigens to the cells involved in acquired immunity (Brown, 2001). However, in 1996, Hoffmann and colleagues demonstrated that the *Drosophila* protein Toll is required for flies to induce effective immune responses to *Aspergillus fumigatus* (Lemaitre et al., 1996). This study made us aware that the innate immune system functions as a pathogen detector. The targets of innate immune recognition are conserved molecular patterns of microorganisms. Therefore, the receptors involved in innate immunity are called pattern-recognition receptors (Medzhitov and Janeway, 1997). These molecular structures were originally called pathogen-associated molecular patterns (PAMPs). However, it is more appropriate to designate them as microorganism-associated molecular patterns (MAMPs) since they are found not only in pathogenic but also in nonpathogenic microorganisms. MAMPs are generated by microbes and not by the host, suggesting that MAMPs are good targets for innate immunity to discriminate between self and non-self. Furthermore, MAMPs are essential for microbial survival and are conserved structures among a given class, which allows innate immunity to respond to microorganisms with limited numbers of PRRs. There are many PRRs associated with opsonization, phagocytosis, complement and coagulation cascades, proinflammatory signaling pathways, apoptosis, and so on. Among them, Toll receptors and the associated signaling pathways represent the most ancient host defense mechanism found in insects, plants, and mammals (Akira, 2004). Studies of the fruit fly have shown that the Toll family is one of the most crucial signaling receptors in innate immunity.

2.1 Immune Responses in Drosophila

Insects do not have counterparts of mammalian B and T cells and cannot induce acquired immune responses based on producing antibodies to pathogenic organisms. Nonetheless, insects can recognize the invasion of various microorganisms and induce antimicrobial responses. Recent studies using a model organism, *Drosophila melanogaster*, have shown that the induction of antimicrobial peptides, which are important for survival after infection, depends on Toll and immune deficiency (Imd) signaling pathways (Tanji and Ip, 2005). A transmembrane protein, Toll, originally identified as an essential component in dorsal-ventral embryonic development (Wu and Anderson, 1997), is also involved in innate immune responses (Lemaitre et al., 1996). Gram-positive bacterial peptidoglycan might bind directly to extracellular peptidoglycan recognition protein (PGRP)-SD (Michel et al., 2001) and SD (Bischoff et al., 2004), which then stimulate the Toll pathway. Another pattern recognition protein, Gram-negative binding protein-1 (GNBP-1), is also involved in the recognition of Gram-positive bacteria (Gobert et al., 2003; Pili-Floury et al., 2004). Not only Gram-positive bacteria but also fungi stimulate the Toll pathway. Fungi are recognized by a serine protease, Persephone, and a protease inhibitor, Necrotic (Levashina et al., 1999; Ligoxygakis et al., 2002). All upstream cascades lead to the cleavage of pro-Spätzle to Spätzle, and the binding of proteolytically processed Spätzle to Toll induces the dimerization of Toll (Hu et al., 2004; Weber et al., 2003). After activation of Toll, the adapter proteins MyD88 and Tube, and a serine-threonine kinase, Pelle, are recruited to Toll (Sun et al., 2004). Then, activated Pelle acts on the Cactus, a Drosophila IκB. Dif and Dorsal are transcription factors of the Rel protein family and are retained in the cytoplasm by Cactus. By the stimulation of the Toll pathway, Cactus is degraded and Dorsal and Dif translocate into the nucleus, leading to the induction of antimicropeptides (Brennan and Anderson, 2004; Hoffmann, 2003; Hultmark, 2003).

The Imd pathway is responsible for the induction of antimicrobial peptides in response to Gram-negative bacteria (Brennan and Anderson, 2004; Hoffmann, 2003; Hultmark, 2003; Lemaitre, 2004). Imd is an adapter protein for this pathway (Georgel ct al., 2001). Recent reports show that PGRP-LC (Choe et al., 2002; Gottar et al., 2002) and PGRP-LE (Takehana et al., 2004), which have putative transmembrane domains, are the pattern recognition receptors in this pathway. There are at least three branches downstream of Imd (Brennan and Anderson, 2004; Hoffmann, 2003; Hultmark, 2003; Lemaitre, 2004). First is TAK1, which induces the proteolytic cleavage of IKK, followed by activation of the transcription factor, Relish (Lu et al., 2001; Rutschmann et al., 2000; Silverman et al., 2003; Silverman et al., 2000; Stoven et al., 2003; Vidal et al., 2001). Second is the FADD-Dredd pathway that also activates Relish (Balachandran et al., 2004; Chen et al., 1998; Elrod-Erickson et al., 2000; Georgel et al., 2001; Hu and Yang, 2000; Leulier et al., 2000; Leulier et al., 2002). Two new components, Sickie and Dnr-1, have been identified; whereas Sickie positively regulates the Relish activation by Dredd, Dnr-1 inhibits

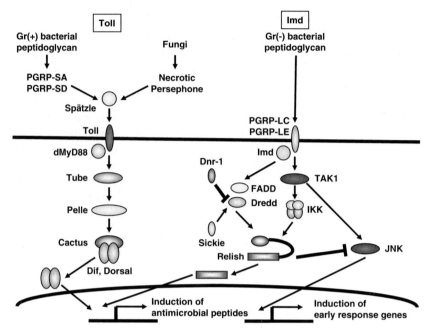

Fig. 1 Toll and Imd pathways in the *Drosophila* innate immune response. The Toll pathway mediates the response to fungal and Gr(+) bacterial infection, whereas the Imd pathway mediates the response to Gr(−) bacterial infection. These pathways are similar to the signaling pathway of the mammalian Toll-like receptor, and are essential for *Drosophila* to survive infection

this pathway (Foley and O'Farrell, 2004; Khush et al., 2002). Third is the JNK pathway that is activated through TAK1. The JNK pathway induces immediate early genes after septic shock, which is negatively regulated by Relish (Boutros et al., 2002; Park et al., 2004).

As stated above, recent genetic and genomic analyses of *D. melanogaster* have shown that insects have an evolutionarily primitive recognition and signaling system (Figure 1). Collectively, these analyses' results provide important insights into the mechanism of pathogen recognition and host responses in mammalian systems.

2.2 Toll-Like Receptors

A mammalian homologue of Toll receptor (now termed TLR4) was identified through database searches and shown to induce expression of the genes involved in inflammatory responses (Medzhitov et al., 1997). Subsequently, a mutation in the *tlr4* gene was identified in C3H/HeJ mice that were hyporesponsive to lipopolysaccharide (LPS) (Poltorak et al., 1998). TLR4-deficient mice confirmed LPS's essential role in the LPS recognition (Hoshino et al., 1999). So far, 13 mammalian members of the TLR family have been identified (Akira, 2004). TLRs are type I integral member glycoproteins characterized by a cytoplasmic signaling domain and extracellular domains. As the cytoplasmic domain of TLRs is similar to that of the interleukin (IL)-1 receptor family, it is called the Toll/IL-1 receptor (TIR) domain. However, the extracellular region of TLRs and IL-1R are markedly different: Whereas IL-1R possesses an Ig-like domain, TLRs contain leucine-rich repeats (LRR) (Akira, 2004). The LRR domains are composed of 19–25 tandem LRR motifs, each of which is 24–29 amino acids in length, containing the motif XLXXLXLXX as well as other conserved amino acid residues (XΦXXΦXXXXFXXLX; Φ = hydrophobic residue). Each LRR consists of a β-strand and an α-helix connected by loops. The LRR domain of TLRs was supposed to form a horseshoe structure with the ligand binding to the concave surface. However, the three-dimensional structure of the human TLR3 LRR motifs suggested that negatively charged dsRNA is more likely to bind to the outside convex surface of TLR3. It is uncertain whether this model fits the other TLR family members. Future crystallographic analysis of other TLRs will be necessary for elucidating the ligand/receptor binding mechanism.

The TLR family is an important group of receptors through which innate immunity recognizes invasive microorganisms. TLRs are key molecules for microbial elimination, such as the recruitment of phagocytes to infected tissues and subsequent microbial killing. Recent gene targeting studies have revealed that TLRs sense organisms ranging from bacteria to fungi, protozoa, and viruses (Tables 1–4).

Table 1 TLRs and bacterial ligands

Bacterial component	Species	TLR usage
LPS	Gram-negative bacteria	TLR4
Diacyl lipopeptides	*Mycoplasma*	TLR2/TLR6
Triacyl lipopeptides	Bacteria	TLR2/TLR1
Peptidoglycans	Gram-positive bacteria	TLR2(?)
Lipoteichoic acid	Gram-positive bacteria	TLR2/TLR6
Phenol-soluble modulin	*Staphylococcus aureus*	TLR2
Glycolipids	*Treponema maltophilum*	TLR2
Atypical LPS	Non-entero bacteria	TLR2(?)
Flagellin	Flagellated bacteria	TLR5
CpG DNA	Bacteria	TLR9
Not determined	Uropathogenic bacteria	TLR11

Table 2 TLRs and fungal ligands

Fugal component	Species	TLR usage
Zymosan	*Saccharomyces cerevisiae*	TLR2/TLR6
Mannan	*Saccharomyces cerevisiae* *Candida albicans*	TLR4
Phospholipomannan	*Candida alibicans*	TLR2
Glucuronoxylomannan	*Cryptococcus neoformans*	TLR4

Table 3 TLRs and protozoan ligands

Protozoan component	Species	TLR usage
(GPI anchors)		
GPI anchor	*Trypanosoma cruzi*	TLR2/TLR6
Glycoinositolphospholipids	*T. cruzi*	TLR4
LPG	*Leishmania major*	TLR2
Galbeta1, 4Manalpha-Po(4)- containing phosphoglycans	*Leishmania donovani*	TLR2
GPI anchor	*Plasmodium falciprum*	TLR2,TLR4
Native GPI anchors	*Toxoplasma gondii*	TLR2, TLR4
(Non-GPI anchors)		
Tc52	*Trypanosoma cruzi*	TLR2
Genomic DNA	*Babesia bovis,* *T. cruzi and T. brucei*	TLR9
Hemozoin	*P. falciparum*	TLR9
Profilin-like protein	*T. gondii*	TLR11

Table 4 TLRs and viral ligands

TLRs (localization)	Virus and components
(cell surface)	
TLR2	envelope proteins of Measles virus, human cytomegalovirus and herpes simplex virus type I
TLR4	F protein of respiratory syncytial virus (RSV) Envelope protein of mouse mammary tumor virus (MMTV)
(endosome)	
TLR3	Viral dsRNA, synthetic dsRNA (Poly(I:C))
TLR7/TLR8	ssRNA, synthetic imidazoquinoline derivatives (anti-viral drugs)
TLR9	CpG DNA

3 Pathogen Recognition by TLR

3.1 Bacteria

Lipopolysaccharide is a cell wall component of Gram-negative bacteria and a strong immunostimulant. As described above, TLR4 is essential for recognition of LPS, which is composed of lipid A (endotoxin), core oligosaccharide, and O-antigen. TLR4 recognizes lipid A of LPS. For LPS recognition, a complex formation of TLR4, MD2, and CD14 on various cells, such as macrophages and dendritic cells, is necessary (Shimazu et al., 1999). LPS is associated with an accessory protein, LPS-binding protein (LBP) in serum, which converts oligomeric micelles of LPS to monomers for delivery to CD14, which is a glycosyl phosphatidylinositol

(GPI)-anchored, high-affinity membrane protein. CD14 concentrates LPS for binding to the TLR4/MD2 complex (Takeda et al., 2003).

TLR2 recognizes various bacterial components, such as lipoproteins/lipopeptides and peptidoglycans from Gram-positive and Gram-negative bacteria, and lipoteichoic acid from Gram-positive bacteria, a phenol-soluble modulin from *Staphylococcus aureus*, and glycolipids from *Treponema maltophilum* (Takeda et al., 2003; Takeuchi et al., 1999a). TLR2 is also reported to be involved in the recognition of LPS from non-enterobacteria, including *Leptospira interrogans, Porphyromonas gingivalis*, and *Helicobacter pylori* (Takeda and Akira, 2005). These are atypical LPSs whose structures are different from typical LPSs of Gram-negative bacteria (Netea et al., 2002b). However, a recent report has indicated that lipoproteins contaminated in LPS preparation from *P. gingivalis* stimulated TLR2 and that LPS from *P. gingivalis* itself had poor TLR4 stimulation activity (Hashimoto et al., 2004). There are also controversial reports regarding peptidoglycan recognition by TLR2. Careful analyses are needed to ensure the exclusion of any possible contaminants.

TLR1 and TLR6 are structural relatives of TLR2 (Takeuchi et al., 1999b). TLR2 and TLR1 or TLR6 form a heterodimer that is involved in the discrimination of subtle changes in the lipid portion of lipoproteins. TLR6-deficient macrophages do not produce inflammatory cytokines in response to diacyl lipopeptides from mycoplasma; however, they normally produce inflammatory cytokines in response to triacyl lipopeptides derived from a variety of bacteria (Takeuchi et al., 2001). Contrarily, TLR1-deficient macrophages show normal responses to triacyl lipopeptides but not to diacyl lipopeptides (Alexopoulou et al., 2002; Takeuchi et al., 2002). These results suggest that TLR2 interacts not only physically but also functionally with TLR1 and TLR6.

CD36 is a member of the class II scavenger family of proteins. A recent report has shown that CD36 serves as a facilitator or co-receptor for diacyl lipopeptide recognition through the TLR2/6 complex (Hoebe et al., 2005).

Bacterial flagellin is a structural protein that forms the major portion of flagella that contribute to virulence through chemotaxis, adhesion to, and invasion of host surfaces. TLR5 is responsible for the recognition of flagellin (Hayashi et al., 2001; Uematsu et al., 2006). Unlike other TLRs, TLR5 is not expressed on conventional dendritic cells or macrophages in mice (Uematsu et al., 2006). Gewirtz et al. reported that TLR5 is expressed on the basolateral surface, but not the apical side of intestinal epithelial cells, suggesting that flagellin is detected when bacteria invade across the epithelium (Gewirtz et al., 2001). However, the expression of TLR5 in mouse intestinal epithelial cells is not high (Uematsu et al., 2006). By contrast, TLR5 is expressed mainly on intestinal CD11c[+] lamina propria cells (LPCs). CD11c[+] LPCs detected pathogenic bacteria and secreted proinflammatory cytokines in a TLR5-dependent way (Uematsu et al., 2006). A common stop codon polymorphism in the ligand-binding domain of TLR5 (TLR5 392STOP SNP) is unable to mediate flagellin signaling and is associated with susceptibility to pneumonia caused by *Legionella pneumophila* (Hawn et al., 2003). However, researchers in Vietnam reported that TLR5 392STOP SNP is not associated with susceptibility to typhoid fever (Dunstan et al., 2005). Although TLR5 initially induced host defenses against flagellated bacteria, TLR5-deficient mice were resistant to oral *Salmonella typhimurium* infection. The transport of *S. typhimurium* from the intestinal tract to the mesenteric lymph nodes (MLNs) was impaired in TLR5-deficient mice. These results suggest that *S. typhimurium* utilizes TLR5 on CD11c$^+$ LPCs for systemic infection (Uematsu et al., 2006). α and ε *Proteobacteria*, including *Helicobacter pylori* and *Campylobacter jejuni*, change the TLR5 recognition site of flagellin without losing flagellar motility (Andersen-Nissen et al., 2005). This modification may contribute to the persistence of these bacteria on mucosal surfaces.

Bacterial DNA is a potent stimulator of the host immune response. This immune stimulation is mediated by unmethylated CpG motifs. In vertebrates, the frequency of CpG motifs is severely reduced and the cytosine residues of CpG motifs are highly methylated, which leads to abrogation of the immunostimulatory activity. Analysis of TLR9-deficient mice showed that CpG DNA recognition is mediated by TLR9 (Hemmi et al., 2000).

Mouse TLR11, a relative of TLR5, is expressed abundantly in the kidney and bladder. TLR11-deficient mice are susceptible to uropathogenic bacterial infections, indicating that TLR11 senses the component of uropathogenic bacteria. However, the human *Tlr11* gene appears to contain a stop codon that would prevent expression of the protein (Zhang et al., 2004) (Table 1).

3.2 Fungi

TLRs have been implicated in the recognition of the fungal pathogens such as *Candida albicans, Aspergillus fumigatus, Cryptococcus neoformans* and *Pneumocystis carinii* (Netea et al., 2004; Takeda et al., 2003). Several components located in the cell wall or cell surface of fungi have been identified as potential ligands. Yeast zymosan, derived from *Saccharomyces cerevisiae*, activates TLR2/TLR6 heterodimers, whereas mannan, derived from *S. cerevisiae* and *C. albicans*, are detected by TLR4. TLR4-deficient mice show increased susceptibility to disseminated candidasis due to the decreased release of chemokines and the impaired recruitment of nutrophils to infected sites (Netca et al., 2002a).

Phospholipomannan, present on the cell surface of *C. albicans*, is also recognized by TLR2, while TLR4 mainly interacts with glucuronoxylomannan, the major capsular polysaccharide of *C. neoformans* (Netea et al., 2004).

Dectin-1 is a lectin family receptor for the fungal cell wall component, β-glucan, which is a major component of zymosan (Brown et al., 2002). Dectin-1 has been reported to functionally collaborate with TLR2 in response to yeast (Netea et al., 2004). The Dectin-1-mediated signaling pathway uses spleen tyrosine kinase (Syk), and interactions with Syk directly induce cellular responses such as the respiratory burst and IL-10 production. Destin-1 is also reported to collaborate with TLR2 and to induce proinflammatory responses such as the induction of TNF-α and IL-12 (Gantner et al., 2003; Rogers et al., 2005; Underhill et al., 2005). Gross et al. reported that Card9 is required to link Dectin-1/Syk activation to Bcl10-Malt1-dependent NF-kB activation by zymosan (Gross et al., 2006). Recently, two groups generated Dectin-1-deficient mice (Saijo et al., 2007; Torok et al., 2004). When stimulated with zymosan, IL-10 production was completely dependent on Dectin-1. However, TNF-α production was not impaired in Dectin-1-deficient mice but was dependent on TLR-mediated signaling pathway. When stimulated with purified β-glucan, both IL-10 and TNF-α production was dependent on Dectin-1, though the total amount of TNF-α production markedly decreased compared with zymosan stimulation. Thus, Dectin-1 is the sole receptor for β-glucan, and most inflammatory cytokine production by zymosan might be the result of TLR recognition of their ligands, except for β-glucan contained in zymosan (Saijo et al., 2007). Experimental infection models of disseminated candidasis in Dectin-1-deficient mice showed different phenotypes between the two research groups. Taylor et al. (2007) reported that Dectin-1-deficient mice were more susceptible to *C. albicans* infection than wild-type mice. These results were inconsistent with the study of Saijo et al. (2007), who found Dectin-1-deficient mice and wild-type mice equally susceptible to candida infection. Interestingly, Dectin-1-deficient mice were more susceptible than wild-type mice to pneumocystis infection (Saijo et al., 2007). Further study is obviously necessary to clarify the *in vivo* function of Dectin-1.

3.3 Protozoa

3.3.1 Protozoan GPI Anchors

Several studies have shown that glycosylphosphatidylinositol (GPI) anchors (or their fragments) from protozoan parasites activate cells of both lymphoid and myeloid lineages (Camargo et al., 1997; de Veer et al., 2003; Debierre-Grockiego et al., 2003; Magez et al., 1998; Schofield and Hackett, 1993). GPI moieties are abundantly expressed by many protozoan parasites and function as anchors to the surface of eukaryotic cells. GPI anchors consist of a glycan core and a lipid component. GPI anchors are featured with variations in the carbohydrate branches, the lipid inositol portion (glycerol versus ceramide), and the number, length, and degree of saturation in the hydrocarbon chains (Gazzinelli and Denkers, 2006). Although GPI anchors are expressed on mammarian cells, they do not initiate host immune responses. The expression levels of GPI anchors on mammarian cells are much lower than those of protozoan parasites. Moreover, the structure of protozoan-derived GPI anchors is different from mammarian-derived ones in the length of the glycan core and lipid component. All these differences may determine the activation of host immunity (Gazzinelli and Denkers, 2006).

TLRs sense GPI anchors of protozoa including *Trypanosoma cruzi, Leishmania* spp., *Toxoplasma gondii* and *Plasmodium falciparum. T. cruzi*-derived GPI anchors were shown to activate host cells through TLR2 (Campos et al., 2001). Also, recognition of the GPI anchors requires a host cell surface molecule, CD14, which is involved in the recognition of LPS by TLR4 (Campos et al., 2001). As mentioned earlier, TLR2 functionally associates with either TLR2 or TLR6. TLR6-deficient macrophages failed to respond to *T. cruzi* GPI anchors, suggesting that a complex of TLR2/TLR6/CD14 is involved in the recognition of these molecules (Ropert and Gazzinelli, 2004). Glycoinositolphospholipids, a subset of free GPI anchors of *T. cruzi*, also activated CHO cells transfected with TLRs. These molecules are recognized by TLR4 and CD14 but not TLR2 (Oliveira et al., 2004). Thus, *T. cruzi* contains two types of ligands that are recognized by TLR2/TLR6 or TLR4.

Leishmania major is an obligate intracellular eukaryotic pathogen of mononuclear phagocytes. Promastigotes invade target cells by receptor-mediated phagocytosis, transform into nonmotile amastigotes, and establish in the phagolysosome. Glycosylphosphatidylinositol-anchored lipophosphoglycan (LPG) is a virulence factor and a major parasite molecule involved in this internalization process. LPG from *L. major* has been shown to activate natural killer cells and macrophages through TLR2 (Becker et al., 2003; de Veer et al., 2003). In addition, *in vivo* studies in mice revealed an important role for TLR4 in the control of *L. major* infection, possibly through the regulation of inducible NO synthase expression. However, it is unclear which molecule of *L. major* is a ligand for TLR4 (Kropf et al., 2004). A recent study of RNA interference showed that TLR3 and TLR2 are involved in the secretion of NO and TNF-α induced by *L. donovani* promastigotes. TLR2-mediated responses are dependent on Galbeta1,4Manalpha-PO(4)-containing phosphoglycans, whereas TLR3-mediated responses are independent of these glycoconjugates. TLR2 and TLR3 participated in the phagocytosis of *L. donovani* promastigotes and TLR3 plays a role in the leishmanicidal activity of the IFN-γ-primed macrophages.

GPI anchors of *P. falciparum* are the major factors that contribute to malaria pathogenesis, doing so through their ability to induce proinflammatory responses. *P. falciparum* GPIs are structurally distinct from those of *T. cruzi*; the former contain a diacylated glycerol moiety and fatty acid acylation at C-2 of inositol, whereas the latter have sn-1-alkyl-sn-2-acylglycerol and lack inositol acylation (Channe Gowda, 2002; Gerold et al., 1994; Naik et al., 2000). The proinflammatory responses to *P. falciparum* GPIs by macrophages are mediated mainly through TLR2 and to a lesser but still significant extent also through TLR4. Interestingly, *P. falciparum* GPIs are degraded by macrophage surface phospholipase A2 and phospholipase D; in addition, intact GPIs and sn-2-lyso-GPIs are differentially recognized by TLR2/TLR1 and TLR2/TLR6 heterodimers (Krishnegowda et al., 2005).

Native GPI anchors purified from *Toxoplasma gondii* tachyzoites, as well as synthetic fragments of the proposed structure of these GPI anchors, activate NF-κB and induced TNF-α in a mouse macrophage cell line, and these responses also appeared mediated through TLR2 and TLR4 (Gazzinelli and Denkers, 2006).

3.3.2 Other Protozoan TLR Ligand

Other protozoan molecules also serve as important mediators of proinflammatory responses except for GPI anchors and their related molecules. The *T. cruzi*-released protein Tc52 contains a tandemly repeated structure characteristic of GSTs, notably of the θ group, and a set of small heat shock proteins, and it is a crucial factor for parasite survival and virulence. Tc52 also plays a central role in innate and adaptive immunity through TLR2 on human and murine dendritic cells (DCs) (Ouaissi et al., 2002).

TLR9, a receptor for unmethylated bacterial CpG DNA motifs, is also important for resistance to protozoan parasite infections. DNA from the protozoan parasites *Babesia bovis*, *T. cruzi*, and *T. brucei* activate macrophages and DCs, leading to the induction of inflammatory responses (Brown and Corral, 2002; Harris et al., 2006; Shoda et al., 2001). A recent study demonstrates that DNA from *T. cruzi* stimulates cytokine production by APCs in a TLR9-dependent manner. *T. cruzi*-infected TLR9-deficient mice show elevated parasitemia and decreased survival, suggesting that TLR9 plays a crucial role for the protection to *T. cruzi* infection (Bafica et al., 2006).

Plasmodium parasites within erythrocytes digest host hemoglobin into a hydrophobic heme polymer, known as hemozoin (HZ) (Arese and Schwarzer, 1997; Sullivan, 2002). Intracellular HZ is released into the bloodstream during schizont rupture and is phagocytosed by myeloid cells resulting in the concentration of HZ in the reticulo-endothelial system (Arese and Schwarzer, 1997). Several studies have shown that HZ purified from *P. falciparum* activates macrophages to produce proinflammatory cytokines, chemokines, and nitric oxide, and it enhances human myeloid DC maturation (Coban et al., 2002; Sherry et al., 1995). A recent report demonstrated that HZ purified from *P. falciparum* is a novel ligand for TLR9 (Coban et al., 2005). Synthetic HZ, which is free of the other contaminants, also activated innate immune responses *in vivo* in a TLR9-dependent manner (Coban et al., 2005). This work is interesting as it provides the first evidence of a non-DNA ligand as recognized by TLR9.

Cerebral malaria is a lethal complication of malaria caused by *P. falciparum* in humans. Besides the high mortality rates, persistent neurocognitive deficits after recovery have become an increasing concern (Aikawa, 1988; Idro et al., 2005; Miller et al., 2002). *Plasmodium berghei* ANKA (PbA) infection in mice is a good experimental model of cerebral malaria (CM) (Engwerda et al., 2005; Good et al., 2005; Schofield and Grau, 2005). Recently, the role of TLRs in the pathogenesis of cerebral malaria was investigated by using this PbA infection model. A significant number of MyD88 (myeloid differentiation primary response gene 88; adapter molecule of TLRs)-deficient mice compared with wild-type mice survived CM caused by PbA infection. Although systemic parasitemia was comparable, sequestration of parasite and HZ load in blood vessels in the brain was significantly lower in MyD88-deficient mice than wild-type mice. Furthermore, brain-specific pathological changes were associated with MyD88-dependent infiltration of CD8[+], CCR5[+] T cells, and CD11c[+] dendritic cells, including CD11c[+], NK1.1[+], and B220[+] cells, and up-regulation of genes such as Granzyme B, Lipocalin 2, Ccl3 and Ccr5. TLR2- and TLR9-deficient mice, but not TLR4-, TLR5-, and TLR7-deficient mice, have decreased susceptibility to cerebral malaria, suggesting that TLR2- and/or TLR9-mediated brain pathogenesis may play a critical role in CM, a lethal complication during PbA infection (Coban et al., 2007).

A profilin-like protein of *T. gondii* (PFTG) is a relatively conserved molecule in a number of apicomplexans. Profilins are small actin-binding proteins that in other eukaryotic cells regulate actin polymerization. Mammalian cell profilins also interact with a number of different proteins and regulate a variety of biological processes, such as membrane trafficking, receptor clustering, as well as small GT-Pase and phosphoinositide signaling pathways. Thus, profilins are thought to play critical roles in governing a number of motility-related functions for eukaryotic cells. Although PFTG is a phylogenetical relative of profilin, the profilins in apicomplexan parasites are quite distinct from those present in mammals, plants, and other microorganisms, including other protozoan species (Yarovinsky and Sher, 2006). The exact function of PFTG is unclear but it seems to be involved in parasite motility and invasion of host cells (Gazzinelli and Denkers, 2006). Murine TLR11 senses PFTG (Yarovinsky et al., 2005). TLR11-deficient mice showed increased susceptibility to infection of *T. gondii*, whose phenotype is associated with decreased IL-12 production *in vivo* (Yarovinsky et al., 2005). In addition, PFTG is an immunodominant protein in the CD4$^+$ T cell response to a soluble extract of the tachyzoite stage of the parasite as well as to live *T. gondii* infection. The immunodominance of PFTG depends on TLR11 both *in vivo* and *in vitro* (Yarovinsky et al., 2006). As TLR11 is non-functional in humans, it would seem that PFTG does not activate human DCs (Gazzinelli and Denkers, 2006).

3.4 Virus

3.4.1 Viral Protein

TLR4 recognizes not only bacterial components but also viral envelope proteins. The fusion (F) protein from respiratory syncytial virus (RSV) is sensed by TLR4 (Kurt-Jones et al., 2000). C3H/HeJ mice were sensitive to RSV infection (Haynes et al., 2001). The envelope protein of mouse mammary tumor virus (MMTV) directly activates B cells via TLR4 (Rassa et al., 2002).

TLR2 has also been reported to be involved in the recognition of envelope proteins of measles virus, human cytomegalovirus, and HSV-1 (Bieback et al., 2002; Compton et al., 2003; Kurt-Jones et al., 2004).

3.4.2 Viral Nucleic Acid

Double-stranded (ds) RNA is generated during viral replication. TLR3 is involved in the recognition of a synthetic analog of dsRNA, polyinosine-deoxycytidylic acid (poly I:C), a potent inducer of type I interferons (IFNs) (Alexopoulou et al., 2001; Yamamoto et al., 2003). Consistent with this result, TLR3-deficient mice were hyper susceptible to mouse cytomegalovirus (Tabeta et al., 2004). Contrarily, TLR3-deficient mice showed more resistance to West Nile virus (WNV) infection. WNV triggers inflammatory responses via TLR3, which results in a disruption of the blood brain barrier, followed by enhanced brain infection (Wang et al., 2004). These findings suggested that WNV utilizes TLR3 to efficiently enter the brain.

Mouse splenic DCs are divided into CD11c high B220- and CD11c dull B220+ cells. The latter contain plasmacytoid DCs (pDCs), which induce large amounts of IFN-α during viral infection. CpG DNA motifs are also found in genomes of DNA viruses, such as Herpes simplex virus type 1 (HSV-1), HSV-2, and murine cytomegalovirus (MCMV). Mouse pDCs produce IFN-α by recognizing CpG DNA of HSV-2 via TLR9 (Lund et al., 2003). TLR9-deficient mice were also shown to be susceptible to MCMV infection, suggesting that TLR9 induces anti-viral responses by sensing CpG DNA of DNA virus (Krug et al., 2004a; Krug et al., 2004b; Tabeta et al., 2004). However, in the case of macrophages, HSV-2-induced IFN-α production is not dependent on TLRs. Mice lacking TLR9 or the adapter molecule MyD88 can still control HSV-1 infection (Hochrein et al., 2004). Thus, TLR9-mediated IFN-α response to DNA virus is limited to pDCs, and the TLR-independent system plays an important role in DNA viral infection.

TLR7 and TLR8 are structurally highly conserved proteins (Akira, 2004). The synthetic imidazoquinoline-like molecules imiquimod (R-837) and resiquimod (R-848) have potent antiviral activities and are used clinically for treatment of viral infections. Analysis of TLR7-deficient mice showed that TLR7 recognizes these synthetic compounds (Hemmi et al., 2002). Human TLR7 and TLR8, but not murine TLR8, recognize imidazoquinoline compounds (Ito et al., 2002). Murine TLR7 has also been shown to recognize guanosine analogs such as loxoribine, which has antiviral and antitumor activities (Akira and Hemmi, 2003). Since all these compounds are structurally similar to ribonucleic acids, TLR7 and human TLR8 are predicted to recognize a nucleic acid-like structure of a virus. TLR7 and human TLR8 have been shown to recognize guanosine- or uridine-rich single-stranded RNA (ssRNA) from viruses such as human immunodeficiency virus (HIV), vesicular stomatitis virus (VSV), and influenza virus (Diebold et al., 2004; Heil et al., 2004). Although ssRNA is abundant in hosts, host-derived ssRNA is not usually detected by TLR7 or TLR8. As TLR7 and TLR8 are expressed in the endosome, host-derived ssRNA is not delivered to the endosome and so is not recognized by TLR7 and TLR8.

Besides TLR7 and TLR8, TLR3 and TLR9 are exclusively expressed in endosomal compartments not on cell surfaces (Latz et al., 2004). After phagocytes internalize viruses or virus-infected apoptotic cells, viral nucleic acids are released in phagolysosomes and are recognized by TLRs. However, intracellular localization of TLR9 is not required for ligand recognition but prevents recognition of self DNA. Localization of nucleic acid-sensing TLRs is critical for discriminating between self and non-self nucleic acids. Clarification of these mechanisms should lead to a comprehensive understanding of the immune system and so contribute to the development of new therapies for infection and immune disorders.

4 Conclusion

The function of TLRs has been extensively clarified in recent decades. TLRs are critically involved in bacterial infection as well as fungal, protozoan, and viral infections. Some TLR ligands, especially nucleic acids, are synthesized *in vitro* and have already been applied to treatment of viral infections and allergic diseases. Also, TLR-independent pathogen recognition has been demonstrated.

Acknowledgements We thank our colleagues in our lab for helpful discussions. This work is supported in part by grants from the Special Coordination Funds of the Japanese Ministry of Education, Culture, Sports, Science and Technology.

References

Akira Aikawa M (1988) Human cerebral malaria. Am J Trop Med Hyg 39: 3–10

S (2004) Toll receptor families: structure and function. Semin Immunol 16: 1–2

Akira S, Hemmi H (2003) Recognition of pathogen-associated molecular patterns by TLR family. Immunol Lett 85: 85–95

Alexopoulou L, Holt AC, Medzhitov R, and Flavell RA (2001) Recognition of double-stranded RNA and activation of NF-kappaB by Toll-like receptor 3. Nature 413: 732–738

Alexopoulou L, Thomas V, Schnare M, Lobet Y, Anguita J, Schoen RT, Medzhitov R, Fikrig E, and Flavell RA (2002) Hyporesponsiveness to vaccination with *Borrelia burgdorferi* OspA in humans and in TLR1- and TLR2-deficient mice. Nat Med 8: 878–884

Andersen-Nissen E, Smith KD, Strobe KL, Barrett SL, Cookson BT, Logan SM, Aderem A (2005) Evasion of Toll-like receptor 5 by flagellated bacteria. Proc Natl Acad Sci USA 102: 9247–9252

Arese P, Schwarzer E (1997) Malarial pigment (haemozoin): A very active 'inert' substance. Ann Trop Med Parasitol 91: 501–516

Bafica A, Santiago HC, Goldszmid R, Ropert C, Gazzinelli RT, Sher A (2006) Cutting edge: TLR9 and TLR2 signaling together account for MyD88-dependent control of parasitemia in *Trypanosoma cruzi* infection. J Immunol 17: 3515–3519

Balachandran S, Thomas E, Barber GN (2004) A FADD-dependent innate immune mechanism in mammalian cells. Nature 432: 401–405

Becker I, Salaiza N, Aguirre M, Delgado J, Carrillo-Carrasco N, Kobeh LG, Ruiz A, Cervantes R Torres AP, Cabrera N, et al. (2003) Leishmania lipophosphoglycan (LPG) activates NK cells through Toll-like receptor-2. Mol Biochem Parasitol 130: 65–74

Bieback K, Lien E, Klagge IM, Avota E, Schneider-Schaulies J, Duprex WP, Wagner H, Kirschning CJ, Ter Meulen V, Schneider-Schaulies S (2002) Hemagglutinin protein of wild-type measles virus activates Toll-like receptor 2 signaling. J Virol 76: 8729–8736

Bischoff V, Vignal C, Boneca IG, Michel T, Hoffmann JA, Royet J (2004) Function of the *Drosophila* pattern-recognition receptor PGRP-SD in the detection of Gram-positive bacteria. Nat Immunol 5: 1175–1180

Boutros M, Agaisse H, Perrimon N (2002) Sequential activation of signaling pathways during innate immune responses in *Drosophila*. Dev Cell 3: 711–722

Brennan CA, Anderson KV (2004) *Drosophila*: The genetics of innate immune recognition and response. Annu Rev Immunol 22: 457–483

Brown GD, Taylor PR, Reid DM, Willment JA, Williams DL, Martinez-Pomares L, Wong SY, Gordon S (2002) Dectin-1 is a major beta-glucan receptor on macrophages. J Exp Med 196: 407–412

Brown, P (2001) Cinderella goes to the ball. Nature 410: 1018–1020

Brown WC, Corral RS (2002) Stimulation of B lymphocytes, macrophages, and dendritic cells by protozoan DNA Microbes Infect 4: 969–974

Camargo MM, Andrade AC, Almeida IC, Travassos LR, Gazzinelli RT (1997) Glycoconjugates isolated from *Trypanosoma cruzi* but not from *Leishmania* species membranes trigger nitric oxide synthesis as well as microbicidal activity in IFN-gamma-primed macrophages. J Immunol 159: 6131–6139

Campos MA, Almeida IC, Takeuchi O, Akira S, Valente EP, Procopio DO, Travassos LR, Smith JA, Golenbock DT, Gazzinelli RT (2001) Activation of Toll-like receptor-2 by glycosylphosphatidylinositol anchors from a protozoan parasite. J Immunol 167: 416–423

Channe Gowda D (2002) Structure and activity of glycosylphosphatidylinositol anchors of *Plasmodium falciparum*. Microbes Infect 4: 983–990

Chen P, Rodriguez A, Erskine R, Thach T, Abrams JM (1998) Dredd, a novel effector of the apoptosis activators reaper, grim, and hid in *Drosophila*. Dev Biol 201: 202–216

Choe KM, Werner T, Stoven S, Hultmark D, Anderson KV (2002) Requirement for a peptidoglycan recognition protein (PGRP) in Relish activation and antibacterial immune responses in *Drosophila*. Science 296: 359–362

Coban C, Ishii KJ, Kawai T, Hemmi H, Sato S, Uematsu S, Yamamoto M, Takeuchi O, Itagaki S, Kumar N, et al. (2005) Toll-like receptor 9 mediates innate immune activation by the malaria pigment hemozoin. J Exp Med 201: 19–25

Coban C, Ishii KJ, Sullivan DJ, Kumar N (2002) Purified malaria pigment (hemozoin) enhances dendritic cell maturation and modulates the isotype of antibodies induced by a DNA vaccine. Infect Immun 70: 3939–3943

Coban C, Ishii KJ, Uematsu S, Arisue N, Sato S, Yamamoto M, Kawai T, Takeuchi O, Hisaeda H, Horii T, Akira S (2007) Pathological role of Toll-like receptor signaling in cerebral malaria. Int Immunol 19: 67–79

Compton T, Kurt-Jones EA, Boehme KW, Belko J, Latz E, Golenbock DT, Finberg RW (2003) Human cytomegalovirus activates inflammatory cytokine responses via CD14 and Toll-like receptor 2. J Virol 77: 4588–4596

de Veer MJ, Curtis JM, Baldwin TM, DiDonato JA, Sexton A, McConville MJ, Handman E, Schofield L (2003) MyD88 is essential for clearance of *Leishmania* major: Possible role for lipophosphoglycan and Toll-like receptor 2 signaling. Eur J Immunol 33: 2822–2831

Debierre-Grockiego F, Azzouz N, Schmidt J, Dubremetz, JF, Geyer H, Geyer R, Weingart R, Schmidt RR, Schwarz RT (2003) Roles of glycosylphosphatidylinositols of *Toxoplasma gondii*. Induction of tumor necrosis factor-alpha production in macrophages. J Biol Chem 278: 32987–32993

Diebold SS, Kaisho T, Hemmi H, Akira S, Reis E, Sousa C (2004) Innate antiviral responses by means of TLR7-mediated recognition of single-stranded RNA Science 303: 1529–1531

Dunstan SJ, Hawn TR, Hue NT, Parry CP, Ho VA, Vinh H, Diep TS, House D, Wain J, Aderem A, et al. (2005) Host susceptibility and clinical outcomes in Toll-like receptor 5-deficient patients with typhoid fever in Vietnam. J Infect Dis 191: 1068–1071

Elrod-Erickson M, Mishra S, Schneider D (2000) Interactions between the cellular and humoral immune responses in *Drosophila*. Curr Biol 10: 781–784

Engwerda C, Belnoue E, Gruner AC, Renia L (2005) Experimental models of cerebral malaria. Curr Top Microbiol Immunol 297: 103–143

Foley E, O'Farrell PH (2004) Functional dissection of an innate immune response by a genome-wide RNAi screen. PLoS Biol 2: E203

Gantner BN, Simmons RM, Canavera SJ, Akira S, Underhill DM (2003) Collaborative induction of inflammatory responses by Dectin-1 and Toll-like receptor 2. J Exp Med 197: 1107–1117

Gazzinelli RT, Denkers EY (2006) Protozoan encounters with Toll-like receptor signalling pathways: implications for host parasitism. Nat Rev Immunol 6: 895–906

Georgel P, Naitza S, Kappler C, Ferrandon D, Zachary D, Swimmer C, Kopczynski C, Duyk G, Reichhart JM, Hoffmann JA (2001) Drosophila immune deficiency (IMD) is a death domain protein that activates antibacterial defense and can promote apoptosis. Dev Cell 1: 503–514

Gerold P, Dieckmann-Schuppert A, Schwarz RT (1994) Glycosylphosphatidylinositols synthesized by asexual erythrocytic stages of the malarial parasite, Plasmodium falciparum. Candidates for plasmodial glycosylphosphatidylinositol membrane anchor precursors and pathogenicity factors. J Biol Chem 269: 2597–2606

Gewirtz AT, Navas TA, Lyons S, Godowski PJ, Madara JL (2001) Cutting edge: bacterial flagellin activates basolaterally expressed TLR5 to induce epithelial proinflammatory gene expression. J Immunol 167: 1882–1885

Gobert V, Gottar M, Matskevich AA, Rutschmann S, Royet J, Belvin M, Hoffmann JA, Ferrandon D (2003) Dual activation of the *Drosophila* toll pathway by two pattern recognition receptors. Science 302: 2126–2130

Good MF, Xu H, Wykes M, Engwerda CR (2005) Development and regulation of cell-mediated immune responses to the blood stages of malaria: implications for vaccine research. Annu Rev Immunol 23: 69–99

Gottar M, Gobert V, Michel T, Belvin M, Duyk G, Hoffmann JA, Ferrandon D, Royet J (2002) The *Drosophila* immune response against Gram-negative bacteria is mediated by a peptidoglycan recognition protein. Nature 416: 640–644

Gross O, Gewies A, Finger K, Schafer M, Sparwasser T, Peschel C, Forster I, Ruland J (2006) Card9 controls a non-TLR signalling pathway for innate anti-fungal immunity. Nature 442: 651–656

Harris TH, Cooney NM, Mansfield JM, Paulnock DM (2006) Signal transduction, gene transcription, and cytokine production triggered in macrophages by exposure to trypanosome DNA Infect Immun 74: 4530–4537

Hashimoto M, Asai Y, Ogawa T (2004) Separation and structural analysis of lipoprotein in a lipopolysaccharide preparation from *Porphyromonas gingivalis*. Int Immunol 16: 1431–1437

Hawn TR, Verbon A, Lettinga KD, Zhao LP, Li SS, Laws RJ, Skerrett SJ, Beutler B, Schroeder L, Nachman A, et al. (2003) A common dominant TLR5 stop codon polymorphism abolishes flagellin signaling and is associated with susceptibility to legionnaires' disease. J Exp Med 198: 1563–1572

Hayashi F, Smith KD, Ozinsky A, Hawn TR, Yi EC, Goodlett DR, Eng JK, Akira S, Underhill DM, Aderem A (2001) The innate immune response to bacterial flagellin is mediated by Toll-like receptor 5. Nature 410: 1099–1103

Haynes LM, Moore DD, Kurt-Jones EA, Finberg RW, Anderson LJ, Tripp RA (2001) Involvement of toll–like receptor 4 in innate immunity to respiratory syncytial virus. J Virol 75: 10730–10737

Heil F, Hemmi H, Hochrein H, Ampenberger F, Kirschning C, Akira S, Lipford G, Wagner H, Bauer S (2004) Species-specific recognition of single-stranded RNA via Toll-like receptor 7 and 8. Science 303: 1526–1529

Hemmi H, Kaisho T, Takeuchi O, Sato S, Sanjo H, Hoshino K, Horiuchi T, Tomizawa H, Takeda K, Akira S (2002) Small anti-viral compounds activate immune cells via the TLR7 MyD88-dependent signaling pathway. Nat Immunol 3: 196–200

Hemmi H, Takeuchi O, Kawai T, Kaisho T, Sato S, Sanjo H, Matsumoto M, Hoshino K, Wagner H, Takeda K, Akira S (2000) A Toll-like receptor recognizes bacterial DNA Nature 408: 740–745

Hochrein H, Schlatter B, O'Keeffe M, Wagner C, Schmitz F, Schiemann M, Bauer S, Suter M, Wagner H (2004) Herpes simplex virus type-1 induces IFN-alpha production via Toll-like receptor 9-dependent and -independent pathways. Proc Natl Acad Sci USA 101: 11416–11421

Hoebe K, Georgel P, Rutschmann S, Du X, Mudd S, Crozat K, Sovath S, Shamel L, Hartung T, Zahringer U, Beutler B (2005) CD36 is a sensor of diacylglycerides. Nature 433: 523–527

Hoffmann JA (2003) The immune response of *Drosophila*. Nature 426: 33–38

Hoshino K, Takeuchi O, Kawai T, Sanjo H, Ogawa T, Takeda Y, Takeda K, Akira S (1999) Cutting edge: Toll-like receptor 4 (TLR4)-deficient mice are hyporesponsive to lipopolysaccharide: Evidence for TLR4 as the Lps gene product. J Immunol 162: 3749–3752

Hu S, Yang X (2000) dFADD, a novel death domain-containing adapter protein for the *Drosophila* caspase DREDD J Biol Chem 275: 30761–30764

Hu X, Yagi Y, Tanji T, Zhou S, Ip YT (2004) Multimerization and interaction of Toll and Spätzle in *Drosophila*. Proc Natl Acad Sci USA 101: 9369–9374

Hultmark D (2003) *Drosophila* immunity: paths and patterns. Curr Opin Immunol 15: 12–19

Idro R, Jenkins NE, Newton CR (2005) Pathogenesis, clinical features, and neurological outcome of cerebral malaria. Lancet Neurol 4: 827–840

Ito T, Amakawa R, Kaisho T, Hemmi H, Tajima K, Uehira K, Ozaki Y, Tomizawa H, Akira S, Fukuhara S (2002) Interferon-alpha and interleukin-12 are induced differentially by Toll-like receptor 7 ligands in human blood dendritic cell subsets. J Exp Med 195: 1507–1512

Khush RS, Cornwell WD, Uram JN, Lemaitre B (2002) A ubiquitin-proteasome pathway represses the *Drosophila* immune deficiency signaling cascade. Curr Biol 12: 1728–1737

Krishnegowda G, Hajjar AM, Zhu J, Douglass EJ, Uematsu S, Akira S, Woods AS, Gowda DC (2005) Induction of proinflammatory responses in macrophages by the glycosylphosphatidylinositols of *Plasmodium falciparum*: cell signaling receptors, glycosylphosphatidylinositol (GPI) structural requirement, and regulation of GPI activity. J Biol Chem 280: 8606–8616

Kropf P, Freudenberg MA, Modolell M, Price HP, Herath S, Antoniazi S, Galanos C, Smith DF, Muller I (2004) Toll-like receptor 4 contributes to efficient control of infection with the protozoan parasite *Leishmania* major. Infect Immun 72: 1920–1928

Krug A, French AR, Barchet W Fischer, JA, Dzionek A, Pingel JT, Orihuela MM, Akira S, Yokoyama WM, Colonna M (2004a) TLR9-dependent recognition of MCMV by IPC and DC generates coordinated cytokine responses that activate antiviral NK cell function. Immunity 21: 107–119

Krug A, Luker GD, Barchet W, Leib DA, Akira S, Colonna M (2004b) Herpes simplex virus type 1 activates murine natural interferon–producing cells through Toll-like receptor 9. Blood 103: 1433–1437

Kurt-Jones EA, Chan M, Zhou S, Wang J, Reed G, Bronson R, Arnold MM, Knipe DM, Finberg RW (2004) Herpes simplex virus 1 interaction with Toll-like receptor 2 contributes to lethal encephalitis. Proc Natl Acad Sci USA 101: 1315–1320

Kurt-Jones EA, Popova L, Kwinn L, Haynes LM, Jones LP, Tripp RA, Walsh EE, Freeman MW, Golenbock DT, Anderson LJ, Finberg RW (2000) Pattern recognition receptors TLR4 and CD14 mediate response to respiratory syncytial virus. Nat Immunol 1: 398–401

Latz E, Schoenemeyer A, Visintin A, Fitzgerald KA, Monks BG, Knetter CF, Lien E, Nilsen NJ, Espevik T, Golenbock DT (2004) TLR9 signals after translocating from the ER to CpG DNA in the lysosome. Nat Immunol 5:190–198

Lemaitre B (2004) The road to Toll. Nat Rev Immunol 4: 521–527

Lemaitre B, Nicolas E, Michaut L, Reichhart JM, Hoffmann JA (1996) The dorsoventral regulatory gene cassette Spätzle/Toll/Cactus controls the potent antifungal response in *Drosophila* adults. Cell 86: 973–983

Leulier F, Rodriguez A, Khush RS, Abrams JM, Lemaitre B (2000) The *Drosophila* caspase Dredd is required to resist Gram-negative bacterial infection. EMBO Rep 1: 353–358

Leulier F, Vidal S, Saigo K, Ueda R, Lemaitre B (2002) Inducible expression of double-stranded RNA reveals a role for dFADD in the regulation of the antibacterial response in *Drosophila* adults. Curr Biol 12: 996–1000

Levashina EA, Langley E, Green C, Gubb D, Ashburner M, Hoffmann JA, Reichhart JM (1999) Constitutive activation of toll-mediated antifungal defense in serpin-deficient *Drosophila*. Science 285. 1917–1919

Ligoxygakis P, Pelte N, Hoffmann JA, Reichhart JM (2002) Activation of *Drosophila* Toll during fungal infection by a blood serine protease. Science 297: 114–116

Lu Y, Wu LP, Anderson KV (2001) The antibacterial arm of the *Drosophila* innate immune response requires an IkappaB kinase. Genes Dev 15: 104–110

Lund J, Sato A, Akira S, Medzhitov R, Iwasaki A (2003) Toll-like receptor 9-mediated recognition of Herpes simplex virus-2 by plasmacytoid dendritic cells. J Exp Med 198: 513–520

Magez S, Stijlemans B, Radwanska M, Pays E, Ferguson MA, De Baetselier P (1998) The glycosyl-inositol-phosphate and dimyristoylglycerol moieties of the glycosylphosphatidylinositol anchor of the trypanosome variant-specific surface glycoprotein are distinct macrophage-activating factors. J Immunol 160: 1949–1956

Medzhitov R, Janeway CJ (1997) Innate immunity: the virtues of a nonclonal system of recognition. Cell 91: 295–298

Medzhitov R, Preston-Hurlburt P, Janeway CJ (1997) A human homologue of the *Drosophila* Toll protein signals activation of adaptive immunity. Nature 388: 394–397

Michel T, Reichhart JM, Hoffmann JA, Royet J (2001) *Drosophila* Toll is activated by Gram-positive bacteria through a circulating peptidoglycan recognition protein. Nature 414: 756–759

Miller LH, Baruch DI, Marsh K, Doumbo OK (2002) The pathogenic basis of malaria. Nature 415: 673–679

Naik RS, Branch OH, Woods AS, Vijaykumar M, Perkins DJ, Nahlen BL, Lal AA, Cotter RJ, Costello CE, Ockenhouse CF et al. (2000) Glycosylphosphatidylinositol anchors of Plasmodium falciparum: Molecular characterization and naturally elicited antibody response that may provide immunity to malaria pathogenesis. J Exp Med 192: 1563–1576

Netea MG, Van der Graaf C, Van der Meer JW, Kullberg BJ (2004) Recognition of fungal pathogens by Toll-like receptors. Eur J Clin Microbiol Infect Dis 23: 672–676

Netea MG, Van Der Graaf CA, Vonk AG, Verschueren I, Van Der Meer JW, Kullberg BJ (2002a) The role of Toll-like receptor (TLR) 2 and TLR4 in the host defense against disseminated candidiasis. J Infect Dis 185: 1483–1489

Netea MG, van Deuren M, Kullberg BJ, Cavaillon JM, Van der Meer JW (2002b) Does the shape of lipid A determine the interaction of LPS with Toll-like receptors? Trends Immunol 23: 135–139

Oliveira AC, Peixoto JR, de Arruda LB, Campos MA, Gazzinelli RT, Golenbock DT, Akira S, Previato JO, Mendonca-Previato L, Nobrega A, Bellio M (2004) Expression of functional TLR4 confers proinflammatory responsiveness to *Trypanosoma cruzi* glycoinositolphospholipids and higher resistance to infection with *T cruzi*. J Immunol 173: 5688–5696

Ouaissi A, Guilvard E, Delneste Y, Caron G, Magistrelli G, Herbault N, Thieblemont N, Jeannin P (2002) The *Trypanosoma cruzi* Tc52-released protein induces human dendritic cell maturation, signals via Toll-like receptor 2: and confers protection against lethal infection. J Immunol 168: 6366–6374

Park JM, Brady H, Ruocco MG, Sun H, Williams D, Lee SJ, Kato T Jr, Richards N, Chan K, Mercurio F et al. (2004) Targeting of TAK1 by the NF-kappa B protein Relish regulates the JNK-mediated immune response in *Drosophila*. Genes Dev 18: 584–594

Pili-Floury S, Leulier F, Takahashi K, Saigo K, Samain E, Ueda R, Lemaitre B (2004) *In vivo* RNA interference analysis reveals an unexpected role for GNBP1 in the defense against Grampositive bacterial infection in *Drosophila* adults. J Biol Chem 279: 12848–12853

Poltorak A, He X, Smirnova I, Liu MY, Van Huffel C, Du X, Birdwell D, Alejos E, Silva M, Galanos C et al. (1998) Defective LPS signaling in C3H/HeJ and C57BL/10ScCr mice: Mutations in Tlr4 gene. Science 282: 2085–2088

Rassa JC, Meyers JL, Zhang Y, Kudaravalli R, Ross SR (2002) Murine retroviruses activate B cells via interaction with Toll-like receptor 4. Proc Natl Acad Sci USA 99: 2281–2286

Rogers NC, Slack EC, Edwards AD, Nolte MA, Schulz O, Schweighoffer E, Williams DL, Gordon S, Tybulewicz VL, Brown GD, Reis ESC (2005) Syk-dependent cytokine induction by Dectin-1 reveals a novel pattern recognition pathway for C type lectins. Immunity 22: 507–517

Ropert C, Gazzinelli RT (2004) Regulatory role of Toll-like receptor 2 during infection with *Trypanosoma cruzi*. J Endotoxin Res 10: 425–430

Rutschmann S, Jung AC, Zhou R, Silverman N, Hoffmann JA, Ferrandon D (2000) Role of *Drosophila* IKK gamma in a Toll-independent antibacterial immune response. Nat Immunol 1: 342–347

Saijo S, Fujikado N, Furuta T, Chung SH, Kotaki H, Seki K, Sudo K, Akira S, Adachi Y, Ohno N et al. (2007) Dectin-1 is required for host defense against *Pneumocystis carinii* but not against *Candida albicans*. Nat Immunol 8: 39–46

Schofield L, Grau GE (2005) Immunological processes in malaria pathogenesis. Nat Rev Immunol 5: 722–735

Schofield L, Hackett F (1993) Signal transduction in host cells by a glycosylphosphatidylinositol toxin of malaria parasites. J Exp Med 177: 145–153

Sherry BA, Alava G, Tracey KJ, Martiney J, Cerami A, Slater AF (1995) Malaria-specific metabolite hemozoin mediates the release of several potent endogenous pyrogens (TNF, MIP-1 alpha, and MIP-1 beta) *in vitro*, and altered thermoregulation *in vivo*. J Inflamm 45: 85–96

Shimazu R, Akashi S, Ogata H, Nagai Y, Fukudome K, Miyake K, Kimoto M (1999) MD-2: A molecule that confers lipopolysaccharide responsiveness on Toll-like receptor 4. J Exp Med 189: 1777–1782

Shoda LK, Kegerreis KA, Suarez CE, Roditi I, Corral RS, Bertot GM, Norimine J, Brown WC (2001) DNA from protozoan parasites *Babesia bovis, Trypanosoma cruzi*, and *T brucei* is mitogenic for B lymphocytes and stimulates macrophage expression of interleukin-12: tumor necrosis factor alpha, and nitric oxide. Infect Immun 69: 2162–2171

Silverman N, Zhou R, Erlich RL, Hunter M, Bernstein E, Schneider D, Maniatis T (2003) Immune activation of NF-kappaB and JNK requires *Drosophila* TAK1. J Biol Chem 278: 48928–48934

Silverman N, Zhou R, Stoven S, Pandey N, Hultmark D, Maniatis T (2000) A *Drosophila* IkappaB kinase complex required for Relish cleavage and antibacterial immunity. Genes Dev 14: 2461–2471

Stoven S, Silverman N, Junell A, Hedengren-Olcott M, Erturk D, Engstrom Y, Maniatis T Hultmark, D (2003) Caspase-mediated processing of the *Drosophila* NF-kappaB factor Relish. Proc Natl Acad Sci USA 100: 5991–5996

Sullivan DJ (2002) Theories on malarial pigment formation and quinoline action. Int J Parasitol 32: 1645–1653

Sun H, Towb P, Chiem DN, Foster BA, Wasserman SA (2004) Regulated assembly of the Toll signaling complex drives *Drosophila* dorsoventral patterning. EMBO J 23: 100–110

Tabeta K, Georgel P, Janssen E, Du X, Hoebe K, Crozat K, Mudd S, Shamel L, Sovath S, Goode J et al. (2004) Toll-like receptors 9 and 3 as essential components of innate immune defense against mouse cytomegalovirus infection. Proc Natl Acad Sci USA 101: 3516–3521

Takeda K, Akira S (2005) Toll-like receptors in innate immunity. Int Immunol 17:1–14

Takeda K, Kaisho T, Akira, S (2003) Toll-like receptors. Annu Rev Immunol 21: 335–376

Takehana A, Yano T, Mita S, Kotani A, Oshima Y, Kurata S (2004) Peptidoglycan recognition protein (PGRP)-LE and PGRP-LC act synergistically in *Drosophila* immunity. EMBO J 23: 4690–4700

Takeuchi O, Hoshino K, Kawai T, Sanjo H, Takada H, Ogawa T, Takeda K, Akira S (1999a) Differential roles of TLR2 and TLR4 in recognition of Gram-negative and Gram-positive bacterial cell wall components. Immunity 11: 443–451

Takeuchi O, Kawai T, Muhlradt PF, Morr M, Radolf JD, Zychlinsky A, Takeda K, Akira S (2001) Discrimination of bacterial lipoproteins by Toll-like receptor 6. Int Immunol 13: 933–940

Takeuchi O, Kawai T, Sanjo H, Copeland NG, Gilbert DJ, Jenkins NA, Takeda K, Akira S (1999b) TLR6: a novel member of an expanding Toll-like receptor family. Gene 231: 59–65

Takeuchi O, Sato S, Horiuchi T, Hoshino K, Takeda K, Dong Z, Modlin RL, Akira S (2002) Cutting edge: role of Toll-like receptor 1 in mediating immune response to microbial lipoproteins. J Immunol 169: 10–14

Tanji T, Ip YT (2005) Regulators of the Toll and Imd pathways in the *Drosophila* innate immune response. Trends Immunol 26: 193–198

Taylor PR, Tsoni SV, Willment JA, Dennehy KM, Rosas M, Findon H, Haynes K, Steele C, Botto M, Gordon S, and Brown GD (2007) Dectin-1 is required for beta-glucan recognition and control of fungal infection. Nat Immunol 8: 31–38

Torok HP, Glas J, Tonenchi L, Mussack T, and Folwaczny C (2004) Polymorphisms of the lipopolysaccharide-signaling complex in inflammatory bowel disease: Association of a mutation in the Toll-like receptor 4 gene with ulcerative colitis. Clin Immunol 112: 85–91

Uematsu S, Jang MH, Chevrier N, Guo Z, Kumagai Y, Yamamoto M, Kato H, Sougawa N, Matsui H, Kuwata H, et al. (2006) Detection of pathogenic intestinal bacteria by Toll-like receptor 5 on intestinal CD11c(+) lamina propria cells. Nat Immunol 7: 868–874

Underhill DM, Rossnagle E, Lowell CA, Simmons RM (2005) Dectin-1 activates Syk tyrosine kinase in a dynamic subset of macrophages for reactive oxygen production. Blood 106: 2543–2550

Vidal S, Khush RS, Leulier F, Tzou P, Nakamura M, Lemaitre B (2001) Mutations in the *Drosophila* dTAK1 gene reveal a conserved function for MAPKKKs in the control of Rel/NF-kappaB-dependent innate immune responses. Genes Dev 15: 1900–1912

Wang T, Town T, Alexopoulou L, Anderson JF, Fikrig E, Flavell RA (2004) Toll-like receptor 3 mediates West Nile virus entry into the brain causing lethal encephalitis. Nat Med 10: 1366–1373

Weber AN, Tauszig-Delamasure S, Hoffmann JA, Lelievre E, Gascan H, Ray KP, Morse MA, Imler JL, Gay, NJ (2003) Binding of the *Drosophila* cytokine Spätzle to Toll is direct and establishes signaling. Nat Immunol 4: 794–800

Wu LP, Anderson KV (1997) Related signaling networks in *Drosophila* that control dorsoventral patterning in the embryo and the immune response. Cold Spring Harb Symp Quant Biol 62: 97–103

Yamamoto M, Sato, S Hemmi H, Hoshino K, Kaisho T, Sanjo H, Takeuchi O, Sugiyama M, Okabe M, Takeda K, and Akira S (2003) Role of adaptor TRIF in the MyD88-independent Toll-like receptor signaling pathway. Science 301: 640–643

Yarovinsky F, Kanzler H, Hieny S, Coffman RL, Sher A (2006) Toll-like receptor recognition regulates immunodominance in an antimicrobial CD4+ T cell response. Immunity 25: 655–664

Yarovinsky F, Sher A (2006) Toll-like receptor recognition of *Toxoplasma gondii*. Int J Parasitol 36: 255–259

Yarovinsky F, Zhang D, Andersen JF, Bannenberg GL, Serhan CN, Hayden MS, Hieny S, Sutter-wala FS, Flavell RA, Ghosh S, Sher A (2005) TLR11 activation of dendritic cells by a protozoan Profilin-like protein. Science 308: 1626–1629

Zhang D, Zhang G, Hayden MS, Greenblatt MB, Bussey C, Flavell RA, Ghosh S (2004) A Toll-like receptor that prevents infection by uropathogenic bacteria. Science 303: 1522–1526

Signalling of Toll-Like Receptors

Constantinos Brikos and Luke A.J. O'Neill(⊠)

Abstract Since Toll-like receptor (TLR) signaling was found crucial for the activation of innate and adaptive immunity, it has been the focus of immunological research. There are at least 13 identified mammalian TLRs, to date, that share similarities in their extracellular and intracellular domains. A vast number of ligands have been identified that are specifically recognized by different TLRs. As a response the TLRs dimerize and their signaling is initiated. The molecular basis of that signaling depends on the conserved part of their intracellular domain; namely the Toll/IL-1 receptor (TIR) domain. Upon TLR dimerization a TIR-TIR structure is formed that can recruit TIR-containing intracellular proteins that mediate their signaling. For this reason these proteins are named adapters. There are five adapters identified so far named myeloid differentiation primary response protein 88 (MyD88), MyD88-adapter like (Mal) or TIR domain-containing adapter (TIRAP), TIR domain-containing adapter inducing interferon-β (IFN-β) (TRIF) or TIR-containing adapter molecule-1 (TICAM-1), TRIF-related adapter molecule (TRAM) or TICAM-2, and sterile α and HEAT-Armadillo motifs (SARM). The first four play a fundamental role in TLR-signaling, defining which pathways will be activated, depending on which of these adapters will be recruited by each TLR. Among these adapter proteins MyD88 and TRIF are now considered as the signaling ones and hence the TLR pathways can be categorized as MyD88-dependent

Luke A.J. O'Neill

School of Biochemistry and Immunology, Trinity College Dublin, Dublin 2, Ireland

`laoneill@tcd.ie`

S. Bauer, G. Hartmann (eds.), *Toll-Like Receptors (TLRs) and Innate Immunity.*
Handbook of Experimental Pharmacology 183.
© Springer-Verlag Berlin Heidelberg 2008

and TRIF-dependent. Mal and TRAM have recently been shown to be required for the recruitment of MyD88 and TRIF, respectively, to TLR(s) and are therefore called bridging adapters. The MyD88- and TRIF-dependent pathways activate not only the transcription factor nuclear factor-kappaB (NF-κB), mitogen-activated protein kinases (MAPKs) but also certain interferon-regulated factors (IRFs). Recently, it was discovered that the remaining adapter SARM has an inhibitory role in TRIF-dependent signaling by binding to TRIF. Apart from SARM there are several proteins of the host that target the adapters in order to suppress their signaling. In addition, some viral proteins have been identified that inhibit TLR-signaling via their interaction with the TLRs, preventing in that way the activation of the immune system of the host and acting beneficially for the survival of the virus.

1 Introduction

The discovery of Toll-like receptors (TLRs) altered significantly our understanding on the initiation and activation of the innate immune response. It is now clear that innate immunity is more specific than it was originally thought. When an organism-host is invaded by several types of microbes such as bacteria, yeast, viruses, fungi, and parasites, they are sensed by the TLRs that are expressed in a wide range of different cell types such as those involved in innate and adaptive immunity. Examples are macrophages, dendritic cells (DCs), B- and certain types of T-cells.

   TLRs recognize a wide variety of molecules from the invaders and initiate various signal transduction cascades that activate and regulate the host's immune response. All the members of this family of receptors as well as the interleukin-1 receptor type I (IL-1RI) members share homology in their cytoplasmic part. In particular, they contain a domain called the Toll/IL-1 receptor (TIR) domain. TIR also exists in intracellular proteins that are called adapters because they can bind via this domain to the liganded receptors, thereby transmitting signaling inside the cells. One of these adapters, which not only binds to almost all signaling TLRs but also associates with IL-1RI, is MyD88. Thus, TLRs and IL-1RI share some similar pathways that induce the activation of the transcription factor nuclear factor-κB (NF-κB) and the mitogen-activated protein kinases (MAPKs), p38, and the c-Jun N-terminal kinase (JNK). As a result a common set of genes are expressed which produce essential molecules for the activation and the regulation of both innate and adaptive immunity, such as cytokines, chemokines and co-stimulatory molecules.

   However, apart from MyD88 there are another four adapter molecules: the MyD88–adapter-like or TIR domain-containing adapter (Mal/TIRAP); the TIR domain-containing adapter-inducing interferon-β (IFN-β) or TIR-containing adapter molecule-1 (TRIF/TICAM-1); the TRIF-related adapter molecule (TRAM), also known as TICAM-2; and the protein that contains sterile α and HEAT-Armadillo motifs (SARM). The existence of adapter molecules explains to some extent the separate signaling cascades that are initiated and regulated by different TLRs. The reason is that not all the members of the TLR family bind the same adapter(s) which specifically mediate certain pathways. For example, some of these proteins are essential for the activation of various members of the family of transcription factors called (IFN) regulatory factors (IRFs) in response to TLR activation. These transcription factors are responsible for the induction of type I IFNs and IFN-induced genes. This is also a main difference between IL-1RI and some TLRs, with IL-1RI being unable to activate IRFs.

In general, it is not certain if all the signaling pathways activated by the TLRs have been discovered yet. In addition, the exact molecular mechanisms by which the known TLR signal transduction pathways are initiated and regulated have not been completely uncovered. However, a lot has already been understood regarding the TLR signaling cascades and their specificity in terms of which genes they induce to ensure that the host will respond efficiently to a certain invasion.

In this chapter, we discuss the current knowledge on TLRs in terms of their signaling pathways. In particular, we describe TLR-signaling on the basis of which adapter molecules—the first intracellular proteins in the cascade known to specify which cascades are initiated—are used.

2 TLRs and Their Ligands

The first receptor belonging to the family of TLRs to be discovered was the *Drosophila melanogaster* protein Toll (or dToll). Initially, its only identified function was its essential role for the formation of the dorsoventral axis of the fly embryo (Hashimoto et al. 1988). Later, it was found that Toll had a cytosolic portion homologous to that of IL-1RI (Dower et al., 1985; Bird et al., 1988; Urdal, et al., 1988; Gay and Keith, 1991), the active receptor for IL-1, a cytokine that plays a very significant role in innate and adaptive immunity by mediating a variety of local and systemic effects (reviewed in (Dinarello, 1994; 1996)). Subsequently, Toll was found to be important for the antifungal defense of the adult fly (Lemaitre et al., 1996).

Since that discovery, at least 13 mammalian TLRs have been identified, which identification is based on their shared sequence similarities. Most of these TLRs have already been shown to recognize pathogen-associated molecular patterns (PAMPs) from a wide range of invading agents.

In general, TLRs can be categorized into two main groups, according to their ligands. One group consists of TLR1, 2, 4, and 6 that recognize PAMPS from lipids, and the other group consists of TLR3, 7, 8, and 9 that recognize PAMPS from nucleic acids.

Very briefly, as the TLR ligands have already been discussed in more detail in Chapter of this volume, TLR2 binds lipopeptides from the cell wall of Gram-positive bacteria, lipomannans from mycobacteria, phospholipomannan from fungi, and glycosylphosphatidylinositolmucin from protozoan parasites. TLR2 is also activated by proteins. Such examples are porins from the cell wall of Gram-negative bacteria and other proteins derived from viruses. TLR2 can actually heterodimerize with TLR1 or TLR6. The TLR1/TLR2 complex is responsible for the recognition of bacterial and mycobacterial diacyl lipopeptides and bacterial tria-cylated lipoproteins; such as the synthetic compound Pam3Cys. The TLR2/TLR6 complex recognizes diacylated lipoproteins from mycoplasma, such as the my-coplasma lipoprotein-2, and the bacterial glycolipid lipotechoic acid.

TLR4 is activated by endotoxin also known as lipopolysaccharide (LPS), which is derived from the cell wall of Gram-negative bacteria (Poltorak et al., 1998; Hoshino et al., 1999; Qureshi et al., 1999; Arbour et al., 2000; Agnese et al., 2002; Lorenz et al., 2002), mannan from fungi, glycoinositolphospholipids from protozoan parasites, and several viral proteins, such as the fusion protein of the res-piratory syncytial virus.

TLR3, TLR7, and TLR8 are key receptors for antiviral responses. TLR3 initiates signaling for double-stranded RNA. TLR7 and TLR8 are induced by single-stranded RNA (Alexopoulou et al., 2001). Furthermore, TLR3 recognizes polyriboinosinic: polyribocytidylic acid (poly(I:C)) (a synthetic analogue of dsRNA) and TLR7, sev-eral imidazoquinolines (e.g., imiquimod and R-848). Other ligands for TLR7 in-clude guanosine analogues (e.g., Loxoribin). R-848 also activates the human TLR8 (Hemmi et al., 2002; Lee et al., 2003; Heil et al., 2004; Lund et al., 2004). The mouse TLR8 has been shown to be unable to initiate signal transduction. Last, TLR9 recognizes unmethylated CpG-DNA motifs from bacteria and mycobacteria. It also senses genomic DNA from parasites (Hemmi et al., 2000; Bauer et al., 2001). It has to be mentioned that, as in the case of TLR2 that forms a complex with either TLR1 or TLR6, TLR8 can interact with TLR7 or TLR9 (Wang et al., 2006). Furthermore, TLR9 can also interact with TLR7. However, in contrast to the formation of the TLR1/2 and TLR2/6 complexes, which initiate signaling, the TLR9-TLR7 interac-tion antagonizes TLR7 signaling. In addition, the TLR8 ligands act as antagonists for the signaling cascades induced by TLR7 and 9.

Apart from these two main groups of TLRs there are also the TLR5 and the murine TLR11 (its human homologue is inactive) that recognize the protein flagellin from bacteria (Hayashi et al., 2001) and a profilin-like molecule (Yarovinsky et al., 2005), respectively. Ligands for the remaining TLRs—TLR10, 12, and 13—have not been identified yet. TLR10 has been found to be expressed in humans but not in mice, and the other two in mice instead of humans.

Except from the mentioned exogenous ligands, TLRs are also activated by sev-eral endogenous molecules. For example, TLR2 and TLR4 have been reported to be activated by heat shock proteins (Ohashi et al., 2000; Vabulas et al., 2001; Vabulas et al., 2002) and fragments of the polysaccharide hyaluronan (Termeer et al., 2002; Jiang et al., 2005; Scheibner et al., 2006). Last, TLR3 and TLR9 have been shown to recognize host mRNA (Kariko et al., 2004) and DNA, respectively (Leadbetter, 2002).

The structural basis that explains the wide variety of ligands recognized by the TLRs and how exactly their signaling is initiated has not been completely elucidated yet. The main reason is that no liganded TLR or TLR-adapter structures have been solved so far. However, a small number of TLR structures are available and several studies on the conserved regions among the TLRs (e.g., identification of mutations that make them inactive) enable us to have a good understanding of the first events in TLR signaling.

3 Structure and Signaling of TLRs

3.1 Structural Characteristics of the TLRs and Initiation of Signaling

The structure of TLRs and the recognition of their ligands will be described concisely as they are discussed in more detail in other chapters of this volume. Briefly, TLRs are type 1 transmembrane receptors that contain an extracellular domain consisting of leucine-rich repeat (LRR) motifs that recognize the ligands. The crystal structure of the LRR domain of TLR3 has been solved at 2.3 Å (Bell et al., 2005; Choe et al., 2005). It contains 23 LRR motifs that build a horseshoe-shaped solenoid structure that is highly glycosylated. Binding of the monomeric TLR3 ligand dsRNA is believed to occur at a surface of the LRR domain that is free of glycosylation. Liganding of TLR3 causes symmetrical dimerization of its ectodomains (Bell et al., 2006). As a result, conformational changes occur that bring the intracellular part of two TLR3 molecules that contain the highly conserved TIR domain into close proximity, thereby forming a TIR-TIR structure. It is believed that in general, liganded TLRs form dimers in order to signal (Ozinsky et al., 2000). These dimers are either homodimers, as in the case of TLR3 and the *Drosophila* Toll (Weber et al., 2003; Weber et al., 2005); or heterodimers, like those of TLR2 with TLR1 or TLR6; or that of IL-1RI with its accessory protein (IL-1RAcP), which also contains a TIR domain.

The TIR domains are between 135 and 160 amino acids in length. The molecular structures of the TIR domains of TLR1 and TLR2 have been resolved. They contain a central, five-stranded, parallel β-sheet which is surrounded by a total of 5 α-helices on both sides (Xu et al., 2000). In terms of its sequence, each TIR domain contains three conserved regions named Box 1, Box 2, and Box 3. Box 1 is the signature sequence of all TLRs; Box 2 contains a loop termed the "BB loop," which is important for signaling, and Box 3 contains certain amino acids that have been identified as important for signaling, at least in the case of IL-1RI. The BB loop contains a conserved proline. When a missense mutation in the *tlr4* gene changed this proline to histidine, the expressed TLR4 protein was unable to signal (Poltorak et al., 1998; Qureshi et al., 1999). There is also another important loop that has been identified as essential for signaling, named the "DD loop." It has been shown that the DD loop of TLR2 interacts with the BB loop of TLR1 (Gautam et al., 2006). Thus, a possible model for the formation of a TIR-TIR structure could be based on an interaction between the DD loop of one TIR domain, with the BB loop of the other. Such a model is also supported by the TIR-TIR interactions among certain TLRs and their adapter molecules. In general, it is now believed that the formation of a TIR-TIR structure at the receptor level provides the place of association with the TIR domain-containing adapters that mediate signaling by linking the receptors to downstream intracellular proteins.

3.2 MyD88

3.2.1 Recruitment of MyD88 by the TLRs

The first adapter to be found essential for the TLR signaling cascades was MyD88. MyD88 had already been identified as a protein expressed in myeloid tissues, and its mRNA levels were used as markers for differentiation (Lord et al., 1990a; Lord et al., 1990b). In particular, MYD88 was induced when M1D+ myeloid precursors were differentiated in response to IL-6. This is why it was named MyD88: "MyD" stands for myeloid differentiation and "88" is the number of the genes induced expressing the MyD88 protein. Four years later, MyD88 was identified as a member of the Toll/IL-1 receptor family (Hultmark, 1994; Yamagata et al., 1994) and consequently, its function was found to be crucial for signaling induced by IL-1, as well as several TLRs (Bonnert et al., 1997; Muzio et al., 1997; Wesche et al., 1997; Burns, 1998; Medzhitov et al., 1998; Muzio et al., 1998). The development of MyD88 knock out mice was normal but their cells were completely unresponsive to IL-1, IL-18 (Adachi et al., 1998), and endotoxin (Kawai et al., 1999; Takeuchi et al., 2000). In general, MyD88 mediates the signaling of all TLRs, apart from TLR3.

The basic characteristics of its structure are a death domain "DD" and a TIR domain at positioned at its N- and C-terminals, respectively. These two domains are linked by an intermediate domain "ID."

The recruitment of MyD88 to TLR2 is based on the DD loop of its TIR domain. In particular, both the BB loop of the TLR2 and the DD loop of the MyD88 are required for the interaction of these two proteins (Xu et al., 2000; Dunne et al., 2003). In addition, site-directed mutagenesis of the amino acids 195–197 in the Box 2 of MyD88 impaired its recruitment to IL-1RI (Li et al., 2005), whereas the conserved proline in its the BB loop (see Section 3.1) is not required for its interaction with TLR2 or TLR4 (Dunne et al., 2003).

In 2006 germ-line mutagenesis offered further insight into the interactions between MyD88 and the TLRs (Jiang et al., 2006). The TLR phenovariant produced in that way was named Pococurante (Poc) and resulted in the MyD88 I179N mutation. Abolished was the ability of the mice of that phenotype to respond to TLR ligands that in turn require MyD88 in order to signal. Only the TLR2/6 signaling heterodimer was active in these mice as they could respond to diacyl lipopeptides. Thus, it was suggested that I179 in MyD88 (Poc site) is required for its interaction with the BB loop of all TLRs apart from those of the TLR2/6 complex. Moreover, the mice having the Poc mutation were different than the MyD88-deficient ones in terms of their susceptibility to infection from *Streptococcus pyogenes*. In particular, the mice that were not expressing MyD88 were highly susceptible to such an infection, in contrast to the mice carrying the Poc mutation. Thus, it can be concluded that the TLR2/6 complex is essential in the host's defence against *Streptococcus pyogenes*.

3.2.2 MyD88-Dependent Pathways

MyD88-Dependent Activation of NF-κB, p38, and JNK

All TLRs that recruit MyD88 signal in a MyD88-dependent manner, which is very similar to the IL-1RI pathway in its activation of NF-κB and the MAPKs. Employment of MyD88 to liganded IL-1RI or TLRs results in the association of the interleukin-1 receptor-associated kinases (IRAKs) to the receptor signaling complexes (Figure 1).

It was first observed that although IL-1RI, IL-1RacP, and MyD88 were not protein kinases an IL-1RI-associated kinase activity could be co-precipitated with the receptor from cells stimulated by IL-1 (Martin et al., 1994). The associated kinase could phosphorylate the exogenous substrate myelin basic protein *in vitro* and an endogenous substrate of approximately 60 kDa (referred to as p60). This kinase activity seemed necessary for IL-1 responsiveness (Croston et al., 1995). Subsequently, a serine/threonine kinase associated with the receptor was purified from a human embryonic kidney (HEK) 293-cell line, which had been stably transfected to overexpress IL-1RI. This enzyme was named IRAK (Cao et al., 1996a). Its murine homologue was also identified (Trofimova et al., 1996) and named mouse Pelle-like protein kinase, based on its similarity to the kinase Pelle of the Toll pathway in the *Drosophila melanogaster*.

IRAK-1 seemed to possess a very important role in IL-1RI signaling. Its overexpression resulted in activation of downstream signaling events (Knop et al., 1998) and mutant HEK 293 cells not expressing IRAK-1 did not respond to IL-1 (Li et al., 1999c). In addition, fibroblasts from IRAK-1 knock out mice showed impaired IL-1 response *in vivo* (Thomas et al., 1999). Upon IL-1 stimulation, IRAK-1 associates with the receptor complex and becomes multiply phosphorylated. Initially, it was thought that this phosphorylation was very likely an autophosphorylation because a kinase-defective IRAK-1 (IRAK-1-Asp^{340}Asn) was not phosphorylated *in vitro* (Maschera et al., 1999). However, when the ATP binding site of IRAK-1 was mutated (K239A) to prevent its autophosphorylation, and transfected into IRAK-1$^{-/-}$ cells, the mutant became phosphorylated. It was thus proposed that IRAK-1 was phosphorylated by another kinase (Li et al., 1999c). Furthermore, the kinase activity of IRAK-1 was not necessary for IL-1RI signaling because kinase-dead IRAK-1 restored IL-1 responsiveness to IRAK-1$^{-/-}$ cells (Knop and Martin 1999; Li et al., 1999c; Maschera et al., 1999; Vig et al., 1999). Later, another kinase was identified based on its similarity to IRAK-1 and named IRAK-4 (Li et al., 2002). The discovery of this kinase could explain the observations regarding the phosphorylation and function of IRAK-1. It was shown that recombinant IRAK-4 could be autophosphorylated and also phosphorylate recombinant IRAK-1 *in vitro*. In contrast, recombinant IRAK-1 was able to become autophosphorylated, but could not phosphorylate IRAK-4 *in vitro*. IRAK-4 knock out mice presented a stronger phenotype than the IRAK-1 ones. IL-1 and TLR downstream signaling was severely impaired (Suzuki et al., 2002). Furthermore, IRAK-4-deficient humans were identified and they were susceptible to pyogenic bacterial infections (Picard et al., 2003). Thus the

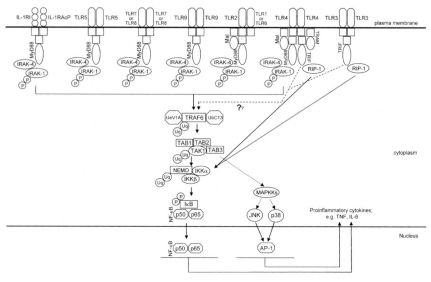

Fig. 1 TLR signaling pathways leading to the activation of NF-κB, p38, and JNK. IL-1RI and all the functional TLRs apart from TLR3, employ the adapter MyD88 in order to signal via intracellular proteins and activate NF-κB and MAPKs. MyD88 recruits IRAK-4 and IRAK-1 in the complex. IRAK-4 is the crucial serine/threonine kinase of the complex. It phosphorylates IRAK-1, which also becomes autophosphorylated to become completely activated. The IRAKs link the receptor complexes with TRAF6, which interacts with the ubiquitin-conjugating enzymes Uev1A and Ubc13 and becomes polyubiquitinated in order to become activated. This TRAF6 complex interacts with the TAK1/TAB1/TAB2/TAB3 complex. TAK1 seems to be the main kinase that phosphorylates and activates the NEMO/IKKα/IKKβ complex. The activation of the IKK complex also requires NEMO to become polyubiquitinated by the TRAF6/Uev1A/Ubc13 complex. In its turn, the IKKs phosphorylates IκB, which is pre-associated with NF-κB consisting of the subunits p50 and p65. This phosphorylation leads to proteosomal degradation of IκB, which enables NF-κB to translocate to the nucleus and bind to genes that contain NF-κB binding motifs; this leads to their transcription and expression. In this way, proinflammatory cytokines such TNFα and IL-6 are produced. TAK1 is also linked to the MAPK cascades. Two main proteins of these cascades that become activated are p38 and JNK. In their turn, they activate the transcription factor AP-1, that, like NF-κB, leads to production of proinflammatory cytokines. In the case of TLR4 signaling, MyD88 is not able to directly associate with the receptor. It requires Mal, which acts as a bridging adapter, bringing MyD88 to the membrane and allowing its downstream signaling. TLR4 utilizes all four signaling adapters. Apart from MyD88 and Mal, it can associate with TRIF and TRAM. TRAM is the bridging adapter that enables the association of TRIF with the receptor. TLR4 also activates the IKK complex through TRIF that can interact with RIP1. The same proteins are used by TLR3 in order to activate NF-κB. TLR3 only utilizes TRIF from the four signaling adapters. Some major inhibiting proteins at the adapter level are MyD88s, , IRAK-M, and RIP3, which are not shown in the figure, for simplicity sake (see text for details)

role of IRAK-4 protein in innate immunity was proved to be essential. However, the role of the kinase activity of IRAK-4 in IL-1RI/TLR signaling had not been completely understood until very recently. Initially, one study showed by reconstituting IRAK-4-deficient cells with kinase inactive IRAK-4 that its kinase activity was not necessary for IL-1RI-induced signaling and for the activation of IRAK-1 *in vivo* (Qin et al., 2004). On the contrary, another study showed that such a reconstitution partially restored the activation of IRAK-1 and signaling induced by IL-1 (Lye et al., 2004). Two very recent studies finally clarified the contradiction between the previous observations (Kawagoe et al., 2007; Koziczak-Holbro et al., 2007). In both studies "knock in" mice were generated; these carry a kinase-dead variant of IRAK-4 instead of the wild type. Comparison of these knock in mice with wild-type IRAK-4 mice and IRAK-4-deficient ones showed that the kinase activity of IRAK-4 is required for IL-1RI/TLR-induced responses and the phosphorylation of IRAK-1.

Thus, in the MyD88-dependent IL-1RI-TLR signaling (Figure 1), recruited IRAK-4 was the missing kinase required to phosphorylate IRAK-1. The protein IRAK-1 is subsequently autophosphorylated to become fully activated (Kollewe et al., 2004), leaves the receptor(s), and eventually is degraded by proteosomes (Yamin and Miller, 1997). Very recently, using a proteomic approach, it was shown that the originally phosphorylated *in vitro* endogenous substrate p60 observed in the IL-1RI signaling complex was actually autophosphorylated IRAK-4 (Brikos et al., 2007). Thus, the initially discovered IL-1RI-associated kinase activity (Martin et al., 1994) was partially or totally due to IRAK-4. This finding clarified the contradiction between the studies showing that the IL-1RI-associated kinase activity was essential for NF-κB activation (Croston et al., 1995) and those claiming that the kinase activity of IRAK-1 was not necessary for signaling (Knop and Martin 1999; Li et al., 1999c; Maschera et al., 1999; Vig et al., 1999).

Apart from IRAK-1 and IRAK-4, two additional members in the family of IRAKs—IRAK-2 and IRAK-M—have been identified (Muzio et al., 1997; Wesche et al., 1999). They are both inactive kinases because a critical aspartate residue in the catalytic site of IRAK-1 (D340) is replaced by a serine or asparagine, respectively. Overexpression of human IRAK-2 restored IL-1 and LPS responsiveness to cells that lack IRAK-1 (Li et al., 1999c; Wesche et al., 1999) and dominant negative forms of IRAK-2 inhibited IL-1RI activity. A murine homologue of IRAK-2 was also identified (Rosati and Martin, 2002) and later it was discovered that there are four murine alternative spliced isoforms of IRAK-2, two of which induce and two that inhibit signaling that leads to activation of NF-κB (Table 1). No IRAK-2 knock out mice have been reported, so the exact role of IRAK-2 in signaling remains to be resolved. IRAK-M (Wesche et al., 1999), when overexpressed in IRAK-1-deficient HEK 293 cells, could also reconstitute their responsiveness to IL-1. However, the IRAK-M knock out mice showed that this inactive kinase is a negative regulator of IL-1RI and certain TLRs (Kobayashi et al., 2002). It acts by inhibiting the dissociation of IRAK-1 from MyD88 and the formation of the complex of IRAK-1 with the next protein downstream: tumor necrosis factor (TNF) receptor-associated factor 6 (TRAF6) (Table 1).

The exact ways by which the IRAKs are recruited to the receptor complexes via MyD88 are not yet completely clear. All the complexes contain an N-terminal DD like MyD88. It was initially thought that this domain of IRAK-1 was necessary for interaction with the DD of MyD88 (Muzio et al., 1997; Wesche et al., 1997). However, in the case of IL-1RI signaling, mutated IL-1RI that could not recruit MyD88 still associated with IRAK-1. In addition, an alternatively spliced variant

Table 1 TLR signaling-inhibitory proteins at/near the adapter level

Protein	Type of inhibitor/host	Mechanism of inhibition
A20	Endogenous	Removes ubiquitin molecules from TRAF6, inhibiting MyD88- but also TRIF-dependent signaling
A46R	Exogenous/viral	Binds to MyD88, Mal, TRIF and TRAM but to SARM, inhibiting activation of NF-κB, the MAPKs and IRF3
A52R	Exogenous/viral	Interacts with IRAK-2 and TRAF6 inhibiting NF-κB activation
IRAK-2	Endogenous/2 out of the 4 spliced isoforms that exist in mice but not in human	Unknown-possibly they prevent the recruitment of the active IRAKs to MyD88 and IL-1RI or TLR signaling complexes
IRAK-M	Endogenous/shown inhibitory in mice	Prevents IRAK-1/IRAK-4 dissociation from MyD88
IRF4	Endogenous	Associates with MyD88 preventing its interaction with IRF5
MyD88s	Endogenous	Prevents IRAK-4 recruitment
NS3/4A	Exogenous/viral	Serine protease that cleaves TRIF inducing its degradation, thereby inhibiting TLR3-induced IRF3 and NF-κB activation
PIASy	Endogenous	Interacts with TRIF, IRF3 and IRF7 preventing their signaling
RIP3	Endogenous	Associates with RIP1 preventing its interaction with TRIF
SARM	Endogenous	Interacts with TRIF preventing directly or indirectly its signaling
SHP-2	Endogenous	Binds to TBK1 and inhibits TRIF-dependent signalling
SIKE	Endogenous	Prevents interactions of TBK1 and IKKε to TRIF and IRF3, inhibiting TRIF-dependent signalling through IRF3
SOCS1	Endogenous	Important for Mal degradation
ST2	Endogenous	Sequesters MyD88 and Mal competing their interaction with the TLRs
TGF-β	Endogenous	Causes ubiquitination and proteosomal degradation of MyD88
TRAF1	Endogenous	TRIF causes cleavage of TRAF1 (via a caspase) releasing a fragment with inhibitory function for TRIF-dependent signalling
TRAF4	Endogenous	Sequesters TRIF and TRAF6

Abbreviations

DCs, dendritic cells; DD, death domain; ID, intermediate domain; HCV, hepatitis C virus; HEK, human embryonic kidney; IκB, inhibitor of NF-κB; IKK, IκB kinase; IL-1, interleukin-1; IL-1RAcP, IL-1 receptor accessory protein; IL-1RI, interleukin-1 receptor type I; IRAK, IL-1 receptor-associated kinase; IRF, interferon-regulated factor; ISRE, IFN-stimulated response element; JNK, c-Jun N-terminal kinase; LPS, lipopolysaccharide; LRR, leucine-rich repeat; MAPK, mitogen-activated protein kinase; Mal, MyD88-adapter like; MyD88, myeloid differentiation primary response protein 88; NEMO, NF-κB essential modulator; NF-κB, nuclear factor-kappaB; PAMPs, pathogen-associated molecular patterns; Poc, Pococurante; RIP, receptor interacting protein; SARM, sterile α and HEAT-Armadillo motifs; SH2, Src homology 2; SHP-2, SH2-containing tyrosine phosphatase 2; SIKE, suppressor of IKKε; SOCS1, suppressor of cytokine signaling 1; TAB, TAK1-binding protein; TAK-1, TGF-β-activated kinase 1; TBK1, (TANK)-binding kinase 1; TANK, TRAF-family-member-associated NF-κB activator; TGF, transforming growth factor; TICAM, TIR-containing adapter molecule; TIR, Toll/IL-1 receptor; TIRAP, TIR domain-containing adapter; TLR, Toll-like receptor; TNF, tumor necrosis factor; TRAF, tumor necrosis factor receptor-associated factor; TRAM, TRIF-related adapter molecule; TRIF, TIR domain-containing adapter inducing IFN-β.

of MyD88 (MyD88s) which still contains the DD, inhibits IL-1RI/TLR signaling (Burns et al., 2003) (Table 1). MyD88s is shorter than MyD88 because it lacks the ID of MyD88. This domain enables MyD88 to associate with IRAK-4 but not with IRAK-1. The association of IRAK-4 to MyD88 is most likely happening via binding of the IRAK-4 DD to the MyD88 ID. Thus, MyD88s inhibits signaling because it interferes with this interaction, and as a result IRAK-1 cannot bind to IRAK-4 and become phosphorylated and degraded (Burns et al., 2003). In more detail, by using *in vitro* pull down assays it was shown that the parts of MyD88 which are responsible for its association with the IRAK-4 DD are a C-terminal portion of the MyD88 ID and its TIR domain (Lasker and Nair, 2006).

As mentioned, when IRAK-1 becomes multiply phosphorylated, it dissociates from the receptor(s) (in contrast to IRAK-4 (Brikos et al., 2007)) and binds to TRAF6. In IL-1RI signaling, however, TRAF6 has been shown to be recruited to the signaling complex via IRAK-1, which is acting as an adapter (Jiang et al., 2002). Consequently, both IRAK-1 and TRAF6 dissociate from the receptor complex together. TRAF6 (Cao et al., 1996b) is the protein considered to link the IL-1RI/TLR complexes with the activation of the NF-κB and the MAPK cascades (Figure 1). It interacts with the ubiquitin-conjugating enzyme E2 variant 1 (Uev1A) and the ubiquitin-conjugating enzyme 13 (Ubc13), becomes polyubiquitinated, and oligomerizes (Deng et al., 2000; Chen, 2005). In that way TRAF6 becomes activated and associates with the downstream proteins, transforming growth factor (TGF)-β-activated kinase 1 (TAK1) and the TAK1-binding proteins, TAB1, TAB2, and TAB3 (Wang et al., 2001). The series of events continues with TAK1 being ubiquitinated as well. TAK1 phosphorylates the inhibitor of NF-κB (IκB) kinases (IKK) complex, which is also polyubiquinated by Uev1A/Ubc13/TRAF6. The activated IKKs phosphorylate the IκB protein(s) that are pre-associated with NF-κB dimers in the cytoplasm of resting cells. This phosphorylation event leads to the release of NF-κB. The predominating dimer of NF-κB consists of two proteins, p50 and the p65, (also known as RelA). The protein p50 is responsible for the assembly of this dimer with IκBα, whereas p65 is needed for transactivation of gene expression. In MyD88-dependent signaling, IκBα becomes phosphorylated, polyubiquitinated, and then degraded (Brockman et al., 1995; Brown et al., 1995; DiDonato et al., 1995; Traenckner et al., 1995; Whiteside et al., 1995; DiDonato et al., 1996; Karin and Ben-Neriah, 2000). Consequently, NF-κB is able to translocate to the nucleus, where it binds and induces its target genes, which are responsible for inflammatory responses.

In more detail, the IKK complex consists of three subunits: one regulatory subunit IKKγ (Cohen et al., 1998; Rothwarf et al., 1998), also named as NF-κB essential modulator (NEMO) (Yamaoka et al., 1998) and two catalytic ones: IKKα and IKKβ (Verma et al., 1995; Rothwarf et al., 1998; Rottenberg et al., 2002). NEMO is a scaffold protein essential for the assembly of the IKKs (Li et al., 2001). Moreover, it also links the IKKs to the activated downstream molecule IκB (Yamamoto et al., 2001). NEMO is thus essential for the pathway. In cells which do not express it, NF-κB activation did not occur (Yamaoka et al., 1998). In addition, either disrupting the association of NEMO with IKKs or overexpressing a deletion-mutant of NEMO blocks the activation of NF-κB (Le Page et al., 2001; May et al., 2002). The kinases of the complex, IKKα and IKKβ, can both phosphorylate IκBα on serines 32 and 36 (Lee et al., 1998). IKKβ is crucial for NF-κB activation and cannot be substituted by IKKα (Li et al., 1999b). It has been shown that phosphorylation of IKKβ at two sites in its activation loop is important for the activation of IKK (Delhase et al., 1999). In contrast, it has not been clarified whether IKKα, which was found to regulate IKKβ (O'Mahony et al., 2000), is a target for IL-1 (Delhase et al., 1999; Hu et al., 1999; Takeda et al., 1999). Two independent studies of IKKα knock out mice showed that it was not essential for activation of IKK complex and NF-κB by IL-1 (Hu et al., 1999; Takeda et al., 1999), but in another IKKα knock out mice report, a high reduction of activation of NF-κB was observed (Li et al., 1999a).

The TAK1 complex is not only essential for IKK activation. It is also linked to the MAPK kinase (MAPKK) 6 (or MKK6) and other MAPKKs such as MKK3 and MKK7 (Figure 1). Phosphorylation of MKK6 leads to the activation of JNK, whereas MKK3 and MKK7 are responsible for the activation of p38. JNK and p38 culminate in the activation of the transcription factor, activator protein-1 (AP-1), which plays a crucial role in the induction of inflammatory-response genes.

MyD88-Dependent Activation of the IRFs

Among the extremely significant recent discoveries on TLR signaling is that the MyD88-dependent pathway also activates some IRFs. One of them is IRF7, which was shown to participate in TLR7 and TLR9 signaling in a cell-specific manner (Figure 2). Specifically, IRF7 activation in these TLR pathways occurred in plasma-cytoid, but not in conventional DCs. MyD88, IRAK-1, IRAK-4, and TRAF6 have been shown to directly associate with IRF7 (Hochrein et al., 2004; Honda et al., 2004; Kawai et al., 2004; Honda et al., 2005; Uematsu et al., 2005). Consequently, IRF7 translocates into the nucleus where it binds IFN-stimulated response element (ISRE) motifs. As a result, type I IFNs are produced. The role of IRAK-1 in these pathways is essential, as shown by the IRAK-1-deficient mice, which do not produce IFN-α following activation of either the TLR7 or TLR9 signaling pathways (Uematsu et al., 2005). It is therefore likely that IRAK-1 needs to phosphorylate IRF7 to induce its activation. In TLR9 signaling, it has also been shown that MyD88 needs to stably associate with the TIR domain of that receptor in order for the activation of IRF7 to occur (Honda et al., 2005).

Another transcription factor from the same family that is activated via MyD88 is IRF5 (Figure 2). In TLR4 and TLR9 signaling, IRF5 has also been found in a complex with MyD88 and TRAF6 (Takaoka et al., 2005). Consequently, it moves into the nucleus and binds ISRE motifs in the promoter regions of cytokine genes, inducing the production of IL-6, IL-12, and TNFα.

Last, in myeloid DCs, MyD88 has been shown to associate with IRF1 (Figure 2) (Negishi et al., 2006). Following that interaction, IRF1 translocates to the nucleus and activates several TLR-dependent genes. IRF1 is induced by the IFN-γ receptor 1 (IFNγR1), affecting in that way the TLR signaling cascades indirectly. Another

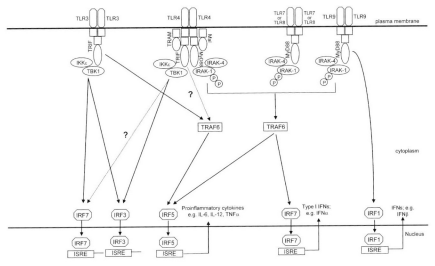

Fig. 2 TLR activation of IRFs. The TLRs that have been found to activate IRFs are TLR3, TLR4, TLR7, TLR8 and TLR9. Apart from the proteins responsible for the NF-κB activation, TRIF that can interact with IKKε and TBK1, which have been shown to induce the activation of IRF3 and IRF7 in the TLR3 and TLR4 signaling cascades (see text for details). IRF3 and IRF7, when activated, translocate into the nucleus, where they bind genes to their ISRE motifs and cause their subscription, leading to production of IFNs type I. TLR3 interacts via TRIF with TRAF6 and activates IRF5, which also translocates into the nucleus and binds to ISRE motifs of genes. However, in that case, instead of IFNs, proinflammatory cytokines are produced. Apart from these pathways, all the other TLR cascades that lead to activation of IRFs are MyD88-dependent. MyD88 and the IRAKs can interact with TRAF6 and IRF5 or IRF7, causing their activation and translocation to the nucleus. MyD88 also acts in a cell-specific way. In myeloid DCs, MyD88 binds to IRF1 in response to TLR7, 8, and 9. (In the figure, for simplicity sake, only the TLR9-recruited MyD88 is linked to IRF1 by an arrow.) MyD88 and IRF1 translocate together into the nucleus, where IRF1 binds to ISRE motifs, inducing the production of IFNs

discovery linking the TLR pathways with that of IFNγR1 is that, although this receptor does not contain a TIR domain, it can recruit MyD88 and thus activate p38 (Sun and Ding, 2006).

Apart from TRAF6, another member of the same family, TRAF3, was also found to participate in MyD88-dependent signaling of some TLRs. In particular, an interaction was observed between TRAF3 and MyD88. Furthermore, TRAF3-deficient mice presented an impaired production of type I IFNs and IL-10 in their TLR4 and TLR9 pathways (Hacker et al., 2006).

Mal—A Bridging Adapter in MyD88-Dependent TLR Signaling

MyD88 is not the only adapter protein required for TLR signal transduction. This notion became evident by the fact that in MyD88-deficient mice, the activation of NF-κB and the MAPKs, was only eliminated in response to IL-1 and the ligands for TLR5, TLR7, TLR8 and TLR9. In response to TLR4 agonists, such activation was only delayed. Eventually, four more adapter molecules homologous to MyD88 were identified that could explain this phenomenon.

The first of these four adapters was Mal/TIRAP (Fitzgerald et al., 2001; Horng et al., 2001). It was discovered based on the similarity of its sequence to that of MyD88. Mal was initially shown to have an important role in TLR4 but not in IL-1RI signaling (Fitzgerald et al., 2001) because when a proline in its Box 2 was mutated to histidine, it blocked the response to endotoxin, but not to IL-1. Similarly, a peptide based on the BB loop of Mal could inhibit TLR4 but not TLR9 signaling. Later, Mal-deficient mice agreed with these original observations (Horng et al., 2002; Yamamoto et al., 2002a). The Mal knock out mice were very similar to the MyD88 ones in terms of TLR4 signaling. In both of these types of knock out mice, the activation of NF-κB and the MAPKs was delayed instead of abolished in response to TLR4. This activation was still induced by IL-1 and various TLR ligands, with an exception of those for TLR2. Interestingly, TLR2 signaling was even more affected than that of TLR4 in the Mal-deficient mice. In particular, NF-κB and p38 activation was completely impaired. Thus, it became clear that Mal is a member of the TLR2 and TLR4 MyD88-dependent pathways. The importance of Mal in the activation of innate immunity was also demonstrated by humans having a single nucleotide polymorphism in the gene encoding the adapter (Khor et al., 2007). This polymorphism results in the S180L Mal phenotype, which attenuates TLR2-induced signaling. It was discovered that the S180L heterozygosity protects its carriers against invasive pneumococcal disease, bacteremia, malaria, and tuberculosis.

The role of Mal in TLR4 signaling was uncovered recently. In contrast to MyD88, Mal has a binding domain for one of the main structural components of the plasma membrane; the phosphatidylinositol-4, 5-bisphosphate (PIP2), (Fitzgerald and Chen, 2006; Kagan and Medzhitov, 2006). Via this domain Mal can interact with PIP2, thereby facilitating the recruitment of MyD88 to the membrane. In that way, Mal and MyD88 can be in close proximity to TLR4 and thus able to associate with it. Thus, Mal is the bridging adapter, enabling MyD88 to be a component of the TLR4 signaling complex, and MyD88 is the signaling adapter, leading to the downstream events. Apart from the PIP2 binding domain, there are several other differences between Mal and MyD88. The first difference that became obvious since the discovery of Mal's sequence is that it does not contain a DD. In addition, in contrast to MyD88, Mal can associate with TRAF6. So it is likely that Mal is responsible for the recruitment of TRAF6 in the TLR2 and TLR4 signaling complexes (Mansell et al., 2004). Last, Mal is able to interact with Bruton's tyrosine kinase (Btk). This protein phosphorylates Mal and makes possible its downstream signaling (Gray et al., 2006). Btk has been shown to participate in TLR2 and TLR4 signaling (Jefferies et al., 2003; Liljeroos et al., 2007) by being involved in the phosphorylation of NF-κB on its p65 subunit (Doyle et al., 2005). However, the tyrosine phosphorylation of Mal is also required for its degradation (Mansell et al., 2006), providing a means of termination of its signaling. An essential protein for the occurrence of this degradation is the suppressor of cytokine signaling 1 (SOCS1) and cells that cannot express SOCS1 respond to endotoxin at a higher extent than SOCS1 wild-type cells (Kinjyo et al., 2002; Nakagawa et al., 2002) (Table 1).

The discovery of Mal was the first evidence that different TLRs recruit different adapter molecules. Furthermore, the generation of Mal-MyD88 double knock out mice showed a delayed instead of abolished response in terms of TLR4 stimulation, indicating the existence of another protein that could lead to downstream signaling (Yamamoto et al., 2002a). Last, the MyD88 knock out mice presented signal transduction that was independent of MyD88 when not only TLR3, but also when TLR4 were liganded (Fitzgerald et al., 2003a; Fitzgerald et al., 2003b). In particular, that pathway culminates in the activation of the transcription factors IRF3 and IRF7, leading to the induction of IFN-α/β and IFN-inducible genes.

3.3 TRIF—The Signaling Adapter for the MyD88-Independent Pathways

3.3.1 TRIF-Dependent Pathways

The adapter that was eventually found to be essential for the MyD88-independent pathway is TRIF (Yamamoto et al., 2002b; Hoebe et al., 2003; Oshiumi et al., 2003a). It was discovered in two independent ways. One was by searching the databases for TIR-containing proteins (Yamamoto et al., 2002b) and the other was by using the yeast two-hybrid system using a part of TLR3 as a bait (Oshiumi et al., 2003a). The TRIF-deficient mice clearly identified the specificity and the role of the adapter. The inflammatory cytokine production was impaired in the TLR4 signaling, but unaffected following activation of TLR2, 7, and 9 (Figure 1). The activation of IRF3 and the following induction of IFN-β was impaired in both the TLR3 and the TLR4 pathways (Yamamoto et al., 2003a) (Figure 2). Thus, TRIF was the missing adapter that was utilized by TLR3 and was also required for TLR4-induced signal transduction. The TRIF/MyD88 double knock out mice shed further light on the function of TRIF in the TLR4 signaling cascades. These mice were unable to activate NF-κB (Hirotani et al., 2005). Thus, TRIF was responsible for the delayed activation of NF-κB that was observed in the MyD88 and Mal knock out mice (discussed in "Mal-A bridging adapter in MyD88-Dependent TLR signaling" under Sect. 2.3.2.2).

In order to signal downstream in both the TLR3 and TLR4 pathways, TRIF forms a complex with an IKK-like kinase named the TRAF-family-member-associated NF-κB activator (TANK)-binding kinase 1 (TBK1) (Fitzgerald et al., 2003a), the IKK homolog IKKε and IRF3. These interactions result in the phosphorylation of IRF3 by TBK1 and IKKε, leading to its activation (Figure 2). Consequently, IRF3 binds to the ISRE on target genes and induces the production of IFN-α/β (Sato et al., 2003). Similar to IRF3, IRF7 becomes activated via its phosphorylation by TBK1 and IKKε, and induces the expression of genes, by binding to their ISREs (Kawai et al., 2004; Honda et al., 2005; Uematsu et al., 2005) (Figure 2).

Furthermore, IRF5-deficient mice showed that IRF5 is also activated via TRIF in TLR3 signaling inducing IL-6, IL-12, and TNFα production (Takaoka et al., 2005) (Figure 2).

In TLR3 signaling, TRIF has also been shown to activate NF-κB (Figure 1). TRIF can bind to the TRAF6-TAK1-TAB2 complex that activates IKK (see Section 2.3.2.3.1) (Jiang et al., 2004). Very likely, this interaction occurs because TRIF contains consensus TRAF6-binding motifs. However, the exact role of TRAF6 in NF-κB activation via TRIF remains unclear, as two studies using TRAF6-deficient mice disagree with each other. In one of them TLR3-induced NF-κB activation from TRAF6-deficient murine embryonic fibroblasts was completely abolished (Jiang et al., 2004), whereas in the other study such signaling was un-affected (Gohda et al., 2004). An explanation for this contradiction could be that there is cell specificity in the usage of TRAF6 in order to activate NF-κB via TRIF.

TRIF also contains a receptor interacting protein (RIP) homotypic interaction motif, and thus it can associate with RIP1 and RIP3 (Meylan et al., 2004). RIP1 is important for TLR3-induced NF-κB activation and RIP3 has an inhibiting ef-fect, preventing the interaction of RIP1 with TRIF (Table 1). In the case of TLR4 signaling, the role of RIP1 is unclear. According to Meylan et al., (2004), in RIP1-deficient murine embryonic fibroblasts the NF-κB activation was completely abolished in response to poly(I:C), but not to endotoxin. However, another study (Cusson-Hermance et al., 2005) showed that the activation was affected in both of the TLR3 and TLR4 pathways.

A difference among the TLR3 and TLR4 pathways that seems clear concerns the activation of NF-κB. In contrast to TLR3 signaling, TLR4 also leads indirectly to NF-κB activation. This is happening via TRIF, which, as previously mentioned, induces TNFα production via the activation of IRF3 (Figure 1). The produced TNFα is then secreted from the stimulated cells and binds to its receptor (TNFR) (Covert et al., 2005). Signaling induced by TNFR also culminates in NF-κB activation. In this way endotoxin can cause a prolonged activation that is important for the defense of the host.

Another difference between TLR3 and TLR4 is evident in the TRIF-dependent pathway that leads to binding of IRF3 to ISRE motifs (Figure 2). In the case of the TLR3 pathway, IRF3 forms homodimers that bind ISRE. In contrast, following activation of TLR4, IRF3 forms a heterocomplex with the p65 subunit of NF-κB which then binds ISRE (Wietek et al., 2003).

Apart from the pathways mentioned above, TRIF in contrast to the other adapter proteins is shown to be important for the induction of apoptosis in response to the activation of TLR3 and TLR4 (Han et al., 2004; Ruckdeschel et al., 2004; De Trez et al., 2005; Kaiser and Offermann, 2005). Along with TRIF this pathway requires involvement of the proteins RIP1, FADD, and caspase-8.

Finally, very recently TRIF was shown to play an important role in the induction of MHCII expression in DCs, which is essential for CD4 T cell activation (Kamon et al., 2006). This process occurs in response to endotoxin and involves the proteins RhoB and the guanine nucleotide exchange factor (GEF)-H1.

3.3.2 TRAM—A Bridging Adapter in TRIF-Dependent TLR Signaling

From the previous section it is clear that TRIF seems to interact with a wider range of proteins in comparison to the other adapters. It is thought that TLR3 associates with TRIF *directly*. On the other hand, TLR4 requires TRAM to *engage* TRIF (Fitzgerald, et al., 2003b; Oshiumi et al., 2003b; Yamamoto et al., 2003b; McGettrick et al., 2006; Rowe et al., 2006). Thus, TRAM is also a bridging adapter like Mal and is different than all the other adapters in the fact that it is strictly utilized by TLR4 (Figure 2). As in the case of Mal, TRAM also associates with the plasma membrane. However, unlike Mal, this depends on myristioylation of the N-terminus of TRAM. Mutation of this myristioylation motif makes TRAM inactive. Furthermore, the activation of TRAM is dependent on the phosphorylation of its serine 16 by protein kinase Cε. Mutant TRAM that cannot be phosphorylated at this site does not function, and inhibition of this phosphorylation impairs TRAM signaling. Thus, this modification is required in order for TRAM to signal, but its exact role is unknown.

3.4 Inhibition of TLR Signaling at the Adapter Level

3.4.1 SARM and Its Role in Suppressing TLR Signaling

The fifth and last adapter is SARM. It was discovered as a human gene that encodes a protein of unknown function with a sterile α-motif (SAM), and it was found to be structurally similar to Armadillo/β-catenin (it contains HEAT/Armadillo repeats) (Mink et al., 2001). It was also shown that SARM was conserved in *Caenorhabditis elegans, Drosophila melanogaster*, and *Mus musculus*. The existence of its TIR domain was observed later (Couillault et al., 2004; Liberati et al., 2004). Initially, the significance of SARM in TLR signaling had not been recognized, as it could not activate NF-κB when overexpressed. In that aspect it is dissimilar to all the other TIR-containing adapters. It was only recently that its role started to be revealed. In contrast to the other adapters, SARM acts as an inhibitor of NF-κB and IRF activation through its interaction with TRIF (Carty et al., 2006) (Table 1). However, exactly how SARM prevents the function of TRIF remains to be identified. It is not clear if SARM forms a complex with TRIF, disabling it to interact with other proteins downstream, or if SARM facilitates the interaction of TRIF with another inhibitory protein. The knockdown of SARM expression using small interfering RNA (siRNA) leads to an increased production of chemokines and cytokines in response to TLR3 and TLR4 activation. Very interestingly, the expression of SARM is increased in response to LPS. It is therefore very likely that this is a negative feedback mechanism used to inhibit prolonged TLR3 and TLR4 activation that could have dangerous effects for the host.

3.4.2 Additional Negative Regulators of TLR Adapter Signaling

Endogenous Inhibitory Proteins at the Adapter Level

Apart from SARM, MyD88s, IRAK-M, SOCS1, and RIP3 mentioned in the previous sections, there are several other proteins of the host that inhibit TLR signaling at the adapter level (Table 1).

One of these proteins is the antiinflammatory cytokine-transforming growth factor-$\beta1$ (TGF-$\beta1$) (Table 1) (Naiki et al., 2005). It has been shown that TGF-$\beta1$ inhibits NF-κB activation via the MyD88-dependent pathway in response to ligands for TLR2, 4, and 5. In particular, it induces ubiquitination of MyD88 and its subsequent proteosomal degradation. Thus, it decreases the levels of MyD88 in the cells of the host without affecting its mRNA levels. TGF-$\beta1$ does not affect the TRIF-dependent pathway of TLR4.

Another inhibitory protein is ST2 (Table 1) (Brint et al., 2004). This transmembrane protein belongs to the IL-1RI/TLR family of receptors because it also contains a TIR domain. When overexpressed, ST2 has been found to inhibit MyD88-dependent signaling induced by IL-1RI and TLR4, but not by TLR3, as it does not utilize that adapter. A recombinant ST2 protein construct is able to interact with Mal and MyD88, but not with TRIF. Thus, the molecular basis of the inhibitory role of ST2 could be its sequestration of the adapters MyD88 and Mal.

Additional adapter-mediated signaling inhibitory proteins belong to the family of TRAFs. In contrast to TRAF6 and TRAF3, which are essential for TLR signaling (see previous sections), TRAF1 and TRAF4 play an inhibitory role (Table 1) (Takeshita et al., 2005; Su et al., 2006). TRAF1 can associate with the adapter TRIF, and its overexpression prevents TLR3 signaling, thereby inhibiting NF-κB, ISRE, and IFN-β promoter activation. In addition, TRIF induces cleavage of TRAF1 (via a caspase), which is essential for its inhibitory function. TRAF4 can interact also not only with TRIF but also with TRAF6. Thus, TRAF4 is able to prevent NF-κB activation induced by TLR2, 3, 4, and 9, and IFN-β promoter activation mediated by both TLR3 and TLR4.

Another inhibitory protein of TLR signal transduction is IRF4 (Table 1) (Negishi et al., 2005). As mentioned in the MyD88-dependent signaling pathways section (2.3.2.2.2), IRF5 and 7 associate with MyD88, which leads to production of type I IFNs and proinflammatory cytokines. IRF4 can bind MyD88, thereby not allowing formation of the MyD88-IRF5 complex. Conversely, the association of IRF4 with MyD88 does not prevent the formation of the MyD88-IRF7 complex. Consequently, IRF4 only inhibits MyD88-IRF5-mediated signaling. In particular, IRF4 suppresses the translocation of IRF5 into the nucleus in response to TLR9. The fact that IRF4 can be a negative feedback regulator is supported by the observation that its mRNA levels are increased following treatment of murine peritoneal macrophages with ligands for TLR4, 7, and 9, all of which activate the MyD88-IRF5 pathway.

At the adapter-IRF level, TLR signaling can be further controlled, by a member of the PIAS family, called PIASy (Table 1) (Zhang et al., 2004). PIAS are protein inhibitors of the activated signal transducer and activator of transcription (STAT) family. PIASy interacts with TRIF, IRF3, and IRF7 and inhibits their activation of ISRE. It also suppresses NF-κB activation and IFN-β production induced by TRIF. It does not, however, affect the apoptotic effects of TRIF (mentioned in the previous section 3.4.1).

Activation of the TRIF-dependent pathway, can also be regulated by the suppressor of IKKε (SIKE) (Table 1) (Huang et al., 2005). Apart from IKKε, SIKE also interacts with TBK1, but not with RIP1 and TRAF6. In fact SIKE is pre-associated with TBK1 in nonstimulated cells, and dissociates from it when the cells are stimulated with TLR3 ligands. As a result, SIKE was shown to inhibit the association of TBK1 and IKKε with TRIF and IRF3, disrupting in that way ISRE and IFN-β promoter activation. On the other hand, as SIKE does not affect the interactions of TRIF with TRAF6 and RIP1, it does not act as an inhibitor of the TLR3-induced NF-κB activation.

Src homology 2 (SH2)-containing tyrosine phosphatase 2 (SHP-2) has been identified as an additional endogenous inhibitor of TRIF-dependent signaling (Table 1) (An et al., 2006). It also, like SIKE, associates with TBK1 and blocks TBK1-induced IFN-β expression. In general, SHP-2 was shown to downregulate IFN-β production in TLR3 and TLR4 signaling. SHP-2 also negatively affected the production of IL-6, TNFα, and the activation of the MAPKs in response to TLR3. This inhibitory function of SHP-2 does not depend on its tyrosine phosphatase activity.

Last, another cytoplasmic protein of the host which is important for terminating TLR signaling is A20 (Table 1) (Boone et al., 2004). This is an enzyme that can remove ubiquitin moieties from TRAF6. As mentioned in a previous section, the ubiquitination of TRAF6 is essential for its signaling resulting in NF-κB activation. In particular, it was shown that A20 is crucial in the termination of NF-κB activation induced by TLR4. However, A20 does not only suppress TLR4 signaling; A20-deficient macrophages express enhanced levels of TNF, IL-6, and nitric oxide in response to ligands for TLR2, TLR3, and TLR9, suggesting that A20 negatively regulates these TLRs as well.

Exogenous Inhibitory Proteins at the Adapter Level

Apart from the previously mentioned endogenous proteins, there are several exogenous proteins of invading agents that are used by them in order to prevent the activation of TLR signaling. Two of these inhibitors, A46R and A52R (Table 1), are expressed by the vaccinia virus. A46R contains a TIR domain and is able to interact with MyD88. In particular, it inhibits NF-κB and MAPKs activation in response to IL-1. A46R also blocks NF-κB activation induced by ligands for TLR2/1, TLR2/6, TLR4, TLR5, TLR7, and TLR9. However, apart from MyD88, A46R can also interact with TLR4, Mal, TRAM, and TRIF, but not with SARM. In that way, the viral protein can completely abolish TLR4 signaling that leads to NF-κB activation, and it can inhibit IRF3 activation mediated by TLR4 and TLR3. The other viral protein, A52R (Harte et al., 2003), can also disrupt MyD88-dependent signaling although it does not contain a TIR domain. A52R can interact with IRAK-2 and TRAF6, and blocks NF-κB activation by TLR1/2, TLR2/6, TLR3, TLR4, and TLR5. In another study, a peptide that was designed based on the sequence of A52R, could suppress TLR signaling and reduce bacterial middle ear inflammation (McCoy et al., 2005).

Last, an additional suppressor of TLR signaling is the serine protease NS3/4A of hepatitis C virus (HCV) (Table 1). NS3/4A cleaves TRIF, causing its degradation and disrupting TLR3-induced IRF3 and NF-κB activation.

4 Final Perspectives

Since the discovery of the essential role that TLRs play for the innate and adaptive immunity, a lot of discoveries have been made regarding their signaling cascades. Continuous research widely increases the number of proteins that participate in the TLR pathways and the interactions that take place during their course. Currently, there is a quite clear understanding on the molecular basis of the initiation of signaling by the TLRs and those sets of genes that they activate in order to activate an immune response.

Several studies have shown that TLRs are activated by a wide spectrum of ligands. As a consequence of this liganding the first step in the initiation of signaling by the TLRs is their homo- or heterodimerization. This pairing provides the structural platform in the cytoplasm of the cells, where the adapter molecules bind and transmit signaling intracellularly.

The existence of these adapters explains, to some extent, the differences in the TLR pathways. The reason is that not all TLRs recruit the same adapter molecule(s). Thus, depending on which adapter or adapters associate with a certain TLR, several different biochemical pathways are activated that culminate in the production of proinflammatory cytokines or IFNs and the genes induced by them. In addition, the adapters link the TLRs to other biochemical pathways by interacting with some of their components. One of the recent discoveries is that TLR signaling leads through TRIF to apoptosis.

However, the adapter molecules are not only responsible for determining which pathways are going to be activated in response to the variety of TLR ligands. The adapters are also essential for the regulation of the TLR cascades.

In fact, one of the very recent discoveries is that one of the adapters—SARM— plays an inhibiting role in TLR signaling. Apart from this adapter, several endogenous proteins have been identified that target the TLR signaling pathways at the adapter level in order to inhibit them and avoid their overactivation that could be extremely dangerous for the host.

This method of inhibiting TLR signaling is also used by certain viruses in order to block the activation of the immune system and survive. In particular, these invaders have evolved to express proteins that are inhibiting the interactions of the adapters with other proteins of the TLR signaling pathways. Furthermore, one of the adapters (TRIF) can also be cleaved by an HCV protease, preventing in that way its signaling.

It is now believed that the adapter molecules provide potential targets for therapeutic intervention. It is hoped that soon new drugs will be designed as adapter-mimetics that could have antimicrobial action or suppress chronic inflammation.

Acknowledgements We thank Science Foundaation Ireland for providing financial support for the research programs in the authors' laboratory, and we thank Pearl Gray for her help in the preparation of this book manuscript.

References

Adachi O, Kawai T, Takeda K, Matsumoto M, Tsutsui H, Sakagami M, Nakanishi K, Akira S (1998) Targeted disruption of the MyD88 gene results in loss of IL-1- and IL-18-mediated function. Immunity 9: 143–150

Agnese DM, Calvano JE, Hahm SJ, Coyle SM, Corbett SA, Calvano SE, Lowry SF (2002) Human TToll-like receptor 4 mutations but not CD14 polymorphisms are associated with an increased risk of GGram-negative infections. J Infect Dis 186: 1522–1525

Alexopoulou L, Holt AC, Medzhitov R, Flavell RA (2001) Recognition of double-stranded RNA and activation of NF-kappaB by Toll-like receptor 3. Nature 413: 732–738

An H, Zhao W, Hou J, Zhang Y, Xie Y, Zheng Y, Xu H, Qian C, Zhou J, Yu Y, Liu S, Feng G, Cao X (2006) SHP-2 phosphatase negatively regulates the TRIF adaptor protein-dependent type I interferon and proinflammatory cytokine production. Immunity 25: 919–928

Arbour NC, Lorenz E, Schutte BC, Zabner J, Kline JN, Jones M, Frees K, Watt JL, Schwartz DA (2000) TLR4 mutations are associated with endotoxin hyporesponsiveness in humans. Nat Genet 25: 187–191

Bauer S, Kirschning CJ, Hacker H, Redecke V, Hausmann S, Akira S, Wagner H, Lipford GB (2001) Human TLR9 confers responsiveness to bacterial DNA via species-specific CpG motif recognition. Proc Natl Acad Sci USA 98: 9237–9242

Bell JK, Askins J, Hall PR, Davies DR, Segal DM (2006) The dsRNA binding site of human Toll-like receptor 3. Proc Natl Acad Sci USA 103: 8792–8797

Bell JK, Botos I, Hall PR, Askins J, Shiloach J, Segal DM, Davies DR (2005) The molecular structure of the Toll-like receptor 3 ligand-binding domain. Proc Natl Acad Sci USA 102: 10976–10980

Bird TA, Gearing AJ, Saklatvala J (1988) Murine interleukin 1 receptor. Direct identification by ligand blotting and purification to homogeneity of an interleukin 1-binding glycoprotein. J Biol Chem 263: 12063–12069

Bonnert TP, Garka KE, Parnet P, Sonoda G, Testa JR, Sims JE (1997) The cloning and characterization of human MyD88: A member of an IL-1 receptor related family. FEBS Lett 402: 81–84

Boone DL, Turer EE, Lee EG, Ahmad RC, Wheeler MT, Tsui C, Hurley P, Chien M, Chai S, Hitotsumatsu O, McNally E, Pickart C, Ma A (2004) The ubiquitin-modifying enzyme A20 is required for termination of Toll-like receptor responses. Nat Immunol 5: 1052–1060

Brikos C, Wait R, Begum S, O'Neill LA, Saklatvala J (2007) Mass spectrometric analysis of the endogenous IL-1RI signalling complex formed after IL-1 binding identifies IL-1RAcP, MyD88 and IRAK-4 as the stable components. Mol Cell Proteomics

Brint EK, Xu D, Liu H, Dunne A, McKenzie AN, O'Neill LA, Liew FY (2004) ST2 is an inhibitor of interleukin 1 receptor and Toll-like receptor 4 signaling and maintains endotoxin tolerance. Nat Immunol 5: 373–379

Brockman JA, Scherer DC, McKinsey TA, Hall SM, Qi X, Lee WY, Ballard DW (1995) Coupling of a signal response domain in I kappa B alpha to multiple pathways for NF-kappaB activation. Mol Cell Biol 15: 2809–2818

Brown K, Gerstberger S, Carlson L, Franzoso G, Siebenlist U (1995) Control of I kappa B-alpha proteolysis by site-specific, signal-induced phosphorylation. Science 267: 1485–1488

Burns K, et al (1998) MyD88, an adapter protein involved in interleukin-1 signalling. J Biol Chem 273: 12203–12209

Burns K, Janssens S, Brissoni B, Olivos N, Beyaert R, Tschopp J (2003) Inhibition of interleukin 1 receptor/Toll-like receptor signaling through the alternatively spliced, short form of MyD88 is due to its failure to recruit IRAK-4. J Exp Med 197: 263–268

Cao Z, Henzel WJ, Gao X (1996a) IRAK: A kinase associated with the interleukin-1 receptor. Science 271: 1128–1131

Cao Z, Xiong J, Takeuchi M, Kurama T, Goeddel DV (1996b) TRAF6 is a signal transducer for interleukin-1. Nature 383: 443–446

Carty M, Goodbody R, Schroder M, Stack J, Moynagh PN, Bowie AG (2006) The human adaptor SARM negatively regulates adaptor protein TRIF-dependent Toll-like receptor signaling. Nat Immunol 7: 1074–1081

Chen ZJ (2005) Ubiquitin signalling in the NF-kappaB pathway. Nat Cell Biol 7: 758–765

Choe J, Kelker MS, Wilson IA (2005) Crystal structure of human Toll-like receptor 3 (TLR3) ectodomain. Science 309: 581–585

Cohen L, Henzel WJ, Baeuerle PA (1998) IKAP is a scaffold protein of the IkappaB kinase complex. Nature 395: 292–296

Couillault C, Pujol N, Reboul J, Sabatier L, Guichou JF, Kohara Y, Ewbank JJ (2004) TLR-independent control of innate immunity in *Caenorhabditis elegans* by the TIR domain adaptor protein TIR-1, an ortholog of human SARM. Nat Immunol 5: 488–494

Covert MW, Leung TH, Gaston JE, Baltimore D (2005) Achieving stability of lipopolysaccharide-induced NF-kappaB activation. Science 309: 1854–1857

Croston GE, Cao Z, Goeddel DV (1995) NF-kappa B activation by interleukin-1 (IL-1) requires an IL-1 receptor-associated protein kinase activity. J Biol Chem 270: 16514–16517

Cusson-Hermance N, Khurana S, Lee TH, Fitzgerald KA, Kelliher MA (2005) Rip1 mediates the Trif-dependent Toll-like receptor 3- and 4-induced NF-kappaB activation but does not contribute to interferon regulatory factor 3 activation. J Biol Chem 280: 36560–36566

De Trez C, Pajak B, Brait M, Glaichenhaus N, Urbain J, Moser M, Lauvau G, Muraille E (2005) TLR4 and Toll-IL-1 receptor domain-containing adapter-inducing IFN-beta, but not MyD88, regulate *Escherichia coli*-induced dendritic cell maturation and apoptosis *in vivo*. J Immunol 175: 839–846

Delhase M, Hayakawa M, Chen Y, Karin M (1999) Positive and negative regulation of IkappaB kinase activity through IKKbeta subunit phosphorylation. Science 284: 309–313

Deng L, Wang C, Spencer E, Yang L, Braun A, You J, Slaughter C, Pickart C, Chen ZJ (2000) Activation of the IkappaB kinase complex by TRAF6 requires a dimeric ubiquitin-conjugating enzyme complex and a unique polyubiquitin chain. Cell 103: 351–361

DiDonato J, Mercurio F, Rosette C, Wu-Li J, Suyang H, Ghosh S, Karin M (1996) Mapping of the inducible IkappaB phosphorylation sites that signal its ubiquitination and degradation. Mol Cell Biol 16: 1295–1304

DiDonato JA, Mercurio F, Karin M (1995) Phosphorylation of I kappa B alpha precedes but is not sufficient for its dissociation from NF-kappa B. Mol Cell Biol 15: 1302–1311

Dinarello CA (1994) The interleukin-1 family: 10 years of discovery. Faseb J 8: 1314–1325

Dinarello CA (1996) Biologic basis for interleukin-1 in disease. Blood 87: 2095–2147

Dower SK, Kronheim SR, March CJ, Conlon PJ, Hopp TP, Gillis S, Urdal DL (1985) Detection and characterization of high affinity plasma membrane receptors for human interleukin 1. J Exp Med 162: 501–515

Doyle SL, Jefferies CA, O'Neill LA (2005) Bruton's tyrosine kinase is involved in p65-mediated transactivation and phosphorylation of p65 on serine 536 during NFkappaB activation by lipopolysaccharide. J Biol Chem 280: 23496–23501

Dunne A, Ejdeback M, Ludidi PL, O'Neill LA, Gay NJ (2003) Structural complementarity of Toll/interleukin-1 receptor domains in Toll-like receptors and the adaptors Mal and MyD88. J Biol Chem 278: 41443–41451

Fitzgerald KA, Chen ZJ (2006) Sorting out Toll signals. Cell 125: 834–836

Fitzgerald KA, McWhirter SM, Faia KL, Rowe DC, Latz E, Golenbock DT, Coyle AJ, Liao SM, Maniatis T (2003a) IKKepsilon and TBK1 are essential components of the IRF3 signaling pathway. Nat Immunol 4: 491–496

Fitzgerald KA, Palsson-McDermott EM, Bowie AG, Jefferies CA, Mansell AS, Brady G, Brint E, Dunne A, Gray P, Harte MT, McMurray D, Smith DE, Sims JE, Bird TA, O'Neill LA (2001) Mal (MyD88–adapter-like) is required for Toll-like receptor-4 signal transduction. Nature 413: 78–83

Fitzgerald KA, Rowe DC, Barnes BJ, Caffrey DR, Visintin A, Latz E, Monks B, Pitha PM, Golenbock DT (2003b) LPS-TLR4 signaling to IRF-3/7 and NF-kappaB involves the Toll adapters TRAM and TRIF. J Exp Med 198: 1043–1055

Gautam JK, Ashish, Comeau LD, Krueger JK, Smith MF, Jr. (2006) Structural and functional evidence for the role of the TLR2 DD loop in TLR1/TLR2 heterodimerization and signaling. J Biol Chem 281: 30132–30142

Gay NJ, Keith FJ (1991) *Drosophila* Toll and IL-1 receptor. Nature 351: 355–356

Gohda J, Matsumura T, Inoue J (2004) Cutting edge: TNFR-associated factor (TRAF) 6 is essential for MyD88-dependent pathway but not Toll/IL-1 receptor domain-containing adaptor-inducing IFN-beta (TRIF)-dependent pathway in TLR signaling. J Immunol 173: 2913–2917

Gray P, Dunne A, Brikos C, Jefferies CA, Doyle SL, O'Neill LA (2006) MyD88 adapter-like (Mal) is phosphorylated by Bruton's tyrosine kinase during TLR2 and TLR4 signal transduction. J Biol Chem 281: 10489–10495

Hacker H, Redecke V, Blagoev B, Kratchmarova I, Hsu LC, Wang GG, Kamps MP, Raz E, Wagner H, Hacker G, Mann M, Karin M (2006) Specificity in Toll-like receptor signalling through distinct effector functions of TRAF3 and TRAF6. Nature 439: 204–207

Han KJ, Su X, Xu LG, Bin LH, Zhang J, Shu HB (2004) Mechanisms of the TRIF-induced interferon-stimulated response element and NF-kappaB activation and apoptosis pathways. J Biol Chem 279: 15652–15661

Harte MT, Haga IR, Maloney G, Gray P, Reading PC, Bartlett NW, Smith GL, Bowie A, O'Neill LA (2003) The poxvirus protein A52R targets Toll-like receptor signaling complexes to suppress host defense. J Exp Med 197: 343–351

Hashimoto C, Hudson KL, Anderson KV (1988) The Toll gene of Drosophila, required for dorsal-ventral embryonic polarity, appears to encode a transmembrane protein. Cell 52: 269–279

Hayashi F, Smith KD, Ozinsky A, Hawn TR, Yi EC, Goodlett DR, Eng JK, Akira S, Underhill DM, Aderem A (2001) The innate immune response to bacterial flagellin is mediated by Toll-like receptor 5. Nature 410: 1099–1103

Heil F, Hemmi H, Hochrein H, Ampenberger F, Kirschning C, Akira S, Lipford G, Wagner H, Bauer S (2004) Species-specific recognition of single-stranded RNA via Toll-like receptor 7 and 8. Science 303: 1526–1529

Hemmi H, Kaisho T, Takeuchi O, Sato S, Sanjo H, Hoshino K, Horiuchi T, Tomizawa H, Takeda K, Akira S (2002) Small anti-viral compounds activate immune cells via the TLR7 MyD88-dependent signaling pathway. Nat Immunol 3: 196–200

Hemmi H, Takeuchi O, Kawai T, Kaisho T, Sato S, Sanjo H, Matsumoto M, Hoshino K, Wagner H, Takeda K, Akira S (2000) A Toll-like receptor recognizes bacterial DNA. Nature 408: 740–745

Hirotani T, Yamamoto M, Kumagai Y, Uematsu S, Kawase I, Takeuchi O, Akira S (2005) Regulation of lipopolysaccharide-inducible genes by MyD88 and Toll/IL-1 domain containing adaptor inducing IFN-beta. Biochem Biophys Res Commun 328: 383–392

Hochrein H, Schlatter B, O'Keeffe M, Wagner C, Schmitz F, Schiemann M, Bauer S, Suter M, Wagner H (2004) Herpes simplex virus type-1 induces IFN-alpha production via Toll-like receptor 9-dependent and -independent pathways. Proc Natl Acad Sci USA 101: 11416–11421

Hoebe K, Du X, Georgel P, Janssen E, Tabeta K, Kim SO, Goode J, Lin P, Mann N, Mudd S, Crozat K, Sovath S, Han J, Beutler B (2003) Identification of LPS2 as a key transducer of MyD88-independent TIR signalling. Nature

Honda K, Ohba Y, Yanai H, Negishi H, Mizutani T, Takaoka A, Taya C, Taniguchi T (2005) Spatiotemporal regulation of MyD88-IRF-7 signalling for robust type-I interferon induction. Nature 434: 1035–1040

Honda K, Yanai H, Mizutani T, Negishi H, Shimada N, Suzuki N, Ohba Y, Takaoka A, Yeh WC, Taniguchi T (2004) Role of a transductional-transcriptional processor complex involving MyD88 and IRF-7 in Toll-like receptor signaling. Proc Natl Acad Sci USA 101: 15416–15421

Horng T, Barton GM, Flavell RA, Medzhitov R (2002) The adaptor molecule TIRAP provides signalling specificity for Toll-like receptors. Nature 420: 329–333

Horng T, Barton GM, Medzhitov R (2001) TIRAP: An adapter molecule in the Toll signaling pathway. Nat Immunol 2: 835–841

Hoshino K, Takeuchi O, Kawai T, Sanjo H, Ogawa T, Takeda Y, Takeda K, Akira S (1999) Cutting edge: Toll-like receptor 4 (TLR4)-deficient mice are hyporesponsive to lipopolysaccharide: Evidence for TLR4 as the LPS gene product. J Immunol 162: 3749–3752

Hu Y, Baud V, Delhase M, Zhang P, Deerinck T, Ellisman M, Johnson R, Karin M (1999) Abnormal morphogenesis but intact IKK activation in mice lacking the IKKalpha subunit of IkappaB kinase. Science 284: 316–320

Huang J, Liu T, Xu LG, Chen D, Zhai Z, Shu HB (2005) SIKE is an IKK epsilon/TBK1-associated suppressor of TLR3- and virus-triggered IRF-3 activation pathways. EMBO J 24: 4018–4028

Hultmark D (1994) Macrophage differentiation marker MyD88 is a member of the Toll/IL-1 receptor family. Biochem Biophys Res Commun 199: 144–146

Jefferies CA, Doyle S, Brunner C, Dunne A, Brint E, Wietek C, Walch E, Wirth T, O'Neill LA (2003) Bruton's tyrosine kinase is a Toll/interleukin-1 receptor domain-binding protein that participates in nuclear factor kappaB activation by Toll-like receptor 4. J Biol Chem 278: 26258–26264

Jiang D, Liang J, Fan J, Yu S, Chen S, Luo Y, Prestwich GD, Mascarenhas MM, Garg HG, Quinn DA, Homer RJ, Goldstein DR, Bucala R, Lee PJ, Medzhitov R, Noble PW (2005) Regulation of lung injury and repair by Toll-like receptors and hyaluronan. Nat Med 11: 1173–1179

Jiang Z, Georgel P, Li C, Choe J, Crozat K, Rutschmann S, Du X, Bigby T, Mudd S, Sovath S, Wilson IA, Olson A, Beutler B (2006) Details of Toll-like receptor:adapter interaction revealed by germ-line mutagenesis. Proc Natl Acad Sci USA 103: 10961–10966

Jiang Z, Mak TW, Sen G, Li X (2004) Toll-like receptor 3-mediated activation of NF-kappaB and IRF3 diverges at Toll-IL-1 receptor domain-containing adapter inducing IFN-beta. Proc Natl Acad Sci USA 101: 3533–3538

Jiang Z, Ninomiya-Tsuji J, Qian Y, Matsumoto K, Li X (2002) Interleukin-1 (IL-1) receptor-associated kinase-dependent IL-1-induced signaling complexes phosphorylate TAK1 and TAB2 at the plasma membrane and activate TAK1 in the cytosol. Mol Cell Biol 22: 7158–7167

Kagan JC, Medzhitov R (2006) Phosphoinositide-mediated adaptor recruitment controls Toll-like receptor signaling. Cell 125: 943–955

Kaiser WJ, Offermann MK (2005) Apoptosis induced by the Toll-like receptor adaptor TRIF is dependent on its receptor interacting protein homotypic interaction motif. J Immunol 174: 4942–4952

Kamon H, Kawabe T, Kitamura H, Lee J, Kamimura D, Kaisho T, Akira S, Iwamatsu A, Koga H, Murakami M, Hirano T (2006) TRIF-GEFH1-RhoB pathway is involved in MHCII expression on dendritic cells that is critical for CD4 T-cell activation. EMBO J 25: 4108–4119

Kariko K, Bhuyan P, Capodici J, Weissman D (2004) Small interfering RNAs mediate sequence-independent gene suppression and induce immune activation by signaling through Toll-like receptor 3. J Immunol 172: 6545–6549

Karin M, Ben-Neriah Y (2000) Phosphorylation meets ubiquitination: The control of NF-[kappa]B activity. Annu Rev Immunol 18: 621–663

Kawagoe T, Sato S, Jung A, Yamamoto M, Matsui K, Kato H, Uematsu S, Takeuchi O, Akira S (2007) Essential role of IRAK-4 protein and its kinase activity in Toll-like receptor-mediated immune responses but not in TCR signaling. J Exp Med 204: 1013–1024

Kawai T, Adachi O, Ogawa T, Takeda K, Akira S (1999) Unresponsiveness of MyD88-deficient mice to endotoxin. Immunity 11: 115–122

Kawai T, Sato S, Ishii KJ, Coban C, Hemmi H, Yamamoto M, Terai K, Matsuda M, Inoue J, Uematsu S, Takeuchi O, Akira S (2004) Interferon-alpha induction through Toll-like receptors involves a direct interaction of IRF7 with MyD88 and TRAF6. Nat Immunol 5: 1061–1068

Khor CC, Chapman SJ, Vannberg FO, Dunne A, Murphy C, Ling EY, Frodsham AJ, Walley AJ, Kyrieleis O, Khan A, Aucan C, Segal S, Moore CE, Knox K, Campbell SJ, Lienhardt C, Scott A, Aaby P, Sow OY, Grignani RT, Sillah J, Sirugo G, Peshu N, Williams TN, Maitland K, Davies RJ, Kwiatkowski DP, Day NP, Yala D, Crook DW, Marsh K, Berkley JA, O'Neill LA, Hill AV (2007) A Mal functional variant is associated with protection against invasive pneumococcal disease, bacteremia, malaria, and tuberculosis. Nat Genet 39: 523–528

Kinjyo I, Hanada T, Inagaki-Ohara K, Mori H, Aki D, Ohishi M, Yoshida H, Kubo M, Yoshimura A (2002) SOCS1/JAB is a negative regulator of LPS-induced macrophage activation. Immunity 17: 583–591

Knop J, Martin MU (1999) Effects of IL-1 receptor-associated kinase (IRAK) expression on IL-1 signaling are independent of its kinase activity. FEBS Lett 448: 81–85

Knop J, Wesche H, Lang D, Martin MU (1998) Effects of overexpression of IL-1 receptor-associated kinase on NFkappaB activation, IL-2 production and stress-activated protein kinases in the murine T cell line EL4. Eur J Immunol 28: 3100–3109

Kobayashi K, Hernandez LD, Galan JE, Janeway CA, Jr., Medzhitov R, Flavell RA (2002) IRAK-M is a negative regulator of Toll-like receptor signaling. Cell 110: 191–202

Kollewe C, Mackensen AC, Neumann D, Knop J, Cao P, Li S, Wesche H, Martin MU (2004) Sequential autophosphorylation steps in the interleukin-1 receptor-associated kinase-1 regulate its availability as an adapter in interleukin-1 signaling. J Biol Chem 279: 5227–5236

Koziczak-Holbro M, Joyce C, Gluck A, Kinzel B, Muller M, Tschopp C, Mathison JC, Davis CN, Gram H (2007) IRAK-4 kinase activity is required for interleukin-1 (IL-1) receptor- and Toll-like receptor 7-mediated signaling and gene expression. J Biol Chem 282: 13552–13560

Lasker MV, Nair SK (2006) Intracellular TLR signaling: A structural perspective on human disease. J Immunol 177: 11–16

Le Page C, Popescu O, Genin P, Lian J, Paquin A, Galipeau J, Hiscott J (2001) Disruption of NF-kappa B signaling and chemokine gene activation by retroviral mediated expression of IKK gamma/NEMO mutants. Virology 286: 422–433

Leadbetter EA, Rifkin IR, Hohlbaum AM, Beaudette BC, Shlomchik MJ, Marshak-Rothstein A (2002) Chromatin-IgG complexes activate B cells by dual engagement of IgM and Toll-like receptors. Nature 416: 603–607

Lee FS, Peters RT, Dang LC, Maniatis T (1998) MEKK1 activates both IkappaB kinase alpha and IkappaB kinase beta. Proc Natl Acad Sci USA 95: 9319–9324

Lee J, Chuang TH, Redecke V, She L, Pitha PM, Carson DA, Raz E, Cottam HB (2003) Molecular basis for the immunostimulatory activity of guanine nucleoside analogs: activation of Toll-like receptor 7. Proc Natl Acad Sci USA 100: 6646–6651

Lemaitre B, Nicolas E, Michaut L, Reichhart JM, Hoffmann JA (1996) The dorsoventral regulatory gene cassette Spätzle/Toll/Cactus controls the potent antifungal response in *Drosophila* adults. Cell 86: 973–983

Li C, Zienkiewicz J, Hawiger J (2005) Interactive sites in the MyD88 Toll/interleukin (IL) 1 receptor domain responsible for coupling to the IL1beta signaling pathway. J Biol Chem 280: 26152–26159

Li Q, Lu Q, Hwang JY, Buscher D, Lee KF, Izpisua-Belmonte JC, Verma IM (1999a) IKK1-deficient mice exhibit abnormal development of skin and skeleton. Genes Dev 13: 1322–1328

Li Q, Van Antwerp D, Mercurio F, Lee KF, Verma IM (1999b) Severe liver degeneration in mice lacking the IkappaB kinase 2 gene. Science 284: 321–325

Li S, Strelow A, Fontana EJ, Wesche H (2002) IRAK-4: A novel member of the IRAK family with the properties of an IRAK-kinase. Proc Natl Acad Sci USA 99: 5567–5572

Li X, Commane M, Burns C, Vithalani K, Cao Z, Stark GR (1999c) Mutant cells that do not respond to interleukin-1 (IL-1) reveal a novel role for IL-1 receptor-associated kinase. Mol Cell Biol 19: 4643–4652

Li XH, Fang X, Gaynor RB (2001) Role of IKKgamma/NEMO in assembly of the Ikappa B kinase complex. J Biol Chem 276: 4494–4500

Liberati NT, Fitzgerald KA, Kim DH, Feinbaum R, Golenbock DT, Ausubel FM (2004) Requirement for a conserved Toll/interleukin-1 resistance domain protein in the *Caenorhabditis elegans* immune response. Proc Natl Acad Sci USA 101: 6593–6598

Liljeroos M, Vuolteenaho R, Morath S, Hartung T, Hallman M, Ojaniemi M (2007) Bruton's tyrosine kinase together with PI 3-kinase are part of Toll-like receptor 2 multiprotein complex and mediate LTA induced Toll-like receptor 2 responses in macrophages. Cell Signal 19: 625–633

Lord KA, Abdollahi A, Hoffman-Liebermann B, Liebermann DA (1990a) Dissection of the immediate early response of myeloid leukemia cells to terminal differentiation and growth inhibitory stimuli. Cell Growth Differ 1: 637–645

Lord KA, Hoffman-Liebermann B, Liebermann DA (1990b) Nucleotide sequence and expression of a cDNA encoding MyD88, a novel myeloid differentiation primary response gene induced by IL6. Oncogene 5: 1095–1097

Lorenz E, Mira JP, Frees KL, Schwartz DA (2002) Relevance of mutations in the TLR4 receptor in patients with Gram-negative septic shock. Arch Intern Med 162: 1028–1032

Lund JM, Alexopoulou L, Sato A, Karow M, Adams NC, Gale NW, Iwasaki A, Flavell RA (2004) Recognition of single-stranded RNA viruses by Toll-like receptor 7. Proc Natl Acad Sci USA 101: 5598–5603

Lye E, Mirtsos C, Suzuki N, Suzuki S, Yeh WC (2004) The role of interleukin 1 receptor-associated kinase-4 (IRAK-4) kinase activity in IRAK-4-mediated signaling. J Biol Chem 279: 40653–40658

Mansell A, Brint E, Gould JA, O'Neill LA, Hertzog PJ (2004) Mal interacts with tumor necrosis factor receptor-associated factor (TRAF)-6 to mediate NF-kappaB activation by Toll-like receptor (TLR)-2 and TLR4. J Biol Chem 279: 37227–37230

Mansell A, Smith R, Doyle SL, Gray P, Fenner JE, Crack PJ, Nicholson SE, Hilton DJ, O'Neill LA, Hertzog PJ (2006) Suppressor of cytokine signaling 1 negatively regulates Toll-like receptor signaling by mediating Mal degradation. Nat Immunol 7: 148–155

Martin M, Bol GF, Eriksson A, Resch K, Brigelius-Flohe R (1994) Interleukin-1-induced activation of a protein kinase co-precipitating with the type I interleukin-1 receptor in T cells. Eur J Immunol 24: 1566–1571

Maschera B, Ray K, Burns K, Volpe F (1999) Overexpression of an enzymically inactive interleukin-1-receptor-associated kinase activates nuclear factor-kappa B. Bio chem J 339: 227–231

May MJ, Marienfeld RB, Ghosh S (2002) Characterization of the Ikappa B-kinase NEMO binding domain. J Biol Chem 277: 45992–46000

McCoy SL, Kurtz SE, Macarthur CJ, Trune DR, Hefeneider SH (2005) Identification of a peptide derived from vaccinia virus A52R protein that inhibits cytokine secretion in response to TLR-dependent signaling and reduces *in vivo* bacterial-induced inflammation. J Immunol 174: 3006–3014

McGettrick AF, Brint EK, Palsson-McDermott EM, Rowe DC, Golenbock DT, Gay NJ, Fitzgerald KA, O'Neill LA (2006) TRIF-related adapter molecule is phosphorylated by PKC{varepsilon} during Toll-like receptor 4 signaling. Proc Natl Acad Sci USA 103: 9196–9201

Medzhitov R, Preston-Hurlburt P, Kopp E, Stadlen A, Chen C, Ghosh S, Janeway CA (1998) MyD88 is an adaptor protein in the hToll/IL-1 receptor family signaling pathways. Mol Cell 2: 253–258

Meylan E, Burns K, Hofmann K, Blancheteau V, Martinon F, Kelliher M, Tschopp J (2004) RIP1 is an essential mediator of Toll-like receptor 3-induced NF-kappa B activation. Nat Immunol 5: 503–507

Mink M, Fogelgren B, Olszewski K, Maroy P, Csiszar K (2001) A novel human gene (SARM) at chromosome 17q11 encodes a protein with a SAM motif and structural similarity to Armadillo/beta-catenin that is conserved in mouse, *Drosophila*, and *Caenorhabditis elegans*. Genomics 74: 234–244

Muzio M, Natoli G, Saccani S, Levrero M, Mantovani A (1998) The human Toll signaling pathway: divergence of nuclear factor kappaB and JNK/SAPK activation upstream of tumor necrosis factor receptor-associated factor 6 (TRAF6). J Exp Med 187: 2097–2101

Muzio M, Ni J, Feng P, Dixit VM (1997) IRAK (Pelle) family member IRAK-2 and MyD88 as proximal mediators of IL-1 signaling. Science 278: 1612–1615

Naiki Y, Michelsen KS, Zhang W, Chen S, Doherty TM, Arditi M (2005) Transforming growth factor-beta differentially inhibits MyD88-dependent, but not TRAM- and TRIF-dependent, lipopolysaccharide-induced TLR4 signaling. J Biol Chem 280: 5491–5495

Nakagawa R, Naka T, Tsutsui H, Fujimoto M, Kimura A, Abe T, Seki E, Sato S, Takeuchi O, Takeda K, Akira S, Yamanishi K, Kawase I, Nakanishi K, Kishimoto T (2002) SOCS-1 partic-ipates in negative regulation of LPS responses. Immunity 17: 677–687

Negishi H, Fujita Y, Yanai H, Sakaguchi S, Ouyang X, Shinohara M, Takayanagi H, Ohba Y, Taniguchi T, Honda K (2006) Evidence for licensing of IFN-gamma-induced IFN regulatory factor 1 transcription factor by MyD88 in Toll-like receptor-dependent gene induction program. Proc Natl Acad Sci USA 103: 15136–15141

Negishi H, Ohba Y, Yanai H, Takaoka A, Honma K, Yui K, Matsuyama T, Taniguchi T, Honda K (2005) Negative regulation of Toll-like-receptor signaling by IRF-4. Proc Natl Acad Sci USA 102: 15989–15994

OMahony A, Lin X, Geleziunas R, Greene WC (2000) Activation of the heterodimeric Ikappa B kinase alpha (IKKalpha)-IKKbeta complex is directional: IKKalpha regulates IKKbeta under both basal and stimulated conditions. Mol Cell Biol 20: 1170–1178

Ohashi K, Burkart V, Flohe S, Kolb H (2000) Cutting edge: heat shock protein 60 is a putative endogenous ligand of the Toll-like receptor-4 complex. J Immunol 164: 558–561

Oshiumi H, Matsumoto M, Funami K, Akazawa T, Seya T (2003a) TICAM-1, an adaptor molecule that participates in Toll-like receptor 3–mediated interferon-beta induction. Nat Immunol 4: 161–167

Oshiumi H, Sasai M, Shida K, Fujita T, Matsumoto M, Seya T (2003b) TICAM-2: A bridging adapter recruiting to Toll-like receptor 4 TICAM-1 that induces interferon-beta. J Biol Chem

Ozinsky A, Underhill DM, Fontenot JD, Hajjar AM, Smith KD, Wilson CB, Schroeder L, Aderem A (2000) The repertoire for pattern recognition of pathogens by the innate immune system is defined by cooperation between Toll-like receptors. Proc Natl Acad Sci USA 97: 13766–13771

Picard C, Puel A, Bonnet M, Ku CL, Bustamante J, Yang K, Soudais C, Dupuis S, Feinberg J, Fieschi C, Elbim C, Hitchcock R, Lammas D, Davies G, Al-Ghonaium A, Al-Rayes H, Al-Jumaah S, Al-Hajjar S, Al-Mohsen IZ, Frayha HH, Rucker R, Hawn TR, Aderem A, Tufenkeji H, Haraguchi S, Day NK, Good RA, Gougerot-Pocidalo MA, Ozinsky A, Casanova JL (2003) Pyogenic bacterial infections in humans with IRAK-4 deficiency. Science 299: 2076–2079

Poltorak A, He X, Smirnova I, Liu MY, Van Huffel C, Du X, Birdwell D, Alejos E, Silva M, Galanos C, Freudenberg M, Ricciardi-Castagnoli P, Layton B, Beutler B (1998) Defective LPS signaling in C3H/HeJ and C57BL/10ScCr mice: mutations in Tlr4 gene. Science 282: 2085–2088

Qin J, Jiang Z, Qian Y, Casanova JL, Li X (2004) IRAK4 kinase activity is redundant for interleukin-1 (IL-1) receptor-associated kinase phosphorylation and IL-1 responsiveness. J Biol Chem 279: 26748–26753

Qureshi ST, Lariviere L, Leveque G, Clermont S, Moore KJ, Gros P, Malo D (1999) Endotoxin-tolerant mice have mutations in Toll-like receptor 4 (Tlr4). J Exp Med 189: 615–625

Rosati O, Martin MU (2002) Identification and characterization of murine IRAK-2. Biochem Bio-phys Res Commun 297: 52–58

Rothwarf DM, Zandi E, Natoli G, Karin M (1998) IKK-gamma is an essential regulatory subunit of the IkappaB kinase complex. Nature 395: 297–300

Rottenberg S, Schmuckli-Maurer J, Grimm S, Heussler VT, Dobbelaere DA (2002) Characteriza-tion of the bovine IkappaB kinases (IKK)alpha and IKKbeta, the regulatory subunit NEMO and their substrate IkappaBalpha. Gene 299: 293–300

Rowe DC, McGettrick AF, Latz E, Monks BG, Gay NJ, Yamamoto M, Akira S, O'Neill LA, Fitzgerald KA, Golenbock DT (2006) The myristoylation of TRIF-related adaptor molecule is essential for Toll-like receptor 4 signal transduction. Proc Natl Acad Sci USA 103: 6299–6304

Ruckdeschel K, Pfaffinger G, Haase R, Sing A, Weighardt H, Hacker G, Holzmann B, Heesemann J (2004) Signaling of apoptosis through TLRs critically involves toll/IL-1 receptor domain-containing adapter inducing IFN-beta, but not MyD88, in bacteria-infected murine macrophages. J Immunol 173: 3320–3328

Sato S, Sugiyama M, Yamamoto M, Watanabe Y, Kawai T, Takeda K, Akira S (2003) Toll/IL-1 receptor domain-containing adaptor inducing IFN-beta (TRIF) associates with TNF receptor-associated factor 6 and TANK-binding kinase 1, and activates two distinct transcription factors, NF-kappa B and IFN-regulatory factor-3, in the Toll-like receptor signaling. J Immunol 171: 4304–4310

Scheibner KA, Lutz MA, Boodoo S, Fenton MJ, Powell JD, Horton MR (2006) Hyaluronan fragments act as an endogenous danger signal by engaging TLR2. J Immunol 177: 1272–1281

Su X, Li S, Meng M, Qian W, Xie W, Chen D, Zhai Z, Shu HB (2006) TNF receptor-associated factor-1 (TRAF1) negatively regulates Toll/IL-1 receptor domain-containing adaptor inducing IFN-beta (TRIF)-mediated signaling. Eur J Immunol 36: 199–206

Sun D, Ding A (2006) MyD88–mediated stabilization of interferon-gamma-induced cytokine and chemokine mRNA. Nat Immunol 7: 375–381

Suzuki N, Suzuki S, Duncan GS, Millar DG, Wada T, Mirtsos C, Takada H, Wakeham A, Itie A, Li S, Penninger JM, Wesche H, Ohashi PS, Mak TW, Yeh WC (2002) Severe impairment of interleukin-1 and Toll-like receptor signalling in mice lacking IRAK-4. Nature 416: 750–756

Takaoka A, Yanai H, Kondo S, Duncan G, Negishi H, Mizutani T, Kano S, Honda K, Ohba Y, Mak TW, Taniguchi T (2005) Integral role of IRF-5 in the gene induction programme activated by Toll-like receptors. Nature 434: 243–249

Takeda K, Takeuchi O, Tsujimura T, Itami S, Adachi O, Kawai T, Sanjo H, Yoshikawa K, Terada N, Akira S (1999) Limb and skin abnormalities in mice lacking IKKalpha. Science 284: 313–316

Takeshita F, Ishii KJ, Kobiyama K, Kojima Y, Coban C, Sasaki S, Ishii N, Klinman DM, Okuda K, Akira S, Suzuki K (2005) TRAF4 acts as a silencer in TLR-mediated signaling through the association with TRAF6 and TRIF. Eur J Immunol 35: 2477–2485

Takeuchi O, Takeda K, Hoshino K, Adachi O, Ogawa T, Akira S (2000) Cellular responses to bacterial cell wall components are mediated through MyD88–dependent signaling cascades. Int Immunol 12: 113–117

Termeer C, Benedix F, Sleeman J, Fieber C, Voith U, Ahrens T, Miyake K, Freudenberg M, Galanos C, Simon JC (2002) Oligosaccharides of Hyaluronan activate dendritic cells via Toll-like receptor 4. J Exp Med 195: 99–111

Thomas JA, Allen JL, Tsen M, Dubnicoff T, Danao J, Liao XC, Cao Z, Wasserman SA (1999) Impaired cytokine signaling in mice lacking the IL-1 receptor-associated kinase. J Immunol 163: 978–984

Traenckner EB, Pahl HL, Henkel T, Schmidt KN, Wilk S, Baeuerle PA (1995) Phosphorylation of human I kappa B-alpha on serines 32 and 36 controls I kappa B-alpha proteolysis and NF-kappa B activation in response to diverse stimuli. Embo J 14: 2876–2883

Trofimova M, Sprenkle AB, Green M, Sturgill TW, Goebl MG, Harrington MA (1996) Developmental and tissue-specific expression of mouse pelle-like protein kinase. J Biol Chem 271: 17609–17612

Uematsu S, Sato S, Yamamoto M, Hirotani T, Kato H, Takeshita F, Matsuda M, Coban C, Ishii KJ, Kawai T, Takeuchi O, Akira S (2005) Interleukin-1 receptor-associated kinase-1 plays an essential role for Toll-like receptor (TLR)7– and TLR9–mediated interferon-{alpha} induction. J Exp Med 201: 915–923

Urdal DL, Call SM, Jackson JL, Dower SK (1988) Affinity purification and chemical analysis of the interleukin-1 receptor. J Biol Chem 263: 2870–2877

Vabulas RM, Ahmad-Nejad P, da Costa C, Miethke T, Kirschning CJ, Hacker H, Wagner H (2001) Endocytosed HSP60s use Toll-like receptor 2 (TLR2) and TLR4 to activate the toll/interleukin-1 receptor signaling pathway in innate immune cells. J Biol Chem 276: 31332–31339

Vabulas RM, Ahmad-Nejad P, Ghose S, Kirschning CJ, Issels RD, Wagner H (2002) HSP70 as endogenous stimulus of the Toll/interleukin-1 receptor signal pathway. J Biol Chem 277: 15107–15112

Verma IM, Stevenson JK, Schwarz EM, Van Antwerp D, Miyamoto S (1995) Rel/NF-kappa B/I kappa B family: intimate tales of association and dissociation. Genes Dev 9: 2723–2735

Vig E, Green M, Liu Y, Donner DB, Mukaida N, Goebl MG, Harrington MA (1999) Modulation of tumor necrosis factor and interleukin-1-dependent NF-kappaB activity by mPLK/IRAK. J Biol Chem 274: 13077–13084

Wang C, Deng L, Hong M, Akkaraju GR, Inoue J, Chen ZJ (2001) TAK1 is a ubiquitin-dependent kinase of MKK and IKK. Nature 412: 346–351

Wang J, Shao Y, Bennett TA, Shankar RA, Wightman PD, Reddy LG (2006) The functional effects of physical interactions among Toll-like receptors 7, 8, and 9. J Biol Chem 281: 37427–37434

Weber AN, Moncrieffe MC, Gangloff M, Imler JL, Gay NJ (2005) Ligand-receptor and receptor-receptor interactions act in concert to activate signaling in the Drosophila toll pathway. J Biol Chem 280: 22793–22799

Weber AN, Tauszig-Delamasure S, Hoffmann JA, Lelievre E, Gascan H, Ray KP, Morse MA, Imler JL, Gay NJ (2003) Binding of the Drosophila cytokine Spatzle to Toll is direct and establishes signaling. Natur Immunol 4: 794–800

Wesche H, Gao X, Li X, Kirschning CJ, Stark GR, Cao Z (1999) IRAK-M is a novel member of the Pelle/interleukin-1 receptor-associated kinase (IRAK) family. J Biol Chem 274: 19403–19410

Wesche H, Henzel WJ, Shillinglaw W, Li S, Cao Z (1997) MyD88: an adapter that recruits IRAK to the IL-1 receptor complex. Immunity 7: 837–847

Whiteside ST, Ernst MK, LeBail O, Laurent-Winter C, Rice N, Israel A (1995) N- and C-terminal sequences control degradation of MAD3/I kappa B alpha in response to inducers of NF-kappa B activity. Mol Cell Biol 15: 5339–5345

Wietek C, Miggin SM, Jefferies CA, O'Neill LA (2003) Interferon regulatory factor-3–mediated activation of the interferon-sensitive response element by Toll-like receptor (TLR) 4 but not TLR3 requires the p65 subunit of NF-kappa. J Biol Chem 278: 50923–50931

Xu Y, Tao X, Shen B, Horng T, Medzhitov R, Manley JL, Tong L (2000) Structural basis for signal transduction by the Toll/interleukin-1 receptor domains. Nature 408: 111–115

Yamagata M, Merlie JP, Sanes JR (1994) Interspecific comparisons reveal conserved features of the Drosophila Toll protein. Gene 139: 223–228

Yamamoto M, Sato S, Hemmi H, Hoshino K, Kaisho T, Sanjo H, Takeuchi O, Sugiyama M, Okabe M, Takeda K, Akira S (2003a) Role of adaptor TRIF in the MyD88-independent Toll-like receptor signaling pathway. Science 301: 640–643

Yamamoto M, Sato S, Hemmi H, Sanjo H, Uematsu S, Kaisho T, Hoshino K, Takeuchi O, Kobayashi M, Fujita T, Takeda K, Akira S (2002a) Essential role for TIRAP in activation of the signalling cascade shared by TLR2 and TLR4. Nature 420: 324–329

Yamamoto M, Sato S, Hemmi H, Uematsu S, Hoshino K, Kaisho T, Takeuchi O, Takeda K, Akira S (2003b) TRAM is specifically involved in the Toll-like receptor 4–mediated MyD88–independent signaling pathway. Nat Immunol 4: 1144–1150

Yamamoto M, Sato S, Mori K, Hoshino K, Takeuchi O, Takeda K, Akira S (2002b) Cutting edge: a novel Toll/IL-1 receptor domain-containing adapter that preferentially activates the IFN-beta promoter in the Toll-like receptor signaling. J Immunol 169: 6668–6672

Yamamoto Y, Kim DW, Kwak YT, Prajapati S, Verma U, Gaynor RB (2001) IKKgamma/NEMO facilitates the recruitment of the IkappaB proteins into the IkappaB kinase complex. J Biol Chem 276: 36327–36336

Yamaoka S, Courtois G, Bessia C, Whiteside ST, Weil R, Agou F, Kirk HE, Kay RJ, Israel A (1998) Complementation cloning of NEMO, a component of the IkappaB kinase complex essential for NF-kappaB activation. Cell 93: 1231–1240

Yamin TT, Miller DK (1997) The interleukin-1 receptor-associated kinase is degraded by proteasomes following its phosphorylation. J Biol Chem 272: 21540–21547

Yarovinsky F, Zhang D, Andersen JF, Bannenberg GL, Serhan CN, Hayden MS, Hieny S, Sutter-
    wala FS, Flavell RA, Ghosh S, Sher A (2005) TLR11 activation of dendritic cells by a protozoan
    profilin-like protein. Science 308: 1626–1629
Zhang J, Xu LG, Han KJ, Wei X, Shu HB (2004) PIASy represses TRIF-induced ISRE and NF-
    kappaB activation but not apoptosis. FEBS Lett 570: 97–101

TLR9-Mediated Recognition of DNA

Thomas Müller, Svetlana Hamm, and Stefan Bauer(✉)

Abstract The mammalian immune system senses pathogens through pattern recognition receptors (PRRs) and responds with activation. The Toll-like receptor (TLR) family that consists of 13 receptors plays a critical role in this process. TLR-mediated signaling activates immune cells and leads to an innate immune response with subsequent initiation of an adaptive immune response. Toll-like receptor 9 (TLR9) recognizes deoxyribonucleic acid (DNA) leading to cellular activation and cytokine production influencing the immune response against viruses and bacteria. The stimulation of TLR9 will be exploited for adjuvant therapy and treatment of cancer or allergy. In this review we will discuss TLR9 ligands, TLR9 expression, signaling, and the therapeutic potential of TLR9 ligands in treatment of infectious or allergic diseases and cancer.

Stefan Bauer

Institut für Immunology, Philipps-Universität Marburg, BMFZ, Hans-Meerweinstr. 2, 35043 Marburg, Germany

stefan.bauer@staff.uni-marburg.de

S. Bauer, G. Hartmann (eds.), *Toll-Like Receptors (TLRs) and Innate Immunity.*
Handbook of Experimental Pharmacology 183.
© Springer-Verlag Berlin Heidelberg 2008

1 Introduction

Twenty years ago DNA was considered as immunological inert. Studies in 1984 by Tokunaga et al. (1984) first demonstrated that bacterial DNA itself was the component of Bacillus Calmette-Guerin (BCG), which promoted immunostimulatory and antitumor effects. The stimulatory effect of bacterial DNA is due to the presence of unmethylated CpG dinucleotides in a particular base context named CpG motif (Krieg et al., 1995). In contrast, vertebrate DNA is not—or is less—stimulatory due to methylation of CpG dinucleotides, their low frequency (CpG suppression), and the presence of possibly inhibitory sequences (Krieg et al., 1998). The immunostimulatory effects of bacterial DNA can be mimicked by synthetic oligodeoxynucleotides containing a CpG-motif (CpG-ODN). CpG-DNA activates macrophages and dendritic cells (DC) to initiate immune responses (Krieg, 2002). During the search for the CpG-DNA receptor it was noted that CpG-DNA signaling is abolished in knockout mice deficient in MyD88, which is an essential component in TLR signaling (see Chapter 4 of this volume) (Hacker et al., 2000). This suggested a TLR as receptor for CpG-DNA, and in a seminal study by Hemmi et al. (2000) it was shown that macrophages from TLR9 knockout mice did not respond to CpG-DNA. This observation was consistent with the view that TLR9 is an essential component of the CpG-DNA receptor. Subsequently. it was reported that TLR9 expression in immune cells correlated with responsiveness to CpG-DNA (Bauer et al., 2001). In genetic complementation assays it was further shown that TLR9-deficient and CpG-DNA unresponsive HEK 293 cells gain responsiveness after transfection of either human or murine TLR9 cDNA (Bauer et al., 2001; Chuang et al., 2002; Takeshita et al., 2001). This review focuses on the various ligands of TLR9, TLR9 expression, and potential therapeutic use of TLR9 activation.

2 Ligands for TLR9

2.1 Recognition of Viruses and Bacteria by TLR9

DNA viruses such as murine cytomegalovirus (MCMV) and herpes-simplex viruses 1 and 2 (HSV-1/HSV-2) are recognized by TLR9 and induce production of inflammatory cytokines and type I IFN (Hochrein et al., 2004; Krug et al., 2004a; Krug et al., 2004b; Lund et al., 2003). The TLR9-mediated IFN-α response to HSV-1 and HSV-2 is limited to a subtype of dendritic cells, called plasmacytoid dendritic cell (pDCs) or natural interferon-α producing cells (NIPCs), which secrete high amounts of IFN-α in response to viral infection (Hochrein et al., 2004; Krug et al., 2004a; Krug et al., 2004b; Lund et al., 2003; Siegal et al., 1999). Cellular activation does not require viral infection since live, heat-, or UV-inactivated HSV-1/HSV-2 produce high levels of IFN-α. In contrast, macrophages produce IFN-α upon HSV infection in a TLR9-independent manner suggesting that pDC- and TLR9-independent mechanisms exist that induce an effective immune response against DNA viruses (Hochrein et al., 2004).

TLR9 also recognizes various bacterial genomic DNAs and activates immune cells (Bauer et al., 2001; Dalpke et al., 2006). Surprisingly, the role of TLR9 in fighting bacterial infection has not been eluded in detail. Interestingly, one study shows that TLR9 activation is critical for the production of IFN-γ during infection with *Propionibacterium acnes* (formerly *Corynebacterium parvum*) that is part of the human flora and associated with several human pathologies. TLR9 dependent activation via *P. acnes* primes IFN-γ dependent enhanced resistance to murine typhoid fever which is abolished in TLR9 deficient mice (Kalis et al., 2005).

2.2 Synthetic Mimics of Viral or Bacterial DNA (CpG Motif Containing DNA)

The original CpG-motif within immunostimulatory oligonucleotides (CpG-ODN) was a hexamer motif consisting of a central CpG dinucleotide with 5′ purines and 3′ pyrimidines (Krieg et al., 1995). Meanwhile, three major classes of structurally and phenotypically different CpG-ODN have been described (Table 1) (Hartmann and Krieg, 2000; Krug et al., 2001a; Verthelyi et al., 2001). The A-class CpG-ODNs (also referred to as type D) are potent inducers of IFN-α secretion from plasmacytoid dendritic cells (pDCs), but poor inducers of B-cell stimulation. The structure of A-class ODN include stretches of phosphorothioate-modified poly-G that form complex higher-ordered structures known as G-tetrads and a central phosphodiester

Table 1 TLR9 ligands containing CpG-DNA motifs

CpG-containing DNA as TLR9 ligands	References
Type A ODN (D-type) ODN 2216: 5′-G*G*GGGACGATCGTCG⁺G⁺G*G*G*G*G	(Hartmann and Krieg, 2000; Krug et al., 2001a; Verthelyi et al., 2001)
Type B ODN (K-type) ODN 2006: 5′-T*C*G*T*C*G*T*T*T*T*G*T*C*G*T*T*T*T*G*T*C*G*T*T ODN1668: 5′-T*C*C*A*T*G*A*C*G*T*T*C*C*T* G*A*T*G*C*T	
Type C ODN 5′-T*C*G*T*C*G*T*T*T*T*C*G*G*C*G*C*G*C*G*C*C*G	(Hartmann et al., 2003; Marshall et al., 2003; Vollmer et al., 2004a)
Viral (HSV, CMV) and bacterial DNA (*E. coli* and other bacteria)	(Bauer et al., 2001; Dalpke et al., 2006; Hochrein et al., 2004; Krug et al., 2004a; Krug et al., 2004b; Lund et al., 2003)

* depicts a phosphorothioate linkage

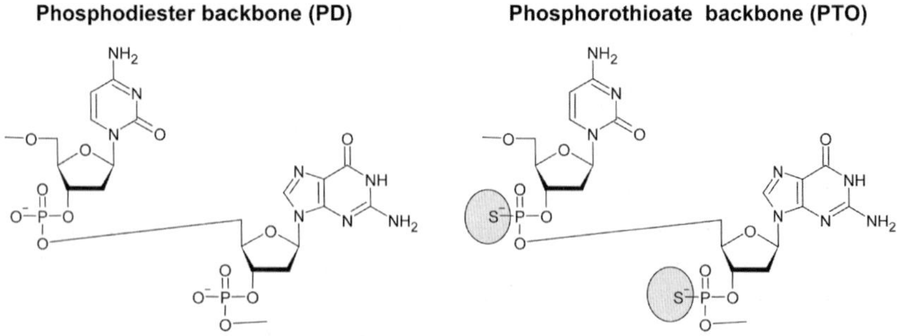

Phosphodiester backbone (PD)   **Phosphorothioate backbone (PTO)**

Fig. 1 Native (phosphodiester) and modified (phosphorothioate) DNA backbone. The change to a sulfur atom from one nonbridging oxygen atom as shown enhances the resistance to nucleases and consequently the half-life of PTO-oligonucleotides. The sulfur is marked by a grey circle

CpG motif (Kerkmann et al., 2005). B-class ODN (also referred to as type K) have a completely phosphorothioate backbone and are strong B cell stimulators but only weakly induce IFN-α secretion (Figure 1). However, if B-class CpG-ODNs are artificially forced into higher-ordered structures with cationic lipid transfection or complexation to polymyxin B, they show the same immune profile as the A-class CpG-ODN (Guiducci et al., 2006; Honda et al., 2005). The C-class CpG-ODN exerts immune properties that are intermediate between the A and B classes, inducing both B cell activation and IFN-α secretion. The unique structure of these ODN with a 5′ CpG motif and a 3′ palindrome may allow duplex formation within the endosomal environment leading to the characteristics of cytokine production (Hartmann et al., 2003; Marshall et al., 2003; Vollmer et al., 2004a).

In the case of the phosphorothioate backbone of class B ODNs, a species-specific CpG-DNA motif for recognition was noted. Accordingly, murine spleen cells respond better to CpG-ODN-containing the core sequence GACGTT (e.g., ODN 1668, Table 1), whereas human peripheral blood mononuclear cells (PBMC) prefer CpG motifs containing more than one CG and the core sequence GTCGTT (e.g., ODN 2006, Table 1) (Bauer et al., 2001; Krieg et al., 1995). Interestingly, the different DNA motifs that are required for optimal stimulation of human and murine immune cells is restricted to phosphorothioate (PS)-modified ODN and is not observed when a natural phosphodiester backbone is used. Thus, human and mouse cells do not recognize different CpG motifs in natural phosphodiester DNA (Roberts et al., 2005).

2.3 Non-CpG Motif-Containing Nucleic Acid

Recently, the strict CpG-dependent recognition of phosphodiester DNA by TLR9 has been questioned, since non-CpG ODNs stimulated FLT3-L-generated DCs in a sequence-independent but TLR9-dependent manner when complexed to the cationic lipid transfection reagent N-[1-(2,3-dioleoyloxy)propyl]-N,N,N trimethylammonium methylsulfate (DOTAP). Supporting this concept, recombinant TLR9 were observed to bind also to non-CpG-ODN in a surface plasmon resonance binding assay (SPR, Biacore) when DNA concentrations were increased (Yasuda et al., 2006; Yasuda et al., 2005). This CpG sequence-independent recognition of DNA by TLR9 upon transfection with DOTAP may be restricted to certain immune cells such as FLT3-L-induced DCs, since murine B-cells, macrophages, conventional DCs, and TLR9 transfected HEK293 fibroblasts respond to PD-DNA in a strictly CpG sequence-dependent manner (Viglianti et al., 2003; unpublished observations). We therefore hypothesize that FLT3-L DC expresses a cofactor that modulates the DNA sequence-dependent recognition by TLR9. The biological function of the CpG DNA-independent recognition in FLT3-L DCs is unclear, but it is known that, as a probably unwanted side effect, nucleic acid recognition by pDCs can sustain certain B-cell-mediated autoimmune diseases such as systemic lupus erythematosus (SLE) (see Chapter 8 of this volume, on autoimmunity).

In addition other non-CpG DNA sequences have been identified as stimuli for TLR9 (Table 2). Further studies on phosphodiester AT-rich ODNs have revealed that a core motif of 5′-ATTTTTAC and a six-base secondary loop structure containing a self-stabilized 5′-C...G-3′ stem sequence stimulate immune cells in a strictly TLR9-dependent way (Shimosato et al., 2006). Additional work on immunostimulatory non-CpG DNA by Vollmer et al., demonstrated that phosphorothioate modified non-CpG ODNs stimulate a TLR9-dependent Th2 type immune response where the 5′-TC and the thymidine content determine the immune stimulatory activity of these DNA sequences (Vollmer et al., 2004b). A synthetic PD-oligonucleotide containing alternating deoxyinosine and deoxycytidine (5′-ICICICICICICICICICICICIC) complexed to the peptide NH_2-KLKLLLLLKLK (IC31) also stimulates the TLR9/Myd88-dependent pathway and its adjuvant properties augment a Th1 immune response against the mycobacterial vaccine antigen Ag85B-ESAT-6. Interestingly this

Table 2 Non-CpG DNA-TLR9 ligands

Non-CpG-containing nucleic acid	References
ODN 1668GC: 5′-TCCATGACGTTCCTGATGCT NAOS-1: 5′-GCTCATGAGCTTCCTGATGCTG AP-1: 5′-GCTTGATGACTCAGCCGGAA	(Yasuda et al., 2006; Yasuda et al., 2005)
PD-AT-rich sequences: AT5ACL: 5′-TATA<u>ATTTTTAC</u>CAACTAGC LGAT243: 5′-TTAACA<u>ATTTTTAC</u>CCAAGA	(Shimosato et al., 2006; Shimosato et al., 2005)
PS-T-rich sequences: ODN 1982: 5′-T*C*C*A*G*G*A*C*T*T*C*T*C*T*C*A*G*G*T*T	(Vollmer et al., 2004b)
PD-IC-rich sequence (IC31): 5′-ICICICICICICICICICICICIC	(Agger et al., 2006; Schellack et al., 2006)
Hemozoin (heme polymer)	(Coban et al., 2005)
Hemozoin + genomic DNA of plasmodium	(Parroche, 2007)

* depicts a phosphorothioate linkage; AT-rich sequences are underlined

formulation confers protective efficacy in a mouse aerosol challenge model of tuberculosis (Agger et al., 2006; Schellack et al., 2006).

Recently, hemozoin (HZ) has been described as the first non-DNA ligand for TLR9 (Coban et al., 2005). HZ is produced during the intraerythrocytic stage of Plasmodium when digestion of hemoglobin leads to the production of potentially toxic heme. In a detoxification process, heme is then converted into insoluble hemozoin which induces inflammatory cytokines *in vitro* and *in vivo* (Coban et al., 2005; Pichyangkul et al., 2004). The identification of TLR9 as receptor for HZ has been challenged by the observation that plasmodium DNA bound to HZ is responsible for TLR9 activation (Parroche et al., 2007). Accordingly, HZ functions as DNA carrier for TLR9 and is superior to synthetic transfection reagents. Interestingly, Plasmodium DNA is very AT-rich, but contains mostly subtelomeric CpG motif sequences that are active when tested as synthetic ODNs. In addition to these CpG motifs, DNA sequences rich in A and T such as 5′-TATAATTTTTACCAACTAGC have been described as TLR9 stimuli (Shimosato et al., 2005). Since both type of sequences (AT-rich and rare CpG motifs) have been identified in the genome of Plasmodium, one might speculate that these motifs mediate TLR9 activation (Parroche et al., 2007).

3 Expression and Localization of TLR9

In humans TLR9 is expressed only in memory B cells (Bernasconi et al., 2003; Bourke et al., 2003) and plasmacytoid dendritic cells (pDC) (Hornung et al., 2002; Kadowaki et al., 2001; Krug et al., 2001b) (Figure 2). Expression of TLR9 and

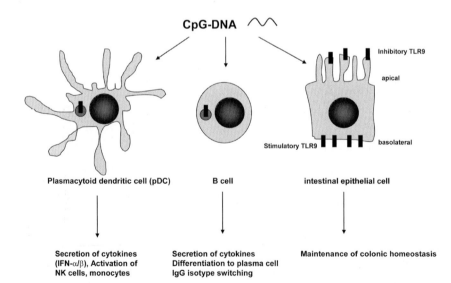

Fig. 2 TLR9 expression and function in various cell types, such as plasmacytoid dendritic cells, B cells, and epithelial cells and intestinal epithelial cells (IECs)

responsiveness to CpG-DNA in other immune cells, such as human monocyte-derived dendritic cells and monocytes, has been reported, but is still a matter of debate (Hoene et al., 2006; Saikh et al., 2004). In contrast, murine TLR9 expression is not limited to B cells and pDC, but is also detected in monocytes, macrophages, and dendritic cells (Edwards et al., 2003; Hemmi et al., 2000). In nonactivated immune cells TLR9 is expressed in the endoplasmic reticulum (ER). Upon cellular activation, TLR9 traffics to endosomal and lysosomal compartments, where it interacts with endocytosed CpG-DNA at acidic pH, a condition that is thought to be necessary for DNA recognition (Latz et al., 2004; Leifer et al., 2004; Rutz et al., 2004). Compounds that interfere with endosomal acidification, such as the weak base chloroquine and bafilomycin A1, an inhibitor of the ATP-dependent acidification of endosomes, consequently, prevent CpG-DNA-driven TLR9 activation (Hacker et al., 1998; Yi et al., 1999). The molecular basis for the retention of TLR9 in the endoplasmic reticulum (ER) in quiescent cells and the subsequent trafficking to the endosome upon cellular stimulation is unclear. Recently the membrane portion of TLR9 has been implied in trafficking (Barton et al., 2006; Kajita et al., 2006), although a recent report challenges this view. Accordingly, this report demonstrates that a tyrosine-based (YNEL) targeting motif in the cytoplasmic domain and the extracellular domain per se regulate TLR9 trafficking independent of the transmembrane domain (Leifer et al., 2006).

Despite these conflicting results on the trafficking-determining domain of TLR9, it is important to note that TLR9 trafficking to the endosome/lysosome does not seem to involve the Golgi apparatus, since the mature protein retains the sensitivity to the glycosidase Endo H, a feature of usually ER-resident proteins. Which alternative route TLR9 uses to reach the endosomal/lysosomal compartment is currently unknown. The recently described ER resident protein unc93b may be involved in TLR9 trafficking since a dominant negative mutant of unc93b leads to nonresponsiveness of TLR9 (together with TLR3, TLR7) accompanied by the disruption of TLR-unc93b interaction (Brinkmann et al., 2007; Tabeta et al., 2006).

Recently TLR9 expression has also been detected on intestinal epithelial cells, and an involvement in the maintenance of colonic homeostasis has been suggested (Ewaschuk et al., 2007; Lee et al., 2006). Interestingly, on epithelial cells TLR9 is expressed on the apical and basolateral membrane, and TLR9 signaling varies in a site-specific manner (Figure 2). Whereas basolateral TLR9 stimulation leads to activation of the nuclear factor-kappa B (NF-κB) pathway, apical TLR9 activation prevents NF-κB activation by accumulation of NF-κB inhibitory protein I kappa B-alpha (IκB − α). Furthermore, apical TLR9 stimulation confers tolerance to subsequent TLR challenges, suggesting that apical exposure to luminal microbial DNA controls intestinal inflammation (Lee et al., 2006).

4 Spatiotemporal Signaling of TLR9

Upon ligand binding, dimerization (or even multimerization) of TLR9 or a conformational change of a preformed dimer occurs leading to the induction of a signaling cascade via adapter molecules. In general, four different adapter molecules

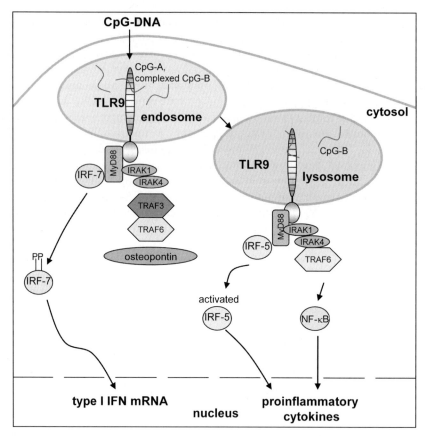

Fig. 3 Spatiotemporal signaling of TLR9. Activation of TLR9 induces secretion of proinflammatory cytokines and type I IFN dependent on ligand localization. CpG-A ODN or CpG-B ODN complexed to transfection agents reside in the endosome and initiate IRF-7 activation leading to type I interferon. In contrast, CpG-B ODN itself traffics to the lysosome and activates IRF-5 and NF-κB. In general, expression of proinflammatory cytokines is induced via IRAK1, IRAK4, TRAF6, and TRAF3. Type I IFN production in plasmacytoid dendritic cells is controlled by TRAF3, TRAF6, osteopontin, and IRF-7

have been identified for TLRs that are recruited after ligand binding: (1) MyD88 (myeloid differentiation protein 88); (2) TIRAP (TIR-associated protein)/MAL (MyD88-adaptor like); (3) TRIF (TIR-domain-containing adapter protein-inducing IFNß/TICAM1 (TIR domain-containing molecule 1); and (4) TRIF-related adapter molecule (TRAM) (see detailed review in Chapter 4). TLR9 solely utilizes MyD88 to induce cytokines (Hacker et al., 2000; Heil et al., 2004; Hemmi et al., 2000) (Figure 3). Usually recruitment of MyD88 is followed by engagement of IL-1 receptor-associated kinase 4 (IRAK-4) and IL-1 receptor-associated kinase 1 (IRAK-1), which is phosphorylated by IRAK-4 and associates with TNF receptor-associated factor-6 (TRAF6) or/and TNF receptor-associated factor-3 (TRAF3)

(Cao et al., 1996; Li et al., 2002; Muzio et al., 1998) (Figure 3). TRAF3 is recruited along with TRAF6 and is essential for the induction of type I IFN but it is dispensable for expression of pro-inflammatory cytokines (Hacker et al., 2006; Oganesyan et al., 2006) (Figure 3). IRF7 is the key component in IFN-α induction which is recruited to a complex consisting of MyD88, IRAK-4, IRAK-1, and TRAF-3 (Honda et al., 2004; Kawai et al., 2004). In addition to IRF7, IRF5 seems to be indispensable for TLR9-mediated induction of proinflammatory cytokines (Takaoka et al., 2005).

The TLR9-MyD88-induced pattern of cytokine production varies among different cell types. For example, pDCs produce large amounts of IFN-α, and it is believed that spatiotemporal regulation of TLR9 signaling accounts for this effect (Honda et al., 2005). Type A CpG-ODN, which induces high amounts of IFN-α, localizes to the endosomal compartment, whereas B-type CpG-ODN is quickly transported to lysosomes and does not induce IFN-α. The lysosomal localization of the CpG-ODN leads to proinflammatory cytokine production instead. Therefore, the endosomal retention of ligands in pDCs probably allows by an unknown mechanism the interactions between MyD88 and IRF7. Interestingly, artificial retention of type B ODN by complexing it to the cationic lipid DOTAP or the circular peptide polymyxin B leads to strong IFN-α production in pDCs (Guiducci et al., 2006; Honda et al., 2005). This establishes that an important determinant of TLR9 signaling is the localization of the ligand (endosome versus lysosome) and demonstrates a strict compartmentalization of the biological response to TLR9 activation in pDCs. This observation still does not explain why localization of the ligand and not TLR9 itself determines the pattern of cytokine production. Presumably, vesicle specific cofactors have to be involved. Recently, osteopontin (Opn) has been identified as a crucial protein for IFN-α production in pDCs (Cao and Liu 2006; Shinohara et al., 2006). Accordingly, Opn deficiency substantially reduced TLR9-dependent IFN-α responses but did not influence expression of transcription factor NF-κB-dependent proinflammatory cytokines. Although it was shown that Opn is targeted to TLR9 and MyD88 after CpG-DNA stimulation, the mechanistic role of Opn still remains elusive (Shinohara et al., 2006).

5 Therapeutic Potential of TLR9 Activation

TLR9 activation induces various effects on immune cells. Since TLR9 is expressed only by B cells and pDCs in humans, TLR9 stimulation can exert direct effects on these cell types, but further cellular immune effects are thought to result from indirect effects (Table 3). In general direct effects involve cytokine production and upregulation of co-stimulatory molecules like CD40 and CD86 on the cell surface. pDC activated by TLR9 produce IFN-α that has antiviral activity but also influences trafficking and clustering of pDCs which is necessary for stimulation of adaptive immune responses in lymph nodes (Asselin-Paturel et al., 2005). Migration is further supported by the TLR9 induced expression of chemokine receptors and the upregulation of co-stimulatory molecules allows for efficient T cell activation.

Table 3 Direct and indirect effects of TLR9 stimulation in humans

	Direct effects	Indirect effects
Human pDCs	• IFN-α • Proinflammatory cytokines (IL-6, IL-12, IL-18, TNF-α)	• Differentiation of Th1 cells • NK cell activation • Monocyte activation • Antiviral activity
Human B cells	• IL-6, IL-10 • Plasma cell differentiation, • IgG class switching	

In addition, pDCs secrete chemokines such as monocytes inflammatory protein 1 (MIP-1) and IFNγ-inducible 10-kDa protein (IP-10) that attract other cell types such as T cells and NK cells (Megjugorac et al., 2004). In B cells TLR9 triggering directly influences activation and antibody production in humans (and mice) (Bernasconi et al., 2003; Jung et al., 2002; Pasare and Medzhitov, 2005). Since B cell receptor (BCR) cross-linking by antigen and cognate interaction with helper T cells is not sufficient to promote survival and differentiation of naive human B cells, B cell proliferation, isotype switch and differentiation to immunoglobulin (Ig)-secreting plasma cells can be induced by activation of TLRs such as TLR9 (Bernasconi et al., 2003; Jung et al., 2002; Ruprecht and Lanzavecchia, 2006).

Overall, TLR9 stimulation induces cell maturation and production of proinflammatory cytokines (TNF-α, IL-1 and IL-6) as well as the regulatory cytokines (IL-12 and IL-18) that induce Th1-biased cellular and humoral effector functions. These properties make TLR9 ligands interesting candidates for therapeutic intervention in infectious diseases and in treatment of cancer and allergies (Krieg, 2006).

5.1 Treatment of Allergies

Since TLR9 stimulation with synthetic CpG motif-containing ODN strongly induces cytokines that promote a Th1 response, it was suggested that CpG-DNA could convert a Th2-driven allergic response and inhibit allergic symptoms. Accordingly, as an allergen-independent therapeutic applied to Th2 sensitized mice just before allergen challenge, CpG-DNA was very effective in a temporary attenuation of hypersensitivity reactions such as asthma, allergic conjunctivitis, and allergic rhinitis (Bohle et al., 1999; Horner et al., 2001; Kline et al., 1998; Magone et al., 2000; Shirota et al., 2000; Sur et al., 1999). CpG-DNA also offers a new antiallergic strategy based on vaccination with allergen-conjugated CpG-DNA. These complexes resulted in an augmented immunotherapeutic effect compared to CpG-DNA alone or a mixture of CpG-DNA and allergen (Horner et al., 2001; Tighe et al., 2000). In general, monotherapy with CpG-ODN suppresses Th2 responses and IgE production. These data suggest that CpG-DNA may be a powerful agent for treatment of allergies. Clinical trials lead by Sanofi-Aventis/Coley Pharmaceuticals or Dynavax for various indications such as asthma and allergy are currently ongoing (Simons et al., 2004).

Recent reports identify an additional mechanism showing how TLR9 activation can influence Th2 immune responses in allergic immune responses. TLR9 stimulation leads to induction of high levels of indoleamine 2,3-dioxygenase (IDO), the rate-limiting enzyme of tryptophan catabolism. IDO degrades the indole moiety of tryptophan, serotonin, and melatonin, and initiates the production of neuroactive and immunoregulatory metabolites. Local depletion of tryptophan and increasing amounts of proapoptotic kynurenines strongly affects T cell proliferation and survival (Grohmann et al., 2003). Accordingly, TLR9 ligand-induced IDO activity in the lung inhibits Th2-driven experimental asthma by suppressing lung inflammation and airway hyperreactivity (Hayashi et al., 2004).

5.2 Treatment of Infectious Diseases

During natural infection with DNA viruses or bacteria, TLR9 presumably stimulates protective immunity against intracellular pathogens. This immune activation can be mimicked by synthetic CpG-containing ODNs and proves useful in a therapeutic and prophylactic treatment of infections. For almost 10 years therapeutic CpG-DNA treatment in mice has been studied. The strong induction of Th1-promoting cytokines can be exploited for therapeutic treatment in a Th2-driven diseases like Leishmania major infections. CpG-DNA treatment, even when administered as late as 20 days after infection, leads to total recovery of a susceptible mouse strain (Zimmermann et al., 1998). This strong Th1-inducing capacity of CpG-DNA also underlines its adjuvant effect during immunization, leading to strong antibody responses and induction of cytotoxic T cells (CTL) even independent of T cell help (Cho et al., 2000; Klinman et al., 1997; Lipford et al., 1997; Moldoveanu et al., 1998; Schwartz et al., 1997). Further studies in mice have demonstrated that application of CpG-DNA protects against a wide range of pathogens such as viruses, bacteria, and parasites (Ashkar et al., 2003; Gramzinski et al., 2001; Juffermans et al., 2002; Krieg, 2006; Ray and Krieg, 2003; Rees et al., 2005). Currently, human clinical trials with B-class ODN 1018 ISS (Dynavax, Phase III) and CpG 7909 (GlaxoSMithKline/Coley Pharmaceuticals) as adjuvant for hepatitis B, influenza, and bacillus anthracis vaccination are ongoing and preliminary results are favorable (Cooper et al., 2005; Cooper et al., 2004a; Cooper et al., 2004b; Halperin et al., 2003; Klinman 2006). The adjuvant effect of CpG-DNA/antigen administration presumably enhances the antigen-specific humoral and cellular immune responses, leading to protection. In contrast, a clinical trial with a type C CpG-ODN as monotherapy (Coley Pharmaceuticals) for increased hepatitis B resistance has been canceled.

5.3 TLR9 Ligands for Cancer Therapy

CpG-ODN shows antitumor activity in numerous mouse models, such as B16 melanoma and human papillomavirus type 16 immortalized tumor cells (Kim et al., 2002; Klinman, 2004; Miconnet et al., 2002; Sharma et al., 2003; Weiner et al., 1997). In humans, CpG monotherapy for small tumors may be successful by inducing a T cell- or NK cell-mediated rejection of established tumors. Accordingly a clinical Phase I/II trial in patients with melanoma or cutaneous T cell lymphoma show some beneficial effect (Link et al., 2006; Molenkamp et al., 2006; Pashenkov et al., 2006). However, eradication of large tumors will depend on combination of multiple strategies such as surgery, chemotherapy, and the use of tumor-specific antibodies. Interestingly, combination of CpG-DNA and chemotherapy, such as Dacarbazine (DTIC) for melanoma (Wagner et al., 2005) and taxane/platin for non-small-cell lung cancer (NSCLC) (Manegold et al., 2005) shows a beneficial effect in a phase II oncology clinical trial. Apart from clinical trials using CpG as monotherapy or in combination with chemotherapy, vaccination has also been considered a therapeutic concept for tumor rejection. In a phase I tumor vaccine trial with type B-ODN and a peptide from MART1 (melanoma antigen recognized by T cells 1) a strong induction of antigen-specific cytotoxic T cells has been measured, although no objective response was observed (Speiser et al., 2005).

6 Safety of CpG-DNA

In the murine system some severe side effects of repeated CpG-DNA administration have been reported. Accordingly, daily injection of 60 μg CpG-ODN alters the morphology and functionality of mouse lymphoid organs. By day 7 follicular dendritic cells (FDC) and germinal center B lymphocytes were suppressed and primary humoral immune responses and immunoglobulin class switching was strongly reduced. Ongoing administration led to multifocal liver necrosis and hemorrhagic ascites (Heikenwalder et al., 2004). In humans and monkeys these side effects have not been observed and therefore these species-specific toxicities presumably depend on the different TLR9 expression pattern (see Section 3). In general, CpG administration in humans is well tolerated, and, in contrast to rodents, which can respond to CpG with increased inflammatory cytokine levels in serum, this response is not observed in humans (Krieg 2007).

Further unwanted side effects of TLR9 stimulation could relate to overshooting Th1 responses combined with autoimmunity. In animal models CpG-DNA treatment can induce and exacerbate autoimmune diseases such as arthritis (Deng et al., 1999; Miyata et al., 2000; Ronaghy et al., 2002), lupus (Hasegawa and Hayashi 2003), multiple sclerosis (Ichikawa et al., 2002), and dextran sulfate sodium (DSS)-induced colitis (Obermeier et al., 2005). For the colitis model the role of TLR9 signaling is still controversial. Whereas Obermeier et al. (2005) demonstrate that CpG-DNA (as well as bacterial DNA) contributes to the perpetuation of chronic intestinal inflammation, while loss of TLR9 or block of TLR9 activation ameliorates chronic inflammation, Katakura et al. show a protective effect of TLR9 activation (2005). In their study TLR9-mediated IFN-α production protects mice from DSS-induced colitis and TLR9-deficient mice develop a more severe colitis after DSS treatment (Katakura et al., 2005; Lee et al., 2006). Overall, the induction of autoimmunity has been reported as a severe side effect for CpG-DNA treatment in mice, although in humans no signs of autoimmunity after CpG-DNA treatment have been observed. Again, the species-specific TLR9 expression may provide an explanation for the lack of autoimmune symptoms in humans. Some caution on the efficiency of CpG treatment may arise from recent studies in mice that have reported a CpG-DNA-dependent activation of indoleamine 2,3-dioxygenase (IDO), the key enzyme of the immunosuppressive pathway of tryptophan catabolism (Mellor and Munn 2004). This suppressive effect is only observed upon systemic application. Subcutaneous injection leads to induction of immunity instead (Manlapat et al., 2007; Mellor et al., 2005; Romani et al., 2006; Wingender et al., 2006). Therefore, the route of CpG-DNA administration has to be carefully evaluated in humans.

7 Conclusion

Overall, recent research in TLR function has illuminated how the innate immune system senses invading pathogens and initiates the adaptive immune response. Intense research on TLR9 focused on its direct function on innate immune cells and cells of the adaptive immune system. Future work should exploit all this knowledge to efficiently manipulate TLR9-mediated immune responses for treatment of allergies, infectious diseases, and cancer. Further effort will focus on the prevention of CpG-DNA side effects and the identification of small molecules as TLR9 agonists.

References

Agger EM, Rosenkrands I, Olsen AW, Hatch G, Williams A, Kritsch C, Lingnau K, von Gabain A, Andersen CS, Korsholm KS, Andersen P (2006) Protective immunity to tuberculosis with Ag85B-ESAT-6 in a synthetic cationic adjuvant system IC31. Vaccine 24: 5452–5460

Ashkar AA, Bauer S, Mitchell WJ, Vieira J, Rosenthal KL (2003) Local delivery of CpG oligodeoxynucleotides induces rapid changes in the genital mucosa and inhibits replication, but not entry, of herpes simplex virus type 2. J Virol 77: 8948–8956

Asselin-Paturel C, Brizard G, Chemin K, Boonstra A, O'Garra A, Vicari A, Trinchieri G (2005) Type I interferon dependence of plasmacytoid dendritic cell activation and migration. J Exp Med 201: 1157–1167

Barton GM, Kagan JC, Medzhitov R (2006) Intracellular localization of Toll-like receptor 9 prevents recognition of self DNA but facilitates access to viral DNA. Nat Immunol 7: 49–56

Bauer S, Kirschning CJ, Hacker H, Redecke V, Hausmann S, Akira S, Wagner H, Lipford GB (2001) Human TLR9 confers responsiveness to bacterial DNA via species-specific CpG motif recognition. Proc Natl Acad Sci U S A 98: 9237–9242

Bernasconi NL, Onai N, Lanzavecchia A (2003) A role for Toll-like receptors in acquired immunity: Up-regulation of TLR9 by BCR triggering in naive B cells and constitutive expression in memory B cells. Blood 101: 4500–4504

Bohle B, Jahn-Schmid B, Maurer D, Kraft D, Ebner C (1999) Oligodeoxynucleotides containing CpG motifs induce IL-12, IL-18 and IFN-gamma production in cells from allergic individuals and inhibit IgE synthesis *in vitro*. Eur J Immunol 29: 2344–2353

Bourke E, Bosisio D, Golay J, Polentarutti N, Mantovani A (2003) The Toll-like receptor repertoire of human B lymphocytes: Inducible and selective expression of TLR9 and TLR10 in normal and transformed cells. Blood 102: 956–963

Brinkmann MM, Spooner E, Hoebe K, Beutler B, Ploegh HL, Kim YM (2007) The interaction between the ER membrane protein UNC93B and TLR3, 7, and 9 is crucial for TLR signaling. J Cell Biol 177: 265–275

Cao W, Liu YJ (2006) Opn: Key regulator of pDC interferon production. Nat Immunol 7: 441–443

Cao Z, Xiong J, Takeuchi M, Kurama T, Goeddel DV (1996) TRAF6 is a signal transducer for interleukin-1. Nature 383: 443–446

Cho HJ, Takabayashi K, Cheng PM, Nguyen MD, Corr M, Tuck S, Raz E (2000) Immunostimulatory DNA-based vaccines induce cytotoxic lymphocyte activity by a T-helper cell-independent mechanism. Nat Biotechnol 18: 509–514

Chuang TH, Lee J, Kline L, Mathison JC, Ulevitch RJ (2002) Toll-like receptor 9 mediates CpG-DNA signaling. J Leukoc Biol 71: 538–544

Coban C, Ishii KJ, Kawai T, Hemmi H, Sato S, Uematsu S, Yamamoto M, Takeuchi O, Itagaki S, Kumar N, Horii T, Akira S (2005) Toll-like receptor 9 mediates innate immune activation by the malaria pigment hemozoin. J Exp Med 201: 19–25

Cooper CL, Davis HL, Angel JB, Morris ML, Elfer SM, Seguin I, Krieg AM, Cameron DW (2005) CPG 7909 adjuvant improves hepatitis B virus vaccine seroprotection in antiretroviral-treated HIV-infected adults. Aids 19: 1473–1479

Cooper CL, Davis HL, Morris ML, Efler SM, Adhami MA, Krieg AM, Cameron DW, Heathcote J (2004a) CPG 7909, an immunostimulatory TLR9 agonist oligodeoxynucleotide, as adjuvant to Engerix-B HBV vaccine in healthy adults: A double-blind phase I/II study. J Clin Immunol 24: 693–701

Cooper CL, Davis HL, Morris ML, Efler SM, Krieg AM, Li Y, Laframboise C, Al Adhami MJ, Khaliq Y, Seguin I, Cameron DW (2004b) Safety and immunogenicity of CPG 7909 injection as an adjuvant to Fluarix influenza vaccine. Vaccine 22: 3136–3143

Dalpke A, Frank J, Peter M, Heeg K (2006) Activation of Toll-like receptor 9 by DNA from different bacterial species. Infect Immun 74: 940–946

Deng GM, Nilsson IM, Verdrengh M, Collins LV, Tarkowski A (1999) Intra-articularly localized bacterial DNA containing CpG motifs induces arthritis. Nat Med 5: 702–705

Edwards AD, Diebold SS, Slack EM, Tomizawa H, Hemmi H, Kaisho T, Akira S, Reis e Sousa C (2003) Toll-like receptor expression in murine DC subsets: Lack of TLR7 expression by CD8 alpha+ DC correlates with unresponsiveness to imidazoquinolines. Eur J Immunol 33: 827–833

Ewaschuk JB, Backer JL, Churchill TA, Obermeier F, Krause DO, Madsen KL (2007) Surface expression of TLR9 is upregulated on intestinal epithelial cells in response to pathogenic bacterial DNA. 75: 2572–2579

Gramzinski RA, Doolan DL, Sedegah M, Davis HL, Krieg AM, Hoffman SL (2001) Interleukin-12- and gamma interferon-dependent protection against malaria conferred by CpG oligodeoxynucleotide in mice. Infect Immun 69: 1643–1649

Grohmann U, Fallarino F, Puccetti P (2003) Tolerance, DCs and tryptophan: Much ado about IDO. Trends Immunol 24: 242–248

Guiducci C, Ott G, Chan JH, Damon E, Calacsan C, Matray T, Lee KD, Coffman RL, Barrat FJ (2006) Properties regulating the nature of the plasmacytoid dendritic cell response to Toll-like receptor 9 activation. J Exp Med 203: 1999–2008

Hacker H, Mischak H, Miethke T, Liptay S, Schmid R, Sparwasser T, Heeg K, Lipford GB, Wagner H (1998) CpG-DNA-specific activation of antigen-presenting cells requires stress kinase activity and is preceded by non-specific endocytosis and endosomal maturation. EMBO J 17: 6230–6240

Hacker H, Redecke V, Blagoev B, Kratchmarova I, Hsu LC, Wang GG, Kamps MP, Raz E, Wagner H, Hacker G, Mann M, Karin M (2006) Specificity in Toll-like receptor signalling through distinct effector functions of TRAF3 and TRAF6. Nature 439: 204–207

Hacker H, Vabulas RM, Takeuchi O, Hoshino K, Akira S, Wagner H (2000) Immune cell activation by bacterial CpG-DNA through myeloid differentiation marker 88 and tumor necrosis factor receptor-associated factor (TRAF)6. J Exp Med 192: 595–600

Halperin SA, Van Nest G, Smith B, Abtahi S, Whiley H, Eiden JJ (2003) A phase I study of the safety and immunogenicity of recombinant hepatitis B surface antigen co-administered with an immunostimulatory phosphorothioate oligonucleotide adjuvant. Vaccine 21: 2461–2467

Hartmann G, Battiany J, Poeck H, Wagner M, Kerkmann M, Lubenow N, Rothenfusser S, Endres S (2003) Rational design of new CpG oligonucleotides that combine B cell activation with high IFN-alpha induction in plasmacytoid dendritic cells. Eur J Immunol 33: 1633–1641

Hartmann G, Krieg AM (2000) Mechanism and function of a newly identified CpG DNA motif in human primary B cells. J Immunol 164: 944–953

Hasegawa K, Hayashi T (2003) Synthetic CpG oligodeoxynucleotides accelerate the development of lupus nephritis during preactive phase in NZB x NZWF1 mice. Lupus 12: 838–845

Hayashi T, Beck L, Rossetto C, Gong X, Takikawa O, Takabayashi K, Broide DH, Carson DA, Raz E (2004) Inhibition of experimental asthma by indoleamine 2,3-dioxygenase. J Clin Invest 114: 270–279

Heikenwalder M, Polymenidou M, Junt T, Sigurdson C, Wagner H, Akira S, Zinkernagel R, Aguzzi A (2004) Lymphoid follicle destruction and immunosuppression after repeated CpG oligodeoxynucleotide administration. Nat Med 10: 187–92

Heil F, Hemmi H, Hochrein H, Ampenberger F, Kirschning C, Akira S, Lipford G, Wagner H, Bauer S (2004) Species-specific recognition of single-stranded RNA via Toll-like receptor 7 and 8. Science 303: 1526–1529

Hemmi H, Takeuchi O, Kawai T, Kaisho T, Sato S, Sanjo H, Matsumoto M, Hoshino K, Wagner H, Takeda K, Akira S (2000) A Toll-like receptor recognizes bacterial DNA. Nature 408: 740–745

Hochrein H, Schlatter B, O'Keeffe M, Wagner C, Schmitz F, Schiemann M, Bauer S, Suter M, Wagner H (2004) Herpes simplex virus type-1 induces IFN-alpha production via Toll-like receptor 9-dependent and -independent pathways. Proc Natl Acad Sci USA 101: 11416–11421

Hoene V, Peiser M, Wanner R (2006) Human monocyte-derived dendritic cells express TLR9 and react directly to the CpG-A oligonucleotide D19. J Leukoc Biol 80: 1328–1336

Honda K, Ohba Y, Yanai H, Negishi H, Mizutani T, Takaoka A, Taya C, Taniguchi T (2005) Spatiotemporal regulation of MyD88-IRF-7 signalling for robust type-I interferon induction. Nature 434: 1035–1040

Honda K, Yanai H, Mizutani T, Negishi H, Shimada N, Suzuki N, Ohba Y, Takaoka A, Yeh WC, Taniguchi T (2004) Role of a transductional-transcriptional processor complex involving MyD88 and IRF-7 in Toll-like receptor signaling. Proc Natl Acad Sci U S A 101: 15416–15421

Horner AA, Van Uden JH, Zubeldia JM, Broide D, Raz E (2001) DNA-based immunotherapeutics for the treatment of allergic disease. Immunol Rev 179: 102–118

Hornung V, Rothenfusser S, Britsch S, Krug A, Jahrsdorfer B, Giese T, Endres S, Hartmann G (2002) Quantitative expression of Toll-like receptor 1-10 mRNA in cellular subsets of human peripheral blood mononuclear cells and sensitivity to CpG oligodeoxynucleotides. J Immunol 168: 4531–4537

Ichikawa HT, Williams LP, Segal BM (2002) Activation of APCs through CD40 or Toll-like receptor 9 overcomes tolerance and precipitates autoimmune disease. J Immunol 169: 2781–7

Juffermans NP, Leemans JC, Florquin S, Verbon A, Kolk AH, Speelman P, van Deventer SJ, van der Poll T (2002) CpG oligodeoxynucleotides enhance host defense during murine tuberculosis. Infect Immun 70: 147–152

Jung J, Yi AK, Zhang X, Choe J, Li L, Choi YS (2002) Distinct response of human B cell subpopulations in recognition of an innate immune signal, CpG DNA. J Immunol 169: 2368–2373

Kadowaki N, Ho S, Antonenko S, Malefyt RW, Kastelein RA, Bazan F, Liu YJ (2001) Subsets of human dendritic cell precursors express different Toll-like receptors and respond to different microbial antigens. J Exp Med 194: 863–869

Kajita E, Nishiya T, Miwa S (2006) The transmembrane domain directs TLR9 to intracellular compartments that contain TLR3. Biochem Biophys Res Commun 343: 578–584

Kalis C, Gumenscheimer M, Freudenberg N, Tchaptchet S, Fejer G, Heit A, Akira S, Galanos C, Freudenberg MA (2005) Requirement for TLR9 in the immunomodulatory activity of *Propionibacterium acnes*. J Immunol 174: 4295–4300

Katakura K, Lee J, Rachmilewitz D, Li G, Eckmann L, Raz E (2005) Toll-like receptor 9-induced type I IFN protects mice from experimental colitis. J Clin Invest 115: 695–702

Kawai T, Sato S, Ishii KJ, Coban C, Hemmi H, Yamamoto M, Terai K, Matsuda M, Inoue J, Uematsu S, Takeuchi O, Akira S (2004) Interferon-alpha induction through Toll-like receptors involves a direct interaction of IRF7 with MyD88 and TRAF6. Nat Immunol 5: 1061–1068

Kerkmann M, Costa LT, Richter C, Rothenfusser S, Battiany J, Hornung V, Johnson J, Englert S, Ketterer T, Heckl W, Thalhammer S, Endres S, Hartmann G (2005) Spontaneous formation of nucleic acid-based nanoparticles is responsible for high interferon-alpha induction by CpG-A in plasmacytoid dendritic cells. J Biol Chem 280: 8086–8093

Kim TY, Myoung HJ, Kim JH, Moon IS, Kim TG, Ahn WS, Sin JI (2002) Both E7 and CpG-oligodeoxynucleotide are required for protective immunity against challenge with human papillomavirus 16 (E6/E7) immortalized tumor cells: involvement of CD4+ and CD8+ T cells in protection. Cancer Res 62: 7234–7240

Kline JN, Waldschmidt TJ, Businga TR, Lemish JE, Weinstock JV, Thorne PS, Krieg AM (1998) Modulation of airway inflammation by CpG oligodeoxynucleotides in a murine model of asthma. J Immunol 160: 2555–2559

Klinman DM (2004) Immunotherapeutic uses of CpG oligodeoxynucleotides. Nat Rev Immunol 4: 249–258

Klinman DM (2006) CpG oligonucleotides accelerate and boost the immune response elicited by AVA, the licensed anthrax vaccine. Expert Rev Vaccines 5: 365–369

Klinman DM, Yamshchikov G, Ishigatsubo Y (1997) Contribution of CpG motifs to the immunogenicity of DNA vaccines. J Immunol 158: 3635–3639

Krieg AM (2002) CpG motifs in bacterial DNA and their immune effects. Annu Rev Immunol 20: 709–760

Krieg AM (2006) Therapeutic potential of Toll-like receptor 9 activation. Nat Rev Drug Discov 5: 471–484

Krieg AM (2007) Development of TLR9 agonists for cancer therapy. J Clin Invest 117: 1184–1194

Krieg AM, Wu T, Weeratna R, Efler SM, Love-Homan L, Yang L, Yi AK, Short D, Davis HL (1998) Sequence motifs in adenoviral DNA block immune activation by stimulatory CpG motifs. Proc Natl Acad Sci U S A 95: 12631–12636

Krieg AM, Yi AK, Matson S, Waldschmidt TJ, Bishop GA, Teasdale R, Koretzky GA, Klinman DM (1995) CpG motifs in bacterial DNA trigger direct B-cell activation. Nature 374: 546–549

Krug A, French AR, Barchet W, Fischer JA, Dzionek A, Pingel JT, Orihuela MM, Akira S, Yokoyama WM, Colonna M (2004a) TLR9-dependent recognition of MCMV by IPC and DC generates coordinated cytokine responses that activate antiviral NK cell function. Immunity 21: 107–119

Krug A, Luker GD, Barchet W, Leib DA, Akira S, Colonna M (2004b) Herpes simplex virus type 1 activates murine natural interferon-producing cells through Toll-like receptor 9. Blood 103: 1433–1437

Krug A, Rothenfusser S, Hornung V, Jahrsdorfer B, Blackwell S, Ballas ZK, Endres S, Krieg AM, Hartmann G (2001a) Identification of CpG oligonucleotide sequences with high induction of IFN-alpha/beta in plasmacytoid dendritic cells. Eur J Immunol 31: 2154–2163

Krug A, Towarowski A, Britsch S, Rothenfusser S, Hornung V, Bals R, Giese T, Engelmann H, Endres S, Krieg AM, Hartmann G (2001b) Toll-like receptor expression reveals CpG DNA as a unique microbial stimulus for plasmacytoid dendritic cells which synergizes with CD40 ligand to induce high amounts of IL-12. Eur J Immunol 31: 3026–3037

Latz E, Schoenemeyer A, Visintin A, Fitzgerald KA, Monks BG, Knetter CF, Lien E, Nilsen NJ, Espevik T, Golenbock DT (2004) TLR9 signals after translocating from the ER to CpG DNA in the lysosome. Nat Immunol 5: 190–198

Lee J, Mo JH, Katakura K, Alkalay I, Rucker AN, Liu YT, Lee HK, Shen C, Cojocaru G, Shenouda S, Kagnoff M, Eckmann L, Ben-Neriah Y, Raz E (2006) Maintenance of colonic homeostasis by distinctive apical TLR9 signalling in intestinal epithelial cells. Nat Cell Biol 8: 1327–1336

Leifer CA, Brooks JC, Hoelzer K, Lopez J, Kennedy MN, Mazzoni A, Segal DM (2006) Cytoplasmic targeting motifs control localization of Toll-like receptor 9. J Biol Chem 281: 35585–35592

Leifer CA, Kennedy MN, Mazzoni A, Lee C, Kruhlak MJ, Segal DM (2004) TLR9 is localized in the endoplasmic reticulum prior to stimulation. J Immunol 173: 1179–1183

Li S, Strelow A, Fontana EJ, Wesche H (2002) IRAK-4: A novel member of the IRAK family with the properties of an IRAK-kinase. Proc Natl Acad Sci USA 99: 5567–5572

Link BK, Ballas ZK, Weisdorf D, Wooldridge JE, Bossler AD, Shannon M, Rasmussen WL, Krieg AM, Weiner GJ (2006) Oligodeoxynucleotide CpG 7909 delivered as intravenous infusion demonstrates immunologic modulation in patients with previously treated non-Hodgkin lymphoma. J Immunother 29: 558–568

Lipford GB, Bauer M, Blank C, Reiter R, Wagner H, Heeg K (1997) CpG-containing synthetic oligonucleotides promote B and cytotoxic T cell responses to protein antigen: A new class of vaccine adjuvants. Eur J Immunol 27: 2340–2344

Lund J, Sato A, Akira S, Medzhitov R, Iwasaki A (2003) Toll-like receptor 9-mediated recognition of Herpes simplex virus-2 by plasmacytoid dendritic cells. J Exp Med 198: 513–520

Magone MT, Chan CC, Beck L, Whitcup SM, Raz E (2000) Systemic or mucosal administration of immunostimulatory DNA inhibits early and late phases of murine allergic conjunctivitis. Eur J Immunol 30: 1841–1850

Manegold C, Mezger J, Peschel C, Leichman G, Haarmann C, Al-Adhami M, Schmalbach T (2005) Combination of a Toll-like receptor 9 (TLR9) agonist, CPG 7909 (CPG) with first line taxane/platinum improves response rate in late stage non-small-cell lung cancer (NSCLC). Ann Oncol 16: 306

Manlapat AK, Kahler DJ, Chandler PR, Munn DH, Mellor AL (2007) Cell-autonomous control of interferon type I expression by indoleamine 2,3-dioxygenase in regulatory CD19(+) dendritic cells. Eur J Immunol 37: 1064–1071

Marshall JD, Fearon K, Abbate C, Subramanian S, Yee P, Gregorio J, Coffman RL, Van Nest G (2003) Identification of a novel CpG DNA class and motif that optimally stimulate B cell and plasmacytoid dendritic cell functions. J Leukoc Biol 73: 781–792

Megjugorac NJ, Young HA, Amrute SB, Olshalsky SL, Fitzgerald–Bocarsly P (2004) Virally stimulated plasmacytoid dendritic cells produce chemokines and induce migration of T and NK cells. J Leukoc Biol 75: 504–514

Mellor AL, Baban B, Chandler PR, Manlapat A, Kahler DJ, Munn DH (2005) Cutting edge: CpG oligonucleotides induce splenic CD19+ dendritic cells to acquire potent indoleamine 2,3-dioxygenase-dependent T cell regulatory functions via IFN type 1 signaling. J Immunol 175: 5601–5605

Mellor AL, Munn DH (2004) IDO expression by dendritic cells: Tolerance and tryptophan catabolism. Nat Rev Immunol 4: 762–774

Miconnet I, Koenig S, Speiser D, Krieg A, Guillaume P, Cerottini JC, Romero P (2002) CpG are efficient adjuvants for specific CTL induction against tumor antigen-derived peptide. J Immunol 168: 1212–1218

Miyata M, Kobayashi H, Sasajima T, Sato Y, Kasukawa R (2000) Unmethylated oligo-DNA containing CpG motifs aggravates collagen-induced arthritis in mice. Arthritis Rheum 43: 2578–2582

Moldoveanu Z, Love-Homan L, Huang WQ, Krieg AM (1998) CpG DNA, a novel immune enhancer for systemic and mucosal immunization with influenza virus. Vaccine 16: 1216–1224

Molenkamp BG, van Leeuwen PA, van den Eertwegh AJ, Sluijter BJ, Scheper RJ, Meijer S, de Gruijl TD (2006) Immunomodulation of the melanoma sentinel lymph node: a novel adjuvant therapeutic option. Immunobiol 211: 651–661

Muzio M, Natoli G, Saccani S, Levrero M, Mantovani A (1998) The human Toll signaling pathway: divergence of nuclear factor kappaB and JNK/SAPK activation upstream of tumor necrosis factor receptor-associated factor 6 (TRAF6). J Exp Med 187: 2097–2101

Obermeier F, Dunger N, Strauch UG, Hofmann C, Bleich A, Grunwald N, Hedrich HJ, Aschenbrenner E, Schlegelberger B, Rogler G, Scholmerich J, Falk W (2005) CpG motifs of bacterial DNA essentially contribute to the perpetuation of chronic intestinal inflammation. Gastroenterology 129: 913–927

Oganesyan G, Saha SK, Guo B, He JQ, Shahangian A, Zarnegar B, Perry A, Cheng G (2006) Critical role of TRAF3 in the Toll-like receptor-dependent and -independent antiviral response. Nature 439: 208–211

Parroche P, Lauw FN, Goutagny N, Latz E, Monks BG, Visintin A, Halmen KA, Lamphier M, Olivier M, Bartholomeu DC, Gazzinelli RT, Golenbock DT (2007) Malaria hemozoin is immunologically inert but radically enhances innate responses by presenting malaria DNA to Toll-like receptor 9. Proc Natl Acad Sci USA 104: 1919–1924

Pasare C, Medzhitov R (2005) Control of B-cell responses by Toll-like receptors. Nature 438: 364–368

Pashenkov M, Goess G, Wagner C, Hormann M, Jandl T, Moser A, Britten CM, Smolle J, Koller S, Mauch C, Tantcheva–Poor I, Grabbe S, Loquai C, Esser S, Franckson T, Schneeberger A, Haarmann C, Krieg AM, Stingl G, Wagner SN (2006) Phase II trial of a Toll-like receptor 9-activating oligonucleotide in patients with metastatic melanoma. J Clin Oncol 24: 5716–5724

Pichyangkul S, Yongvanitchit K, Kum-arb U, Hemmi H, Akira S, Krieg AM, Heppner DG, Stewart VA, Hasegawa H, Looareesuwan S, Shanks GD, Miller RS (2004) Malaria blood stage parasites activate human plasmacytoid dendritic cells and murine dendritic cells through a Toll-like receptor 9-dependent pathway. J Immunol 172: 4926–4933

Ray NB, Krieg AM (2003) Oral pretreatment of mice with CpG DNA reduces susceptibility to oral or intraperitoneal challenge with virulent Listeria monocytogenes. Infect Immun 71: 4398–4404

Rees DG, Gates AJ, Green M, Eastaugh L, Lukaszewski RA, Griffin KF, Krieg AM, Titball RW (2005) CpG-DNA protects against a lethal orthopoxvirus infection in a murine model. Antiviral Res 65: 87–95

Roberts TL, Sweet MJ, Hume DA, Stacey KJ (2005) Cutting edge: Species-specific TLR9-mediated recognition of CpG and non-CpG phosphorothioate-modified oligonucleotides. J Immunol 174: 605–608

Romani L, Bistoni F, Perruccio K, Montagnoli C, Gaziano R, Bozza S, Bonifazi P, Bistoni G, Rasi G, Velardi A, Fallarino F, Garaci E, Puccetti P (2006) Thymosin alpha1 activates dendritic cell tryptophan catabolism and establishes a regulatory environment for balance of inflammation and tolerance. Blood 108: 2265–2274

Ronaghy A, Prakken BJ, Takabayashi K, Firestein GS, Boyle D, Zvailfler NJ, Roord ST, Albani S, Carson DA, Raz E (2002) Immunostimulatory DNA sequences influence the course of adjuvant arthritis. J Immunol 168: 51–56

Ruprecht CR, Lanzavecchia A (2006) Toll-like receptor stimulation as a third signal required for activation of human naive B cells. Eur J Immunol 36: 810–816

Rutz M, Metzger J, Gellert T, Luppa P, Lipford GB, Wagner H, Bauer S (2004) Toll-like receptor 9 binds single-stranded CpG-DNA in a sequence- and pH-dependent manner. Eur J Immunol 34: 2541–2550

Saikh KU, Kissner TL, Sultana A, Ruthel G, Ulrich RG (2004) Human monocytes infected with Yersinia pestis express cell surface TLR9 and differentiate into dendritic cells. J Immunol 173: 7426–7434

Schellack C, Prinz K, Egyed A, Fritz JH, Wittmann B, Ginzler M, Swatosch G, Zauner W, Kast C, Akira S, von Gabain A, Buschle M, Lingnau K (2006) IC31, a novel adjuvant signaling via TLR9, induces potent cellular and humoral immune responses. Vaccine 24: 5461–5472

Schwartz DA, Quinn TJ, Thorne PS, Sayeed S, Yi AK, Krieg AM (1997) CpG motifs in bacterial DNA cause inflammation in the lower respiratory tract. J Clin Invest 100: 68–73

Sharma S, Karakousis CP, Takita H, Shin K, Brooks SP (2003) Intra-tumoral injection of CpG results in the inhibition of tumor growth in murine Colon-26 and B-16 tumors. Biotechnol Lett 25: 149–153

Shimosato T, Kimura T, Tohno M, Iliev ID, Katoh S, Ito Y, Kawai Y, Sasaki T, Saito T, Kitazawa H (2006) Strong immunostimulatory activity of AT-oligodeoxynucleotide requires a six-base loop with a self-stabilized 5′-C...G-3′ stem structure. Cell Microbiol 8: 485–495

Shimosato T, Kitazawa H, Katoh S, Tohno M, Iliev ID, Nagasawa C, Kimura T, Kawai Y, Saito T (2005) Augmentation of T(H)-1 type response by immunoactive AT oligonucleotide from lactic acid bacteria via Toll-like receptor 9 signaling. Biochem Biophys Res Commun 326: 782–787

Shinohara ML, Lu L, Bu J, Werneck MB, Kobayashi KS, Glimcher LH, Cantor H (2006) Osteo-pontin expression is essential for interferon-alpha production by plasmacytoid dendritic cells. Nat Immunol 7: 498–506

Shirota H, Sano K, Kikuchi T, Tamura G, Shirato K (2000) Regulation of murine airway eosinophilia and Th2 cells by antigen-conjugated CpG oligodeoxynucleotides as a novel antigen-specific immunomodulator. J Immunol 164: 5575–5582

Siegal FP, Kadowaki N, Shodell M, Fitzgerald-Bocarsly PA, Shah K, Ho S, Antonenko S, Liu YJ (1999) The nature of the principal type 1 interferon-producing cells in human blood. Science 284: 1835–1837

Simons FE, Shikishima Y, Van Nest G, Eiden JJ, HayGlass KT (2004) Selective immune redirection in humans with ragweed allergy by injecting Amb a 1 linked to immunostimulatory DNA. J Allergy Clin Immunol 113: 1144–1151

Speiser DE, Lienard D, Rufer N, Rubio-Godoy V, Rimoldi D, Lejeune F, Krieg AM, Cerottini JC, Romero P (2005) Rapid and strong human CD8+ T cell responses to vaccination with peptide, IFA, and CpG oligodeoxynucleotide 7909. J Clin Invest 115: 739–746

Sur S, Wild JS, Choudhury BK, Sur N, Alam R, Klinman DM (1999) Long term prevention of allergic lung inflammation in a mouse model of asthma by CpG oligodeoxynucleotides. J Immunol 162: 6284–6293

Tabeta K, Hoebe K, Janssen EM, Du X, Georgel P, Crozat K, Mudd S, Mann N, Sovath S, Goode J, Shamel L, Herskovits AA, Portnoy DA, Cooke M, Tarantino LM, Wiltshire T, Steinberg BE, Grinstein S, Beutler B (2006) The Unc93b1 mutation 3d disrupts exogenous antigen presentation and signaling via Toll-like receptors 3, 7 and 9. Nat Immunol 7: 156–164

Takaoka A, Yanai H, Kondo S, Duncan G, Negishi H, Mizutani T, Kano S, Honda K, Ohba Y, Mak TW, Taniguchi T (2005) Integral role of IRF-5 in the gene induction programme activated by Toll-like receptors. Nature 434: 243–9

Takeshita F, Leifer CA, Gursel I, Ishii KJ, Takeshita S, Gursel M, Klinman DM (2001) Cutting edge: Role of Toll-like receptor 9 in CpG DNA-induced activation of human cells. J Immunol 167: 3555–3558

Tighe H, Takabayashi K, Schwartz D, Marsden R, Beck L, Corbeil J, Richman DD, Eiden JJ, Jr, Spiegelberg HL, Raz E (2000) Conjugation of protein to immunostimulatory DNA results in a rapid, long-lasting and potent induction of cell-mediated and humoral immunity. Eur J Immunol 30: 1939–1947

Tokunaga T, Yamamoto H, Shimada S, Abe H, Fukuda T, Fujisawa Y, Furutani Y, Yano O, Kataoka T, Sudo T, et al. (1984) Antitumor activity of deoxyribonucleic acid fraction from *Mycobacterium bovis* BCG. I. Isolation, physicochemical characterization, and antitumor activity. J Natl Cancer Inst 72: 955–962

Verthelyi D, Ishii KJ, Gursel M, Takeshita F, Klinman DM (2001) Human peripheral blood cells differentially recognize and respond to two distinct CPG motifs. J Immunol 166: 2372–2377

Viglianti GA, Lau CM, Hanley TM, Miko BA, Shlomchik MJ, Marshak–Rothstein A (2003) Activation of autoreactive B cells by CpG dsDNA. Immunity 19: 837–847

Vollmer J, Weeratna R, Payette P, Jurk M, Schetter C, Laucht M, Wader T, Tluk S, Liu M, Davis HL, Krieg AM (2004a) Characterization of three CpG oligodeoxynucleotide classes with distinct immunostimulatory activities. Eur J Immunol 34: 251–262

Vollmer J, Weeratna RD, Jurk M, Samulowitz U, McCluskie MJ, Payette P, Davis HL, Schetter C, Krieg AM (2004b) Oligodeoxynucleotides lacking CpG dinucleotides mediate Toll-like receptor 9 dependent T helper type 2 biased immune stimulation. Immunology 113: 212–223

Wagner S, Weber J, Redman B, Schmalbach T, Bright D, Al-Adhami M, Zarour H, Trefzer U (2005) CPG 7909, a TLR9 agonist immunomodulator in metastatic melanoma: A randomized phase II trial comparing two doses and in combination with DTIC. Journal of Clinical Oncology, 2005 ASCO Annual Meeting Proceedings. Vol 23, No. 16S, Part I of II (June 1 Supplement), 2005: 7526

Weiner GJ, Liu HM, Wooldridge JE, Dahle CE, Krieg AM (1997) Immunostimulatory oligodeoxynucleotides containing the CpG motif are effective as immune adjuvants in tumor antigen immunization. Proc Natl Acad Sci USA 94: 10833–10837

Wingender G, Garbi N, Schumak B, Jungerkes F, Endl E, von Bubnoff D, Steitz J, Striegler J, Moldenhauer G, Tuting T, Heit A, Huster KM, Takikawa O, Akira S, Busch DH, Wagner H, Hammerling GJ, Knolle PA, Limmer A (2006) Systemic application of CpG-rich DNA suppresses adaptive T cell immunity via induction of IDO. Eur J Immunol 36: 12–20

Yasuda K, Rutz M, Schlatter B, Metzger J, Luppa PB, Schmitz F, Haas T, Heit A, Bauer S, Wagner H (2006) CpG motif-independent activation of TLR9 upon endosomal translocation of "natural" phosphodiester DNA. Eur J Immunol 36: 431–436

Yasuda K, Yu P, Kirschning CJ, Schlatter B, Schmitz F, Heit A, Bauer S, Hochrein H, Wagner H (2005) Endosomal translocation of vertebrate DNA activates dendritic cells via TLR9-dependent and -independent pathways. J Immunol 174: 6129–6136

Yi AK, Peckham DW, Ashman RF, Krieg AM (1999) CpG DNA rescues B cells from apoptosis by activating NFkappaB and preventing mitochondrial membrane potential disruption via a chloroquine-sensitive pathway. Int Immunol 11: 2015–2024

Zimmermann S, Egeter O, Hausmann S, Lipford GB, Rocken M, Wagner H, Heeg K (1998) CpG oligodeoxynucleotides trigger protective and curative Th1 responses in lethal murine *leishmaniasis*. J Immunol 160: 3627–3630

RNA Recognition via TLR7 and TLR8

Veit Hornung, Winfried Barchet, Martin Schlee, and Gunther Hartmann(✉)

Abstract In this chapter we focus on immunorecognition of RNA by two members of the family of Toll-like receptors (TLRs), TLR7, and TLR8. While any long single-stranded RNA is readily recognized by both TLR7 and TLR8, sequence-dependent activation of TLR7 and TLR8 becomes more evident when using short RNA oligonucleotides. RNA oligonucleotides containing sequence motifs for TLR7 and TLR8 are termed is RNA (immunostimulatory RNA). Moreover, short double-stranded RNA oligonucleotides as used for siRNA (short interfering RNA) containing such sequences function primarily as ligands for TLR7 but not TLR8. Even in the presence of appropriate sequence motifs, RNA is not detected by TLR7 and TLR8 when certain chemical modifications are present. Both immunological recognition and ignorance are relevant for the development of RNA-based therapeutics, depending on the clinical setting for which they are developed.

1 Introduction

Receptor-mediated detection of pathogen-derived nucleic acids assists in protecting genomic nucleic acid from invading foreign genetic material. A new picture is evolving in which the ability of biological systems to detect foreign nucleic acids

Gunther Hartmann
Institute of Clinical Biochemistry and Pharmacology, University Hospital, University of Bonn, Sigmund-Freud-Str. 25, 53127 Bonn, Germany. Tel: 0049/228/287-16080
gunther.hartmann@ukb.uni-bonn.de

S. Bauer, G. Hartmann (eds.), *Toll-Like Receptors (TLRs) and Innate Immunity.*
Handbook of Experimental Pharmacology 183.
© Springer-Verlag Berlin Heidelberg 2008

via protein receptor/nucleic acid ligand interactions is crucial for maintaining the integrity of the genome and for survival. A number of pattern recognition receptors (PRRs) have evolved that take part in nucleic acid recognition. In general, PRRs can be classified into several families. The Toll-like receptor (TLR) family consists of 10 members (13 in mice), which enable innate immune cells and other specialized cell subsets such as epithelial cells to respond to a variety of pathogen-associated molecular patterns (PAMPs) (Akira et al., 2006). TLR3, TLR7, TLR8, and TLR9 recognize nucleic acid. Based on sequence and structural and functional similarities, TLR3, TLR7, TLR8, and TLR9 form a distinct subgroup of TLRs. In addition, viral RNA with certain characteristics is also detected by members of the RIG-I-like RNA helicase (RLH) family, such as RIG-I and mda-5 (Yoneyama et al., 2004). TLRs and the two RLH members RIG-I and mda-5 differ in their cellular localization, ligand specificity, and downstream signaling pathways; this suggests that host cells employ multiple, nonredundant defense mechanisms to detect invading pathogens: While RIG-I and mda-5 are cytosolic receptors, the four members of the TLR family (TLR3, TLR7, TLR8, and TLR9) involved in viral nucleic acid recognition are all located in the endosomal membrane. The long double-stranded RNA mimic known as polyinosinic:polycytidylic acid [poly(I:C)] is the ligand for mda-5 (Gitlin et al., 2006; Kato et al., 2006); either single- or double-stranded RNA with a triphosphate group at the $5'$ end was recently found to be the ligand for RIG-I (Hornung et al., 2006) (Pichlmair et al., 2006). As for mda-5, the ligand for TLR3 is poly(I:C) (Alexopoulou et al., 2001). The ligands for TLR7 and TLR8 are ssRNA (Diebold et al., 2004; Heil et al., 2004) and short dsRNA with certain sequence motifs (Hornung et al., 2005), and the ligand for TLR9 is DNA-containing CpG motifs (Hemmi et al., 2000; Krieg et al., 1995). While RIG-I and mda-5 are widely expressed in all immune and all nonimmune cells (Kato et al., 2005), TLRs show distinct expression patterns in certain immune cell subsets. For example, expression of human TLR9 is restricted to B cells and plasmacytoid dendritic cells (PDC) (Hornung et al., 2002).

2 RNA Detection by TLR7 and TLR8

Given the fact that many viruses synthesize double-stranded RNA (dsRNA) during their replication cycle (Baltimore et al., 1964; Montagnier and Sanders, 1963), dsRNA was long postulated to be the prime molecular signature of viral infection. In support of this concept the enzymatically generated double-stranded RNA polynucleotide poly(I:C) was found to be a potent inducer of type I IFN (Field et al., 1967). Although the authors at the time were careful to emphasize that all other double-stranded polynucleotides tested were inactive, the notion that long viral double-stranded RNA elicited type I IFN became commonplace, and poly I:C was used as an interferon-inducing mimic of viral dsRNA ever since.

With the advent of efficient RNA stabilization and transfection technologies, the delivery of antigen-specific mRNA into dendritic cells was examined by a number of investigators. While performing such studies researchers noted that single-stranded RNA (mRNA, bacterial RNA, and RNA oligonucleotides) triggered potent innate immune responses when transfected into dendritic cells (Riedl et al., 2002; Weissman et al., 2000). In fact, experiments with MyD88-deficient mice soon pointed to a TLR as the responsible PRR (Scheel et al., 2004). Subsequently, TLR7 and TLR8, initially identified as receptors for antiviral small molecules such as imidazoquinoline derivatives (Heil et al., 2003; Jurk et al., 2002), were found to be responsible for the detection of single-stranded RNA derived from the human immunodeficiency virus (HIV) and the influenza virus (Diebold et al., 2004; Heil et al., 2004). Today, many RNA viruses have been identified that are fully or partially recognized via TLR7 or the closely related TLR8 (Beignon et al., 2005; Lund et al., 2004; Melchjorsen et al., 2005). While gain of function studies in the human system showed that both TLR7 and TLR8 transfer responsiveness to ssRNA, in the mouse system this was true only for TLR7 (Heil et al., 2004; Jurk et al., 2002). Based on these data it was postulated that murine TLR8 was nonfunctional. However, recent studies demonstrate that murine TLR8 is functional, since cells overexpressing murine TLR8 responded to a combination of imidazoquinoline derivatives and poly T oligodeoxynucleotides (Gorden et al., 2006a; Gorden et al., 2006b). Though fully active as single components in the human system, only a combination of imidazoquinoline derivatives and poly T oligodeoxynucleotides showed strong synergy to activate TLR8 (Gorden et al., 2006a; Jurk et al., 2006).

3 TLR7 and TLR8: Expression and Signal Transduction

Expression of TLR7 and TLR8 is largely confined to immune cell subsets. In fact, in the human system, the expression of TLR7 is restricted to PDCs and B cells (Bekeredjian-Ding et al., 2005; Hornung et al., 2002). TLR8 is mainly expressed in cells of the myeloid lineage including monocytes, myeloid dendritic cells, and macrophages (Bekeredjian-Ding et al., 2006; Hornung et al., 2002). In these cell types, activation of the respective TLRs triggers a potent cytokine response leading to secondary responses in immune effector cells (NK cells and T cells). While recent reports proposed that NK cells and T cells also express these TLRs under certain circumstances, the physiological relevance is not completely understood (Caron et al., 2005; Gelman et al., 2004). In the murine system, expression pattern of TLR7 and TLR8 is similar to humans.

Following receptor/ligand interaction, TLR7 and TLR8 recruit the universal TLR adapter protein MyD88, which functions downstream of all TLRs with exception of TLR3. MyD88 recruitment is followed by the formation of a complex with the IRAK family members IRAK1 and IRAK4 and with TRAF6, which results in the activation of NF-κB. While TLR7/8-mediated MyD88 activation does not lead to IFN-α induction in the myeloid lineage, both in human and murine PDCs, the

TLR7/MyD88 axis results in a strong IFN-α response, indicating that PDCs are able to activate a unique pathway that mediates IFN-α induction. Since there is no cell line available to study the signaling cascade in PDCs, most of our knowledge is based on loss-of-functions approaches in the murine system. Given the close relationship between TLR7 and TLR9, studies on TLR9 may be used to predict the signaling of TLR7 in PDC. Type I IFN induction in response to TLR9 ligands was found to be independent of the "classical" IFN-β-inducing transcription factor IRF3, yet dependent of IRF7, which is expressed constitutively in PDC. The groups of Shizuo Akira and Tadatsugu Taniguchi have shown that IRF7 is able to form a signaling complex with MyD88, IRAK1, IRAK4, and TRAF6, and that this complex translocates into the nucleus upon TLR activation (Kawai et al., 2004; Uematsu et al., 2005). In fact, PDCs from mice that are deficient in either MyD88, IRAK4, or TRAF6 show defects in both IRF7- and NF-κB-activation, and thus lack the induction of type I IFN and inflammatory cytokines (Kawai et al., 2004). Mice lacking IRAK1, on the other hand, show an impaired activation of IRF7 while maintaining normal NF-κB activation (Uematsu et al., 2005). Consistent with these findings, IRAK1, but not IRAK4, is capable of phosphorylating IRF7. Similar findings have been reported for the kinase IKKα, and IKKα knockout mice also show a complete defect in type I interferon induction via TLR7 and TLR9 (Hoshino et al., 2006). TRAF3 is a member of the TRAF family that is critical for the induction of type I IFN in response to TLR7- and TLR9-signaling (Hacker et al., 2006; Oganesyan et al., 2006). TRAF3 binds MyD88 and IRAK1, thereby activating IRF7. Further biochemical studies are needed to fully explore the signaling complex that is employed in PDCs to induce type I interferon production in response to TLR7 activation. TLR8, as noted above, is restricted to cells of the myeloid lineage and thus activates the canonical MyD88 pathway following ligand receptor interaction.

4 Sequence Specific Recognition of RNA by TLR7 and TLR8

Specific sequences and certain structural requirements have been reported to impact on the TLR-dependent recognition and of ssRNA and siRNA. Indeed, much of our knowledge on how RNA oligonucleotides are recognized by TLR7 and TLR8 comes from studies that aimed at the understanding of nonspecific immune effects of siRNA molecules. However, experiments assessing the immunostimulatory properties of synthetic RNA oligonucleotides have been carried out in varying species, cell types, or cell systems using different modes of delivery and employing different readouts, which complicates conclusive interpretation. Yet all studies agree that IFN-α production in response to unmodified, synthetic RNA is mediated by PDC that express TLR7. Thus, while IFN-α induced by synthetic RNA in either purified PDC or mixed immune cell populations is dependent on TLR7, the production of other cytokines such as IL-6 or TNF-α by several cell types is influenced by both

TLR7 and TLR8. This should be kept in mind when comparing different reports that appear contradictive at first.

TLR7 activation by ssRNA was initially described as dependent on the base composition of RNA (Diebold et al., 2004; Heil et al., 2004). In our hands, and consistent with this idea, siRNAs showed significant differences in the level of type I IFN-induction in PDCs (Hornung et al., 2005). Further reports confirmed the observation that TLR7-mediated recognition of ssRNA or siRNA was sequence-dependent (Judge et al., 2005; Sioud, 2006). In our search for the stimulatory sequence motifs we demonstrated that the mere frequency of guanosine or uridine bases was not sufficient to predict the stimulatory activity of RNA, as 1) RNAs with identical numbers of GU dinucleotides displayed varying activities, and 2) ssRNAs with low or no GU-residues also showed immunological activity (Sioud, 2006). In our studies the internal 9-mer motif 5'-GUCCUUCAA-3' was identified as a potent stimulus; in addition, others showed that 5'-UGUGU-3' in siRNA duplexes (Judge et al., 2005), or UU dinucleotide repeats in ssRNA constitute additional stimulatory motifs {Barchet, 2005 #51}. These motifs seem to be representatives of a large number of active sequence motifs. While the frequency of adenosines decreases the stimulatory properties of RNA, uridines increase immunorecognition (Sioud, 2006).

A recent study concludes that the mere quantity of uridines correlates with high immunostimulatory activity via TLR7 (Diebold et al., 2006). In fact, a comparison with the previously described highly active TLR7 RNA oligonucleotides RNA40 and RNA9.2DR is used to suggest that a 21-mer poly U RNA oligonucleotide (polyUs21) showed superior activity. However, several important points need to be considered when we compare these ligands: The backbone of the homopolymeric oligonucleotide polyUs21 was phosphorothioate-stabilized, whereas RNA40 and RNA9.2DR were synthesized as common phosphodiesters. The nature of the RNA backbone strongly impacts on the half-life and thus the activity of the oligonucleotide tested. Moreover, different complexation reagents and nucleic acid concentrations were used, further complicating the interpretation of this study.

In the human system TLR8 function can be studied by analyzing the proinflammatory cytokine response cells of the myeloid lineage including MDCs, monocytes, and macrophages. Notably, some RNA sequences were found to preferentially promote activation of myeloid cells while not being recognized by PDCs (Heil et al., 2004; Judge et al., 2005; Sugiyama et al., 2005). In this context it is interesting to note that in at least one instance a G-to-A replacement within an immunostimulatory RNA sequence abrogated IFN-α induction in PDCs, while TNF-α, IL-6, and IL-12 induction in PBMCs was maintained (Heil et al., 2004). Thus, both the type of TLR triggered and the cell subset stimulated critically impact on the cytokine response elicited. Moreover, murine TLR7 has been reported to favor sequence motifs that are distinct from those active on human TLR7 (Heil et al., 2004). This finding is similar to the species-specific CpG motifs described for murine and human TLR9 (Hartmann and Krieg, 2000; Hartmann et al., 2000; Hemmi et al., 2000; Krieg, 2002).

Flanking sequences or the relative positioning within the RNA strand may influence the immunostimulatory properties of a potent RNA motif. In this respect,

CpG-RNA motifs flanked by poly-G tails were reported to induce the up-regulation of co-stimulatory molecules and cytokines within monocytes but not PDCs (Sugiyama et al., 2005). Another important feature of RNA is its natural occurrence in single- or double-stranded conformation. The finding that a stimulatory motif can confer activity in the form of both ssRNA and dsRNA points to a model in which immunostimulatory sequences are equally recognized in the context of either RNA conformation. Yet, the striking observation that monocytes, unlike PDC, seem responsive only to ssRNA but not dsRNA (Sioud, 2006) (Hornung et al., unpublished observation) suggests that a ssRNA conformation is required for the recognition by TLR8, or another yet undefined mechanism of recognition in human monocytes. Taken together, there is indeed evidence for a sequence motif-dependent recognition of RNA by TLR7 and TLR8; however a more systematic study of the cell type-specific contribution and RNA configuration is required for a comprehensive model able to describe RNA recognition by TLRs.

An important step towards this goal was the report on the crystal structure of TLR3 postulating the direct interaction of RNA with TLR domains (Choe et al., 2005). A similar mode of interaction was proposed for CpG and TLR9 (Latz et al., 2004; Rutz et al., 2004). Besides the direct molecular interaction between TLRs and their ligands, the presence of auxiliary proteins or co-receptors may facilitate uptake and recognition in some cell types, while limiting it in others. The presence of a cofactor modifying RNA-responsiveness has recently been proposed based on the observation that addition of autologous plasma enhances the inflammatory response to RNAs (Judge et al., 2005).

5 Discrimination of Self and Foreign RNA

For nonviral pathogens, the recognition strategy of the innate immune system is based on the presence of highly conserved molecular patterns that are unique to microbes but absent in the host. Nucleic acids are an essential constituent of every living organism. Therefore, in order to function as a means to discriminate the presence of viruses, the detection of foreign RNA molecules among the abundance of self RNA appears challenging and raises the following questions: What are the molecular determinants associated with pathogen-derived RNA? and How can host RNA avoid recognition by endogenous RNA receptors?

TLRs that specialize on the detection of viral (and possibly bacterial) nucleic acids are expressed in intracellular organelles. The intracellular expression of TLR3 is controlled by its cytoplasmic linker region; the transmembrane domain regulates localization of TLR7 and TLR9 (Barton et al., 2006; Funami et al., 2004; Leifer et al., 2004; Matsumoto et al., 2003; Nishiya et al., 2005). Such compartmentalization of TLRs serves a dual function: 1) the low pH microenvironment in endosomes favors the uncoating of viral capsids and the release and adequate recognition of RNA or DNA ligands for TLRs; and 2) TLR localization within the endosomal niche may have evolved to scan for viral or bacterial RNA at a location that avoids self RNA encounter. Under homeostatic conditions, host RNA is abundant within the nucleus and in the cytoplasm but absent from endosomes. Notably, a majority of viruses enter host cells via the endosomal route. This latter hypothesis is also supported by the observation that host RNA is not generally ignored by TLRs but can regain the ability to stimulate immune effector cells under pathological circumstances in situations when endogenous RNA enters the endosome (Lau et al., 2005) {Savarese, 2006 #141}. Additional support for the concept that compartmentalization of PRRs is responsible for ignorance of self RNA came from John Rossi's group. In their study (Robbins et al., 2006) it was shown that lipid-delivered, exogenous siRNA-induced IFN in CD34+ progenitor-derived hematopoietic cells in a TLR-dependent manner, whereas the same sequences endogenously expressed via shRNAs were nonstimulatory.

Although sequestration of TLRs in the endosome certainly increases the probability that an immune response is preferentially mounted in the presence of foreign RNA, further reports point to additional features that regulate the immune reactivity of RNA. It has long been appreciated that bacterial DNA contains more unmethylated CpG dinucleotides, which function as TLR9 ligands, as compared to vertebrate DNA, in which the frequency of CpG dinucleotides is markedly diminished (Krieg, 2002). Consequently, certain nucleotide motifs may also be suppressed within the mammalian RNA spectrum. There is some indication that UG sequences occur more frequently in viral RNA (Karlin et al., 1994); however precise information on nucleotide suppression in mammalian RNA is currently not available. Nevertheless, while the role of pathogen RNA sequences is currently unknown, it is well established that RNA recognition by TLR7 and TLR8 is sequence-specific.

Moreover, certain nucleoside modifications within RNA occur more frequently in vertebrates than in evolutionary lower organism, adding an additional aspect for self vs. non-self recognition (Cavaille and Bachellerie, 1998). In fact, RNA derived from prokaryotes has shown to elicit stronger TLR activation as compared to mammalian RNA, correlating with a lower degree of nucleoside modifications in prokaryotic RNA (Kariko et al., 2005). On the other hand, endogenous eukaryotic RNA is subject to numerous modifications (Rozenski et al., 1999). Besides $5'$ capping, eukaryotic RNA undergoes several other posttranscriptional maturation steps, including the modification of various nucleobases of the RNA transcript and the methylation of the backbone ribose at the $2'$-hydroxyl position. Regarding the immunosuppressive effects of nucleobase modifications, TLR7 and TLR8 appear to be particularly sensitive to alterations of the uridine with substitution of this base by pseudouridine, 5-methyluridine, or 2-thiouridine, resulting in a substantial decrease in activation. Interestingly, TLR3 differs from TLR7 and TLR8 in its susceptibility to $2'$-O-methylated RNAs, and the respective activation profile in primary DCs was not identical to TLR-expressing cell lines, suggesting that additional mechanisms of RNA recognition were involved in these cell types (Kariko et al., 2005).

6 Learning from Nature: Bypassing Immunostimulation by RNA

RNA-based therapeutic strategies include gene silencing with siRNA and modulating immunity with immunostimulatory RNA (isRNA). The development of RNA-based drugs needs to address pharmacokinetics, including stability and biodistribution of RNA, and toxicity (Dorsett and Tuschl, 2004). Sequence-dependent TLR7 ligand activity contributes to toxicity associated with the administration of siRNA *in vivo* (Hornung et al., 2005; Judge et al., 2006; Judge et al., 2005; Morrissey et al., 2005). It is important to note that immunostimulation and gene silencing are entirely independent functional activities of siRNA (Hornung et al., 2005; Judge et al., 2005; Sledz et al., 2003). It is agreed that an avoidance of immunorecognition is a key issue for the successful clinical development of siRNA therapeutics.

The TLR7 ligand activity of double-stranded siRNA is due to the immunostimulatory activity of the two single strands (Hornung et al., 2005). Most siRNA molecules designed without addressing the TLR7 ligand activity of the single strands show a nontolerable degree of immunostimulation. The finding that the siRNA sequence itself is the central culprit of immunostimulation pinpoints the design of the primary RNA sequence as an important selection criterion for its safe therapeutic use. In a comprehensive analysis we created a database of stimulatory IFN-inducing RNA sequences. Based on this database we were able to create a mathematical algorithm allowing the prediction of the putative stimulatory value of any given RNA oligonucleotide (Hornung et al., unpublished). On the one hand, such an algorithm would allow the selection of RNA sequences with high immunostimulatory activity including is RNA with no gene silencing activity and siRNA with TLR7 ligand activity on top of gene silencing function. On the other hand, connecting the algorithm predicting TLR7 ligand activity with algorithms that predict optimal gene silencing will provide a valuable platform for effective and safe siRNA design without immunostimulatory side effects. Such siRNAs do not depend on chemical modifications to avoid immunostimulation. This may be advantageous since chemical modifications may cause unpredictable side effects of siRNA *in vivo*.

Chemical RNA modifications that allow avoidance of immunostimulation were initially developed in order to improve pharmacokinetics of RNA therapeutics such as antisense ORNs and ribozymes (Beigelman et al., 1995; Levin, 1999; Pieken et al., 1991). Chemical modifications of RNA include backbone modifications (phosphodiester bond and ribose sugar) and modifications of the nucleobase. In general, backbone modifications do not directly affect Watson-Crick base pairing, yet increase siRNA efficacy by increasing nuclease stability (Amarzguioui et al., 2003). Backbone modifications that enhance nuclease stability of RNA include the phosphorothioate (PS) modification in which one oxygen atom in the phosphodiester bond is replaced by sulfur. PS-modification improves siRNA activity although it has no direct effect on gene silencing nor does it reduce immunostimulatory properties of siRNA (Braasch et al., 2003) (Hornung unpublished observation).

Several studies examined chemical modifications of the 2′ position of the sugar ribose on the gene silencing and the immunostimulatory properties of RNA (Cekaite et al., 2007; Judge et al., 2006; Sioud, 2006; Sugiyama et al., 2005). Introduction of 2′-fluoro, 2′-deoxy or 2′-O-methyl groups in ssRNA abrogated TNF-α in human PBMC (Sioud, 2006). In fact, analyzing the global gene expression profile of human PBMC following ssRNA or siRNA transfection revealed a complete lack of an immune response when 2′-O-methyl-modified RNA oligonucleotides were used. Of note, 2′-O-methyl modification of the sense strand in siRNAs did not alter the gene silencing activity of the siRNA. Ian MacLachlan's group confirmed that as little as two 2′-O-methyl modified uridines rendered siRNA nonstimulatory (Judge et al., 2006). Interestingly, immune inhibition by 2′-O-methyl modification was operational in trans. As a consequence, 2′-O-methyl modification in the sense strand abolished the immunostimulatory activity of the antisense strand and thus the complete double strand. Although completely 2′-O-methyl-modified duplexes lack their silencing ability, the introduction of a limited number of 2′-O-methyl substitutes in the sense strand is well tolerated and induces efficient gene inhibition (Chiu and Rana, 2003; Czauderna et al., 2003; Elbashir et al., 2001; Jackson et al., 2006).

The locked-nucleic acid (LNA) modification is another tool for modulating silencing activity. Containing a methylen linkage between the 2′-oxygen and the 4′-carbon of the ribose ring, LNAs strongly enhance binding affinity (Manoharan, 2004) and thus increase the melting temperature of hybridized RNA. When located in the wing region, LNAs do not compete with mRNA suppression, and introduction of LNAs into either end of the sense strand still maintains the full silencing activity of the siRNA duplex (Hornung et al., 2005; Manoharan, 2004). However, in contrast to 2′-O-methyl modification described above, the introduction of LNA into the ssRNA of an siRNA duplex does not have an inhibitory effect in trans on a stimulatory motif within the same strand or within the complementary strand (Hornung et al., 2005). Altogether, siRNA molecules that combine a high degree of respective backbone modifications (>90%) have been shown to promote effective RNAi-dependent silencing of HBV RNA *in vivo* (Morrissey et al., 2005).

Nucleobase modifications offer additional ways to suppress immunostimulatory activity of nucleic acids. Methylation of cytidines in mammalian DNA inhibits immunostimulatory properties of host DNA, and more recently it has been shown that methylation of cytidines abolished stimulatory activity of RNA in human monocytes (Hemmi et al., 2000; Sugiyama et al., 2005). For RNA, several base modifications, especially of uridines, were shown to alter TLR ligand activity (Kariko et al., 2005). Although nucleobase modifications could be used for the design of nonstimulatory siRNA, nucleobase-modified RNA is less reliable with respect to gene silencing since this type of modification directly interferes with complementary base pairing. In this respect it has been shown that the presence of 6-methyladenosine within RNA markedly destabilizes RNA duplexes (Kierzek and Kierzek, 2003). Further investigation is needed to validate the impact of base modifications on RNAi-mediated mRNA degradation (Manoharan, 2004).

Based on the current knowledge, the prediction of the TLR7/8 ligand activity of a given RNA molecule with modifications of the backbone or the nucleobase is not straightforward for several reasons: While some modifications confer a broad inhibition of the immunostimulatory activity (2′-O-methyl) in cis and trans, other

modifications are only relevant in particular sequence contexts or at defined positions (LNA). Therefore, it is not yet possible to predict how particular alterations
in the chemical structure of a siRNA molecule impacts on gene silencing and immunostimulation. As a consequence, gene silencing activity and immunostimulatory
activity need to be analyzed experimentally for any given siRNA drug candidate.

7 Delivery and TLR7/8 Ligand Activity

As the RNAi machinery is located in the cytosol, exogenous siRNA needs to cross
the cell membrane in order to initiate the gene-silencing process. Two issues need
to be addressed when aiming at siRNA-mediated gene silencing *in vitro* or *in vivo*:
1) RNA is highly susceptible to degradation by RNAses, and 2) siRNA molecules
are not readily taken up into cells. Macromolecular carriers such as cationic polymers (cationic lipids or peptides) are often used to deliver siRNA across the cell
membrane. Of note, cationic lipids do not directly fuse with the plasma membrane
but instead are incorporated into the cellular endocytosis pathway (Almofti et al.,
2003) where TLR3, 7, 8, or 9 are located. The mechanism of TLR9 activation
has been studied in detail and most likely the same pathway also applies to TLR7
and TLR8: nonactivated TLR9 resides in the ER, but is recruited to endosomes
upon stimulation with CpG where TLR9 encounters DNA and subsequently triggers downstream signaling events (Latz et al., 2004; Leifer et al., 2004). Therefore,
if RNA traffics through the endosomal compartments of innate immune cells, it
is predicted to induce TLR stimulation. Thus, the use of cationic lipids does not
bypass endocytosis but rather enhances the immunostimulatory activity of RNA
in endosomes. Of interest, the cationic peptide-driven delivery preferentially activates myeloid immune cells whereas cationic lipid-complexed RNA appears to be a
stronger stimulus for PDCs (Judge et al., 2005) (Hornung et al., unpublished).

An alternative way of siRNA delivery *in vivo* is the administration of naked
siRNA through high pressure tail-vein injection that does not require complexation
to a cationic polymer (Heidel et al., 2004). However, this type of siRNA delivery
requires rapid injection of a large volume of liquid over a short time period, a proce-
dure that can prove lethal for the animals treated. Alternatively, *in vivo* delivery of
siRNA without the need for transfection agents can be achieved by 2'-F modification
of siRNA, rendering siRNA resistant to RNase A (Capodici et al., 2002). Another
remarkable improvement in siRNA administration has been achieved by covalent
conjugation of cholesterol to backbone-modified siRNAs (two PS-linkages and two
2'-O-methyl groups at the 3' end of the siRNA molecule) (Soutschek et al., 2004).
Of note, the covalent linkage of bulky molecules at the 3' end of the sense strand
does not interfere with gene silencing activity (Manoharan, 2004). However, in this
study successful immune evasion was most likely achieved through the chemical
modifications used and not through the cholesterol modification. A novel approach
takes delivery one step further and aims at targeting specific cell types *in vivo*.
Song et al. engineered fusion proteins that contain a positive-charged protamine

domain and a heavy chain antibody fragment F(ab). The positively charged peptide portion noncovalently tethers siRNA, and the antibody fragment serves to carry siRNA specifically to cells of interest, thus bypassing nontargeted immune cells (Song et al., 2005).

8 Concluding Remarks

Numerous protein drugs such as cytokines, growth factors, or antibodies have dramatically expanded and improved our therapeutic repertoire. One could speculate that the next wave of innovation will come from nucleic acid-based drugs. Specifically, two biological properties of short nucleic acids are in the focus of current drug development: gene silencing and the induction of innate antiviral responses. While gene silencing is based on the sequence-specific binding of oligonucleotides to a complementary target sequence such as mRNA, the induction of innate antiviral responses depends on a classical receptor ligand interaction. Due to their distinct molecular mechanism, gene silencing and the induction of antiviral responses are independent properties of oligonucleotides. However, both functional activities need to be considered when oligonucleotides are in contact with biological systems. It is interesting to note that 30 years ago the oligonucleotide field started with aiming at gene silencing (so-called antisense oligodeoxynucleotides), and it took almost 15 years before scientists realized that such compounds have profound interactions with the immune system (recognition of CpG motifs in DNA via TLR9). While initially RNA was considered not stable enough for antisense activity, the breakthrough in gene silencing technology came with RNA interference and the synthetic molecules inducing RNA interference, siRNA. As with DNA, it became clear that RNA oligonucleotides could be recognized by specialized receptors of innate immunity (TLR7 and TLR8).

Today we are in the favorable situation, in that both biological properties of RNA oligonucleotides—gene silencing, and the induction of innate antiviral responses—are well defined, and can be applied separately or in combination depending on the therapeutic goal. Our current knowledge about immunological properties of RNA and the molecular ways to avoid such interaction now provide a sound basis for continued enthusiasm for a future development of siRNA. On the immunostimulatory side of oligonucleotide development, it is important to note that targeting of TLR7 and TLR8 with RNA, unlike CpG-DNA, allows potent virus-like stimulation of myeloid cells such as monocytes, macrophages, and myeloid dendritic cells; due to a distinct expression pattern of TLR9, in humans (but not in mice) CpG-DNA is limited to the activation of plasmacytoid dendritic cells and B cells. This long-desired new window of immunological activities is highly useful for oligonucleotide drug development. Finally, having witnessed the oligonucleotide field moving from DNA to RNA, from gene silencing to immunorecognition first through DNA and then RNA, it will now be exciting to follow the promising future of oligonucleotides into clinical application.

References

Akira S, Uematsu S, Takeuchi O (2006) Pathogen recognition and innate immunity. Cell 124: 783–801

Alexopoulou L, Holt AC, Medzhitov R, Flavell RA (2001) Recognition of double-stranded RNA and activation of NF-kappaB by Toll-like receptor 3. Nature 413: 732–738

Almofti MR, Harashima H, Shinohara Y, Almofti A, Baba Y, Kiwada H (2003) Cationic liposome-mediated gene delivery: Biophysical study and mechanism of internalization. Arch Biochem Biophys 410: 246–253

Amarzguioui M, Holen T, Babaie E, Prydz H (2003) Tolerance for mutations and chemical modifications in a siRNA. Nucleic Acids Res 31: 589–595

Baltimore D, Becker Y, Darnell JE (1964) Virus-Specific Double-Stranded Rna in Poliovirus-Infected Cells. Science 143: 1034–1036

Barton GM, Kagan JC, Medzhitov R (2006) Intracellular localization of Toll-like receptor 9 prevents recognition of self DNA but facilitates access to viral DNA. Nat Immunol 7: 49–56

Beigelman L, McSwiggen JA, Draper KG, Gonzalez C, Jensen K, Karpeisky AM, Modak AS, Matulic-Adamic J, DiRenzo AB, Haeberli P, et al. (1995) Chemical modification of hammerhead ribozymes. Catalytic activity and nuclease resistance. J Biol Chem 270: 25702–25708

Beignon AS, McKenna K, Skoberne M, Manches O, DaSilva I, Kavanagh DG, Larsson M, Gorelick RJ, Lifson JD, Bhardwaj N (2005) Endocytosis of HIV-1 activates plasmacytoid dendritic cells via Toll-like receptor-viral RNA interactions. J Clin Invest 115: 3265–3275

Bekeredjian-Ding I, Roth SI, Gilles S, Giese T, Ablasser A, Hornung V, Endres S, Hartmann G (2006) T cell-independent, TLR-induced IL-12p70 production in primary human monocytes. J Immunol 176: 7438–7346

Bekeredjian-Ding IB, Wagner M, Hornung V, Giese T, Schnurr M, Endres S, Hartmann G (2005) Plasmacytoid dendritic cells control TLR7 sensitivity of naive B cells via type I IFN. J Immunol 174: 4043–4050

Braasch DA, Jensen S, Liu Y, Kaur K, Arar K, White MA, Corey DR (2003) RNA interference in mammalian cells by chemically-modified RNA. Biochem 42: 7967–7975

Capodici J, Kariko K, Weissman D (2002) Inhibition of HIV-1 infection by small interfering RNA-mediated RNA interference. J Immunol 169: 5196–5201

Caron G, Duluc D, Fremaux I, Jeannin P, David C, Gascan H, Delneste Y (2005) Direct stimulation of human T cells via TLR5 and TLR7/8: Flagellin and R-848 up-regulate proliferation and IFN-gamma production by memory CD4 + T cells. J Immunol 175: 1551–1557

Cavaille J, Bachellerie JP (1998) SnoRNA-guided ribose methylation of rRNA: Structural features of the guide RNA duplex influencing the extent of the reaction. Nucleic Acids Res 26: 1576–1587

Cekaite I., Furset G, Hovig E, Sioud M (2007) Gene expression analysis in blood cells in response to unmodified and 2′-modified siRNAs reveals TLR-dependent and independent effects. J Mol Bio 365: 90–108

Chiu YL, Rana TM (2003) siRNA function in RNAi: A chemical modification analysis. Rna 9: 1034–1048

Choe J, Kelker MS, Wilson IA (2005) Crystal structure of human Toll-like receptor 3 (TLR3) ectodomain. Science 309: 581–585

Czauderna F, Fechtner M, Dames S, Aygun H, Klippel A, Pronk GJ, Giese K, Kaufmann J (2003) Structural variations and stabilising modifications of synthetic siRNAs in mammalian cells. Nucleic Acids Res 31: 2705–2716

Diebold SS, Kaisho T, Hemmi H, Akira S, Reis e Sousa C (2004) Innate antiviral responses by means of TLR7-mediated recognition of single-stranded RNA. Science 303: 1529–1531

Diebold SS, Massacrier C, Akira S, Paturel C, Morel Y, Reis ESC (2006) Nucleic acid agonists for Toll-like receptor 7 are defined by the presence of uridine ribonucleotides. Eur J of Immun 36: 3256–3267

Dorsett Y, Tuschl T (2004) siRNAs: applications in functional genomics and potential as therapeutics. Nat Rev Drug Discov 3: 318–329

Elbashir SM, Martinez J, Patkaniowska A, Lendeckel W, Tuschl T (2001) Functional anatomy of siRNAs for mediating efficient RNAi in *Drosophila melanogaster* embryo lysate. EMBO J 20: 6877–6888

Field AK, Tytell AA, Lampson GP, Hilleman MR (1967) Inducers of interferon and host resistance. II. Multistranded synthetic polynucleotide complexes. Proc Natl Acad Sci USA 58: 1004–1010

Funami K, Matsumoto M, Oshiumi H, Akazawa T, Yamamoto A, Seya T (2004) The cytoplasmic 'linker region' in Toll-like receptor 3 controls receptor localization and signaling. Int Immunol 16: 1143–154

Gelman AE, Zhang J, Choi Y, Turka LA (2004) Toll-like receptor ligands directly promote activated CD4 + T cell survival. J Immunol 172: 6065–6073

Gitlin L, Barchet W, Gilfillan S, Cella M, Beutler B, Flavell RA, Diamond MS, Colonna M (2006) Essential role of mda-5 in type I IFN responses to polyriboinosinic:polyribocytidylic acid and encephalomyocarditis picornavirus. Proc Nat Acad Sci USA 103: 8459–8464

Gorden KK, Qiu X, Battiste JJ, Wightman PP, Vasilakos JP, Alkan SS (2006a) Oligodeoxynucleotides differentially modulate activation of TLR7 and TLR8 by imidazoquinolines. J Immunol 177: 8164–8170

Gorden KK, Qiu XX, Binsfeld CC, Vasilakos JP, Alkan SS (2006b) Cutting edge: Activation of murine TLR8 by a combination of imidazoquinoline immune response modifiers and polyT oligodeoxynucleotides. J Immunol 177: 6584–6587

Hacker H, Redecke V, Blagoev B, Kratchmarova I, Hsu LC, Wang GG, Kamps MP, Raz E, Wagner H, Hacker G, Mann M, Karin M (2006) Specificity in Toll-like receptor signalling through distinct effector functions of TRAF3 and TRAF6. Nature 439: 204–207

Hartmann G, Krieg AM (2000) Mechanism and function of a newly identified CpG DNA motif in human primary B cells. J Immunol 164: 944–953

Hartmann G, Weeratna RD, Ballas ZK, Payette P, Blackwell S, Suparto I, Rasmussen WL, Waldschmidt M, Sajuthi D, Purcell RH, Davis HL, Krieg AM (2000) Delineation of a CpG phosphorothioate oligodeoxynucleotide for activating primate immune responses *in vitro* and *in vivo*. J Immunol 164: 1617–1624

Heidel JD, Hu S, Liu XF, Triche TJ, Davis ME (2004) Lack of interferon response in animals to naked siRNAs. Nat Biotechnol 22: 1579–1582

Heil F, Ahmad-Nejad P, Hemmi H, Hochrein H, Ampenberger F, Gellert T, Dietrich H, Lipford G, Takeda K, Akira S, Wagner H, Bauer S (2003) The Toll-like receptor 7 (TLR7)-specific stimulus loxoribine uncovers a strong relationship within the TLR7, 8, and 9 subfamily. Eur J Immunol 33: 2987–2997

Heil F, Hemmi H, Hochrein H, Ampenberger F, Kirschning C, Akira S, Lipford G, Wagner H, Bauer S (2004) Species-specific recognition of single-stranded RNA via Toll-like receptor 7 and 8. Science 303: 1526–1529

Hemmi H, Takeuchi O, Kawai T, Kaisho T, Sato S, Sanjo H, Matsumoto M, Hoshino K, Wagner H, Takeda K, Akira S (2000) A Toll-like receptor recognizes bacterial DNA. Nature 408: 740–745

Hornung V, Guenthner-Biller M, Bourquin C, Ablasser A, Schlee M, Uematsu S, Noronha A, Manoharan M, Akira S, de Fougerolles A, Endres S, Hartmann G (2005) Sequence-specific potent induction of IFN-alpha by short interfering RNA in plasmacytoid dendritic cells through TLR7. Nat Med 11: 263–270

Hornung V, Rothenfusser S, Britsch S, Krug A, Jahrsdorfer B, Giese T, Endres S, Hartmann G (2002) Quantitative expression of Toll-like receptor 1–10 mRNA in cellular subsets of human peripheral blood mononuclear cells and sensitivity to CpG oligodeoxynucleotides. J Immunol 168: 4531–4537

Hoshino K, Sugiyama T, Matsumoto M, Tanaka T, Saito M, Hemmi H, Ohara O, Akira S, Kaisho T (2006) IkappaB kinase-alpha is critical for interferon-alpha production induced by Toll-like receptors 7 and 9. Nature 440: 949–953

Jackson AL, Burchard J, Leake D, Reynolds A, Schelter J, Guo J, Johnson JM, Lim L, Karpilow J, Nichols K, Marshall W, Khvorova A, Linsley PS (2006) Position-specific chemical modification of siRNAs reduces "off-target" transcript silencing. Rna 12: 1197–1205

Judge AD, Bola G, Lee AC, MacLachlan I (2006) Design of noninflammatory synthetic siRNA mediating potent gene silencing *in vivo*. Mol Ther 13: 494–505

Judge AD, Sood V, Shaw JR, Fang D, McClintock K, MacLachlan I (2005) Sequence-dependent stimulation of the mammalian innate immune response by synthetic siRNA. Nat Biotechnol 23: 457–462

Jurk M, Heil F, Vollmer J, Schetter C, Krieg AM, Wagner H, Lipford G, Bauer S (2002) Human TLR7 or TLR8 independently confer responsiveness to the antiviral compound R-848. Nat Immunol 3: 499

Jurk M, Kritzler A, Schulte B, Tluk S, Schetter C, Krieg AM, Vollmer J (2006) Modulating responsiveness of human TLR7 and 8 to small molecule ligands with T-rich phosphorothiate oligodeoxynucleotides. Eur J Immunol 36: 1815–1826

Kariko K, Buckstein M, Ni H, Weissman D (2005) Suppression of RNA recognition by Toll-like receptors: the impact of nucleoside modification and the evolutionary origin of RNA. Immunity 23: 165–175

Karlin S, Doerfler W, Cardon LR (1994) Why is CpG suppressed in the genomes of virtually all small eukaryotic viruses but not in those of large eukaryotic viruses? J Virol 68: 2889–2897

Kato H, Sato S, Yoneyama M, Yamamoto M, Uematsu S, Matsui K, Tsujimura T, Takeda K, Fujita T, Takeuchi O, Akira S (2005) Cell type-specific involvement of RIG-I in antiviral response. Immunity 23: 19–28

Kato H, Takeuchi O, Sato S, Yoneyama M, Yamamoto M, Matsui K, Uematsu S, Jung A, Kawai T, Ishii KJ, Yamaguchi O, Otsu K, Tsujimura T, Koh CS, Reis ESC, Matsuura Y, Fujita T, Akira S (2006) Differential roles of MDA5 and RIG-I helicases in the recognition of RNA viruses. Nature

Kawai T, Sato S, Ishii KJ, Coban C, Hemmi H, Yamamoto M, Terai K, Matsuda M, Inoue J, Uematsu S, Takeuchi O, Akira S (2004) Interferon-alpha induction through Toll-like receptors involves a direct interaction of IRF7 with MyD88 and TRAF6. Nature immunology 5: 1061–1068

Kierzek E, Kierzek R (2003) The thermodynamic stability of RNA duplexes and hairpins containing N6-alkyladenosines and 2-methylthio-N6-alkyladenosines. Nucleic Acids Res 31: 4472–4480

Krieg AM (2002) CpG motifs in bacterial DNA and their immune effects. Annu Rev Immunol 20: 709–760

Krieg AM, Yi AK, Matson S, Waldschmidt TJ, Bishop GA, Teasdale R, Koretzky GA, Klinman DM (1995) CpG motifs in bacterial DNA trigger direct B-cell activation. Nature 374: 546–549

Latz E, Schoenemeyer A, Visintin A, Fitzgerald KA, Monks BG, Knetter CF, Lien E, Nilsen NJ, Espevik T, Golenbock DT (2004) TLR9 signals after translocating from the ER to CpG DNA in the lysosome. Nat Immunol 5: 190–198

Lau CM, Broughton C, Tabor AS, Akira S, Flavell RA, Mamula MJ, Christensen SR, Shlomchik MJ, Viglianti GA, Rifkin IR, Marshak-Rothstein A (2005) RNA-associated autoantigens activate B cells by combined B cell antigen receptor/Toll-like receptor 7 engagement. J Exp Med 202: 1171–1177

Leifer CA, Kennedy MN, Mazzoni A, Lee C, Kruhlak MJ, Segal DM (2004) TLR9 is localized in the endoplasmic reticulum prior to stimulation. J Immunol 173: 1179–1183

Levin AA (1999) A review of the issues in the pharmacokinetics and toxicology of phosphorothioate antisense oligonucleotides. Biochim Biophys Acta 1489: 69–84

Lund JM, Alexopoulou L, Sato A, Karow M, Adams NC, Gale NW, Iwasaki A, Flavell RA (2004) Recognition of single-stranded RNA viruses by Toll-like receptor 7. Proc Nat Acad Sci USA 101: 5598–5603

Manoharan M (2004) RNA interference and chemically modified small interfering RNAs. Curr Opin Chem Biol 8: 570–579

Matsumoto M, Funami K, Tanabe M, Oshiumi H, Shingai M, Seto Y, Yamamoto A, Seya T (2003) Subcellular localization of Toll-like receptor 3 in human dendritic cells. J Immunol 171: 3154–3162

Melchjorsen J, Jensen SB, Malmgaard L, Rasmussen SB, Weber F, Bowie AG, Matikainen S, Paludan SR (2005) Activation of innate defense against a paramyxovirus is mediated by RIG-I and TLR7 and TLR8 in a cell-type-specific manner. J Virol 79: 12944–12951

Montagnier L, Sanders FK (1963) Replicative form of encephalomyocarditis virus ribonucleic acid. Nature 199: 664–667

Morrissey DV, Lockridge JA, Shaw L, Blanchard K, Jensen K, Breen W, Hartsough K, Machemer L, Radka S, Jadhav V, Vaish N, Zinnen S, Vargeese C, Bowman K, Shaffer CS, Jeffs LB, Judge A, MacLachlan I, Polisky B (2005) Potent and persistent *in vivo* anti-HBV activity of chemically modified siRNAs. Nat Biotechnol 23: 1002–1007

Nishiya T, Kajita E, Miwa S, Defranco AL (2005) TLR3 and TLR7 are targeted to the same intracellular compartments by distinct regulatory elements. J Biol Chem 280: 37107–37117

Oganesyan G, Saha SK, Guo B, He JQ, Shahangian A, Zarnegar B, Perry A, Cheng G (2006) Critical role of TRAF3 in the Toll-like receptor-dependent and -independent antiviral response. Nature 439: 208–211

Pichlmair A, Schulz O, Tan CP, Naslund TI, Liljestrom P, Weber F, Reis e Sousa C (2006) RIG-I-mediated antiviral responses to single-stranded RNA bearing $5'$-phosphates. Science 314: 997–1001

Pieken WA, Olsen DB, Benseler F, Aurup H, Eckstein F (1991) Kinetic characterization of ribonuclease-resistant $2'$-modified hammerhead ribozymes. Science 253: 314–317

Riedl P, Stober D, Oehninger C, Melber K, Reimann J, Schirmbeck R (2002) Priming Th1 immunity to viral core particles is facilitated by trace amounts of RNA bound to its arginine-rich domain. J Immunol 168: 4951–4959

Robbins MA, Li M, Leung I, Li H, Boyer DV, Song Y, Behlke MA, Rossi JJ (2006) Stable expression of shRNAs in human CD34+progenitor cells can avoid induction of interferon responses to siRNAs *in vit*ro. Nat Biotechnol 24: 566–571

Rozenski J, Crain PF, McCloskey JA (1999) The RNA modification database: 1999 update. Nucleic Acids Res 27: 196–197

Rutz M, Metzger J, Gellert T, Luppa P, Lipford GB, Wagner H, Bauer S (2004) Toll-like receptor 9 binds single-stranded CpG-DNA in a sequence- and pH-dependent manner. Eur J Immunol 34: 2541–2550

Scheel B, Braedel S, Probst J, Carralot JP, Wagner H, Schild H, Jung G, Rammensee HG, Pascolo S (2004) Immunostimulating capacities of stabilized RNA molecules. Eur J Immunol 34: 537–547

Sioud M (2006) Single-stranded small interfering RNA are more immunostimulatory than their double-stranded counterparts: a central role for $2'$-hydroxyl uridines in immune responses. Eur J Immunol 36: 1222–1230

Sledz CA, Holko M, de Veer MJ, Silverman RH, Williams BR (2003) Activation of the interferon system by short-interfering RNAs. Nat Cell Biol 5: 834–839

Song E, Zhu P, Lee SK, Chowdhury D, Kussman S, Dykxhoorn DM, Feng Y, Palliser D, Weiner DB, Shankar P, Marasco WA, Lieberman J (2005) Antibody mediated *in vivo* delivery of small interfering RNAs via cell-surface receptors. Nat Biotechnol 23: 709–717

Soutschek J, Akinc A, Bramlage B, Charisse K, Constien R, Donoghue M, Elbashir S, Geick A, Hadwiger P, Harborth J, John M, Kesavan V, Lavine G, Pandey RK, Racie T, Rajeev KG, Rohl I, Toudjarska I, Wang G, Wuschko S, Bumcrot D, Koteliansky V, Limmer S, Manoharan M, Vornlocher HP (2004) Therapeutic silencing of an endogenous gene by systemic administration of modified siRNAs. Nature 432: 173–178

Sugiyama T, Gursel M, Takeshita F, Coban C, Conover J, Kaisho T, Akira S, Klinman DM, Ishii KJ (2005) CpG RNA: Identification of novel single-stranded RNA that stimulates human CD14 + CD11c+monocytes. J Immunol 174: 2273–2279

Uematsu S, Sato S, Yamamoto M, Hirotani T, Kato H, Takeshita F, Matsuda M, Coban C, Ishii KJ, Kawai T, Takeuchi O, Akira S (2005) Interleukin-1 receptor-associated kinase-1 plays an essential role for Toll-like receptor (TLR)7- and TLR9-mediated interferon-{alpha} induction. J Exp Med 201: 915–923

Weissman D, Ni H, Scales D, Dude A, Capodici J, McGibney K, Abdool A, Isaacs SN, Cannon G, Kariko K (2000) HIV gag mRNA transfection of dendritic cells (DC) delivers encoded antigen to MHC class I and II molecules, causes DC maturation, and induces a potent human *in vitro* primary immune response. J Immunol 165: 4710–4717

Yoneyama M, Kikuchi M, Natsukawa T, Shinobu N, Imaizumi T, Miyagishi M, Taira K, Akira S, Fujita T (2004) The RNA helicase RIG-I has an essential function in double-stranded RNA-induced innate antiviral responses. Nat Immunol 5: 730–737

Fungal Recognition by TLR2 and Dectin-1

Helen S. Goodridge and David M. Underhill(✉)

Abstract The innate immune system utilizes multiple receptors to recognize fungal pathogens, and the net inflammatory response is controlled by interactions between these receptors. Many fungi are recognized, at least in part, by Toll-like receptor 2 (TLR2) and Dectin-1. Examination of the roles these receptors play together and on their own is a useful model for understanding the interplay between innate immune receptors. This review focuses on the role(s) of TLR2 and Dectin-1 in triggering inflammatory responses, transcription factor activation, phagocytosis, and reactive oxygen production in response to fungi.

1 Introduction

Fungal detection by myeloid phagocytes is achieved by the direct association of components of the fungal cell wall with a variety of phagocyte receptors including Toll-like receptors (TLRs), lectin receptors, and scavenger receptors, as well as by

David M. Underhill
Immunobiology Research Institute, Cedars-Sinai Medical Center, 8700 Beverly Blvd., Los Angeles, CA 90048, USA
david.underhill@cshs.org

S. Bauer, G. Hartmann (eds.), *Toll-Like Receptors (TLRs) and Innate Immunity.*
Handbook of Experimental Pharmacology 183.
© Springer-Verlag Berlin Heidelberg 2008

indirect recognition of complement- and antibody-opsonized fungi by complement receptors and Fc receptors, respectively (Underhill and Ozinsky, 2002; Taylor et al., 2005). While it is important to dissect the mechanisms by which individual receptors detect and respond to pathogen components, it is becoming increasingly clear that effective inflammatory responses are the result of coordinated activation of sets of such receptors. In this chapter we will focus on two of these receptors—the Toll-like receptor TLR2, and the lectin receptor Dectin-1—that have been demonstrated to recognize a range of pathogenic fungi and to collaborate to generate effective antifungal responses.

2 Fungal Receptors—Toll-Like Receptors

The structure and function of TLRs has been described in previous chapters. TLRs are known to mediate immune responses to a wide range of microbes and microbial products, but a role for TLRs in antifungal responses in particular has been clear from the earliest days of mammalian TLR immunology. The demonstration that Toll-deficient *Drosophila* are highly susceptible to *Aspergillus* infection (Lemaitre et al., 1996), combined with the observation that mammals possess homologues of *Drosophila* Toll (Medzhitov et al., 1997), was strongly indicative of a role for TLRs in mammalian antifungal responses. Indeed, we subsequently showed that TLR2 is recruited to macrophage phagosomes containing zymosan, a cell wall preparation of *Saccharomyces cerevisiae*, and that the inflammatory response of macrophages to zymosan exposure could be abrogated by expression of dominant negative TLR2 or dominant negative MyD88 (Underhill et al., 1999a). TLR2 has since been demonstrated to be a key receptor for pathogenic fungi, including *Candida albicans, Aspergillus fumigatus, Aspergillus niger, Cryptococcus neoformans, Pneumocystis carinii*, and *Coccidioides posadasii*.

   The specific role of TLR2 in the detection of fungi and subsequent antifungal responses, in particular its collaboration with Dectin-1, will be discussed in detail below. However, it is important to note at this point that other TLRs have also been implicated in antifungal responses (reviewed by (Netea et al., 2006)). TLR2 forms heterodimers with TLR1 and TLR6, although the precise requirement for these TLRs in fungal recognition is currently unclear. We have demonstrated that TLR1 and TLR6 colocalize with TLR2 on zymosan-containing phagosomes and that expression of a TLR6-dominant negative blocks the inflammatory response of macrophages to zymosan (Ozinsky et al., 2000). In addition, several studies have demonstrated roles for TLR4 (and CD14) in responses to *C. albicans, A. fumigatus, A. niger, C. neoformans*, and *P. carinii*. For example, Netea et al. showed that TLR4 Pro712His mutant (C3H/HeJ) mice display increased susceptibility to disseminated candidiasis due to impaired chemokine (KC and MIP-2) production and reduced neutrophil recruitment, although production of proinflammatory cytokines, including TNF-α, was only marginally influenced, and the ability of phagocytes to kill *Candida* was not affected (Netea et al., 2002). In humans TLR4

Asp299Gly/Thr399Ile polymorphisms are associated with increased susceptibility to *Candida* bloodstream infections, and peripheral blood mononuclear cells from individuals bearing these polymorphisms produce more IL-10 following *in vitro* exposure to *C. albicans* (Van der Graaf et al., 2006). In addition, TLR9-deficient mice with disseminated candidiasis have been reported to produce less IL-12 and more IL-10 and IL-4 than wild-type mice, although they were, surprisingly, no more susceptible to infection, and it is unclear what role TLR9 might play in the antifungal response (Bellocchio et al., 2004). Data also demonstrate that *Aspergillus* conidia and swollen conidia are detected by TLR4 in addition to TLR2 (Meier et al., 2003; Netea et al., 2003; Gersuk et al., 2006).

3 Fungal Receptors—Dectin-1

Dectin-1 was originally cloned as a dendritic cell surface molecule capable of delivering co-stimulatory signals to T cells (Ariizumi et al., 2000). It was subsequently shown to be expressed more widely on myeloid cells including macrophages, dendritic cells, and neutrophils (Taylor et al., 2002), and identified as a receptor for β-glucans (Brown and Gordon, 2001). Dectin-1 specifically recognizes soluble or particulate β-1,3- and/or β-1,6-glucans, which are found primarily in the cell walls of fungi, but also in plants and some bacteria. As discussed below, Dectin-1 has been demonstrated to recognize and mediate responses to a variety of fungi, and, additionally, it has been suggested to be involved in the recognition of mycobacteria (Yadav and Schorey, 2006).

Dectin-1 is a member of the NK-like C-type lectin family and comprises an extracellular carbohydrate recognition domain, a 47 amino acid "stalk," a transmembrane region, and a 40 amino acid N-terminal cytoplasmic tail (Figure 1a). Mouse Dectin-1 has two N-linked glycosylation sites on the C-type lectin domain, while human Dectin-1 has instead a glycosylation site on the stalk region (Willment et al., 2001; Heinsbroek et al., 2006; Kato et al., 2006). Two functional isoforms are produced by humans and mice, the shorter isoform lacking the stalk region. Heinsbroek et al. have demonstrated that binding of the shorter Dectin-1 to yeast cell walls is more sensitive to temperature and is slightly more potent at inducing cellular responses (Heinsbroek et al., 2006).

The intracellular tail of Dectin-1 contains a sequence resembling an immunoreceptor tyrosine-based activation motif (ITAM), which is classically associated with signaling by lymphocyte antigen receptors (TCR and BCR) and Fc receptors. However, the Dectin-1 motif does not conform to the conventional ITAM consensus ($YxxL/Ix_{6-12}YxxL/I$) (Figure 1b). Although two tyrosines are appropriately spaced, the N-terminal tyrosine (tyrosine-3) resides in a YxxxL rather than a YxxL context, suggesting that it may not be functional.

ITAM signaling following antigen receptor ligation is characterized by phosphorylation of the dual ITAM tyrosines by Src family kinases (reviewed in (Barrow and Trowsdale 2006; Fodor et al., 2006)). This allows recruitment of Syk family

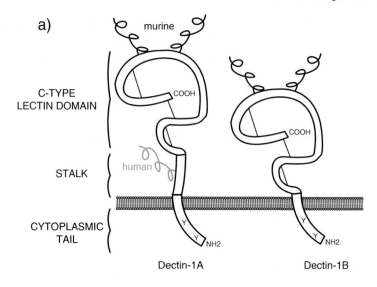

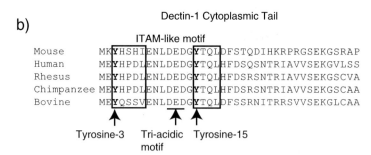

Fig. 1 The structure of Dectin-1. **a** Dectin-1 is a small type II transmembrane protein with a short (40-amino acid) amino-terminal cytoplasmic tail, and an extracellular domain of consisting of a 46-amino acid "stalk" region and a single carboxy-terminal C-type lectin domain. The murine C-type lectin domain has two N-linked glycosylation sites, while the stalk region of the human receptor has one N-linked gylcosylation site. A common splice variant lacking the stalk domain (Dectin-1B) is produced by mice and humans. **b** The amino acid sequences of the cytoplasmic tails of Dectin-1 from a variety of species show conservation of tyrosine-15 and a triacidic motif that are important for signaling by the receptor

kinases, which interact with the dual phosphotyrosines via their dual SH2 domains. Consistent with ITAM-like signaling, the intracellular tail of Dectin-1 is tyrosine phosphorylated upon ligand binding, mutation of the membrane-proximal ITAM tyrosine (tyrosine-15) abolishes its signaling, and a synthetic peptide based on the phosphorylated membrane-proximal YxxL motif of murine Dectin-1 binds to Syk (Gantner et al., 2003; Herre et al., 2004; Rogers et al., 2005; Underhill et al., 2005). Furthermore, Src family kinases and Syk are phosphorylated following ligation of

Dectin-1 on both macrophages and dendritic cells and have been demonstrated to mediate downstream signaling (Rogers et al., 2005; Underhill et al., 2005). However, mutation of the tyrosine in the atypical, membrane-distal repeat (tyrosine-3) does not compromise Dectin-1-mediated responses (Herre et al., 2004; Rogers et al., 2005; Underhill et al., 2005), suggesting that, unlike conventional ITAM signaling, a single phosphorylated tyrosine might be sufficient to recruit Syk to Dectin-1.

An unusual triacidic motif located just upstream of the membrane-proximal tyrosine appears to be required for Dectin-1 signaling and may participate in Syk activation (Underhill et al., 2005).

4 Fungal Recognition by TLR2 and Dectin-1

TLR2 and Dectin-1 recognize components of the fungal cell wall. The cell wall of yeast such as *S. cerevisiae* and *C. albicans* is composed primarily of mannan, chitin, and glucan (Figure 2a). The structural inner face of the wall is a mesh of β-1,3-glucan with β-1,6-glucan branches. Chitin (β-1,4-GlcNAc) is linked directly to the glucan core and is particularly enriched in the ring that forms between mother and daughter cells during division. The outer face of the wall is coated with mannan linked to the β-glucan core through short polypeptides (Kollar et al., 1997). Glycoproteins involved in processes such as cell wall synthesis are found in the perimplasmic space just outside the plasma membrane, and additional mannoproteins are found associated with the outer face of the cell wall. While this structure is largely

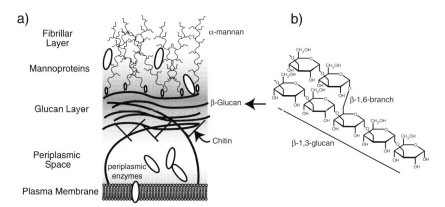

Fig. 2 Yeast cell wall structure. **a** A schematic diagram of the yeast cell wall shows the major layers outside the plasma membrane of the cell. Major carbohydrate components of the cell wall include mannan, glucan, and chitin. Proteins are found within the periplasmic space or attached to mannan on the cell surface. **b** The structure of the major β-glucan, β-1,3-glucan, is shown with a β-1,6 branch. The frequency of β-1,6 branches is highly variable, and β-1,6-glucan polymers are also found in yeast cell walls. Dectin-1 recognizes the β-1,3-glucan, and an oligomer of at least ten glucoses is required for recognition

shared by other fungi, there are important variations. For example, *C. neoformans*, an important human pathogen that can cause fatal meningoencephalitis in immunosuppressed individuals, is surrounded by a thick polysaccharide capsule. This capsule, which is required for pathogenicity, is made primarily of glucuronoxylomannan and has been demonstrated to inhibit phagocytosis of the yeasts (Buchanan and Murphy, 1998).

As discussed above, TLR2 is recruited to zymosan-containing phagosomes (Underhill et al., 1999a) and plays a significant role in mediating the functional response of myeloid phagocytes against a variety of pathogenic fungi (discussed further below). However, the components of the yeast cell wall detected by TLR2 remain to be definitively identified. A variety of glycolipid components of nonfungal microbes have been identified as TLR2 ligands, including mycobacterial lipoarabinomannan, lipoteichoic acid from *Staphylococcus*, glycolipids from *Treponema*, and glycosylphosphatidylinositol from trypanosomes (Underhill et al., 1999b; Campos et al., 2001; Opitz et al., 2001). Hence it would seem most likely that the fungal TLR2 ligand is also a glycolipid. One candidate is phospholipomannan; peritoneal macrophages from TLR2-deficient mice stimulated with phospholipomannan purified from *C. albicans* produce significantly less TNF-α than macrophages from wild-type mice (Jouault et al., 2003). However, it is not clear whether phospholipomannan is a cell wall component of other fungi and thus whether it could be a generic fungal TLR2 ligand.

In contrast, the fungal component detected by Dectin-1 is well established. Brown and Gordon (2001) first demonstrated that Dectin-1 is a receptor for β-1, 3-linked glucans by showing that a variety of fungal and plant β-glucans, but not monosaccharides or other carbohydrates with different linkages, are detected by NIH3T3 cells expressing Dectin-1. Furthermore, binding of fluorescently labeled zymosan, as well as intact *S. cerevisiae* and *C. albicans*, to Dectin-1-expressing NIH3T3 cells or to macrophages was blocked by the soluble β-glucans laminarin (from the brown seaweed, *Laminaria digitata*) and glucan phosphate, but not by mannan (Brown and Gordon, 2001; Brown et al., 2002). A more comprehensive approach to defining the β-glucan structure recognized by Dectin-1 using oligosaccharide microarrays defined the minimum structure recognized as a β-1,3-glucan 10-mer (Palma et al., 2006). β-glucans are not produced by mammalian cells, making them ideal targets for innate immune receptors such as Dectin-1 (Figure 2b).

A variety of clinically important fungal pathogens are now known to be recognized by Dectin-1, although cellular morphology can be a key determinant, due to variation in β-glucan masking at the fungal surface. The ability of *C. albicans* to rapidly and reversibly switch between yeast and filamentous morphologies is crucial to its pathogenicity; the filamentous morphology is thought to provide some advantage during interaction with the mammalian immune system (Lo et al., 1997; Calderone and Fonzi, 2001; Saville et al., 2003). Indeed, *C. albicans* mutants that lack the ability to switch from yeast to filamentous growth are avirulent (Lo et al., 1997). We recently showed that the extracellular domain of Dectin-1 (soluble Dectin-1) detects the budding yeast but not the filamentous form of *C. albicans* (Gantner et al., 2005) (Figure 3a).

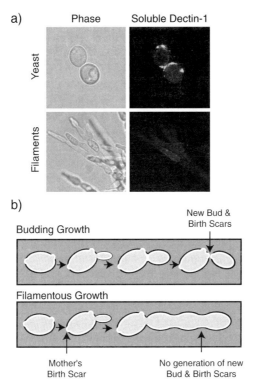

Fig. 3 Dectin-1 recognizes *C. albicans* yeast, but not filaments. **a** *C. albicans* was grown as budding yeast (top) or filaments (bottom), and Dectin-1 binding sites were identified using fluorescently labeled soluble Dectin-1. Dectin-1 recognizes patches of the yeast cell wall, but does not recognize the filament cell wall. Reprinted with permission from Gantner et al., EMBO J. 2005 24:1277. **b** The yeast cell wall consists of a mannan-rich outer coat (black) covering a β-glucan-rich structural core (white). During budding growth, the core β-glucan-rich layer is exposed when mother and daughter cells separate. During filamentous growth, cell separation does not occur and the core β-glucan remains largely inaccessible to recognition by Dectin-1

Interestingly, soluble Dectin-1 bound discrete patches of the yeast cell surface corresponding to bud and birth scars (Figure 3a). These are perturbations of the cell wall architecture that form during yeast cell division as a budding daughter cell separates from the mother cell. The bud and birth scars are permanent and are not repaired during subsequent cell growth. Dectin-1 binding to bud and birth scars was competed by the soluble β-glucan laminarin and could also be blocked by pretreatment of yeast with a β-glucanase enzyme (Gantner et al., 2005). Hence it appears that β-glucan, which is normally buried beneath the outer mannan layer of the yeast cell wall, is exposed upon separation of budding *C. albicans* yeast and becomes accessible to Dectin-1 (Figure 3b). In contrast, soluble Dectin-1 failed to stain *C. albicans* hyphae; this form of the fungus does not undergo division and hence the β-glucan remains concealed beneath the surface. The reader is directed to scanning electron micrographs published by (Osumi, 1998) showing the presence of bud and birth scars on budding yeast, but not on cells undergoing filamentous growth. Thus Dectin-1 can be expected to play a more important role in inflammatory response to the yeast form of *C. albicans* than to the filamentous form.

Another recent report demonstrated that treatment of *C. albicans* with subinhibitory doses of the antifungal drug caspofungin, which targets cell wall biosynthetic pathways, disrupts the cell wall architecture to expose β-glucan and is hence capable of "unmasking" hyphae (Wheeler and Fink, 2006). Furthermore, these investigators used an anti-β-glucan antibody to screen a genome-wide library of approximately 4800 *S. cerevisiae* mutants for increased β-glucan exposure to identify genes involved in β-glucan masking. Of the 79 mutants exhibiting increased β-glucan exposure, 68 (86%) also displayed increased binding to soluble Dectin-1.

Three recent studies have examined the recognition of different morphological forms of *A. fumigatus* by Dectin-1 (Hohl et al., 2005; Steele et al., 2005; Gersuk et al., 2006). *Aspergillus conidia* (resting spores), which are ubiquitous in the environment, are inhaled frequently. In immunocompetent individuals, germinating conidia are phagocytosed and cleared by alveolar macrophages and recruited neutrophils; in immunocompromised individuals, failure to clear *Aspergillus* can result in invasive pneumonia and disseminated infection (Marr et al., 2002). Following inhalation, conidia swell and, if not cleared, produce germ tubes that eventually extend to form filamentous hyphae. Soluble Dectin-1 stained swollen but not resting *Aspergillus* conidia (Steele et al., 2005; Gersuk et al., 2006). Consistent with this, an anti-β-glucan antibody detected β-glucan exposed on the surface of swollen conidia but failed to bind to resting spores (Hohl et al., 2005; Gersuk et al., 2006). Unlike *C. albicans* however, β-glucan was also exposed on the surface of *Aspergillus* germ tubes and hyphae, which could therefore be detected by Dectin-1 (Hohl et al., 2005; Steele et al., 2005; Gersuk et al., 2006).

There is also evidence that Dectin-1 can bind to *P. carinii*, which frequently causes pneumonia in immunocompromised individuals. Binding of *P. carinii* to RAW264.7 macrophages was enhanced by overexpression of Dectin-1, and this could be blocked with an antibody against Dectin-1 (Steele et al., 2003). Immunofluorescence microscopy demonstrated that Dectin-1 on the surface of alveolar macrophages localized to the point where the cells contact *P. carinii* cysts.

5 Phagocytosis of Fungi

Myeloid phagocytes exposed to fungi bind and internalize the organisms through a process called phagocytosis. Binding triggers reorganization of the actin cytoskeleton beneath the particle, extension of membrane ruffles around the particle, and internalization (Underhill and Ozinsky, 2002). Once internalized, the newly formed phagosomal compartment acidifies and matures through a series of fusion and fission events into a phagolysosome. The low pH and hydrolytic enzymes in the compartment assist in killing and degrading the organism.

While TLRs recognize fungi, they are not sufficient to trigger phagocytosis. One widely used method for defining TLR agonists is to express TLRs in model cell lines such as HEK293 cells and to determine whether TLR expression is sufficient for conferring activation of NF-κB upon exposure to a model ligand. TLR2 expression in HEK293 cells is sufficient for conferring some responsiveness to the model yeast cell wall particle zymosan, but TLR2 expression is not sufficient to drive phagocytosis of the particle. Similarly, macrophages lacking TLR2, TLR4, or MyD88 internalize yeast particles normally ((Gantner et al., 2003) and personal observations), suggesting that other receptors play the main role in triggering phagocytosis.

Dectin-1 is one receptor that is sufficient to trigger phagocytosis of β-glucan-containing yeast. In fact, the receptor was originally identified by Brown and coworkers in an expression-cloning scheme designed specifically to identify macrophage receptor(s) capable of triggering phagocytosis of zymosan (Brown and Gordon, 2001). These investigators transfected the non-phagocytic cell line, NIH 3T3, with a macrophage cDNA expression library and screened for cells that gained the ability to bind/internalize fluorescently labeled yeast particles. The clone identified turned out to be Dectin-1.

For macrophages and dendritic cells Dectin-1 is the primary (although certainly not the exclusive) receptor for phagocytosis of zymosan. Investigators established nearly two decades ago that β-glucan recognition is important for macrophage phagocytosis of zymosan since it can be inhibited by the soluble β-glucan, laminarin (Janusz et al., 1986; Giaimis et al., 1993). After the cloning of Dectin-1, monoclonal (Brown et al., 2002) and polyclonal (Gantner et al., 2005) blocking antibodies were generated and shown to specifically inhibit macrophage phagocytosis of zymosan and *C. albicans* yeast. Most recently, two groups have demonstrated that macrophages from Dectin-1-deficient mice are impaired in binding and phagocytosis of zymosan and live fungi (Saijo et al., 2007; Taylor et al., 2007). It is important to note that phagocytosis of fungal cells is not completely blocked under any of these conditions. This is perhaps not too surprising since myeloid phagocytes will, given sufficient time, bind and internalize nearly any foreign particle. There are certainly receptors in addition to Dectin-1 that can bind to yeast and trigger phagocytosis, although the data strongly suggest that for β-glucan-rich yeast cell wall particles Dectin-1 is by far the most efficient phagocytic receptor. Yeast cell walls also contain large amounts of α-mannan, and it has long been established that, like soluble β-glucan, soluble mannan can suppress phagocytosis of yeast cell walls (Giaimis et al., 1993), although there is some concern that even small amounts of β-glucan in commercial mannan preparations might also inhibit Dectin-1. The mannose receptor is expressed on macrophages and dendritic cells and has been reported to be a phagocytic receptor. It is likely that receptors like the mannose receptor participate in binding and internalization of yeast particles, although their relative contributions are likely to vary with cell type and with fungal species and morphotypes.

Although we have noted that TLRs are not sufficient to trigger phagocytosis, there is considerable debate as to whether TLR signaling influences phagocytosis triggered by receptors such as Dectin-1. TLRs could influence phagocytosis by either regulating expression of proteins involved in phagocytosis, or by directly

influencing signaling during phagocytosis. There is ample evidence that TLR signaling modifies expression of genes for proteins involved in phagocytosis (Hume
et al., 2002). Expression of proteins including lysosomal hydrolases, enzymes required for reactive oxygen production, and MHC molecules are regulated by TLR
signaling. Immature dendritic cells stimulated with TLR agonists mature into fully
competent antigen-presenting cells, a process that is coupled to a decrease in phagocytic activity of the cells.

Yates and Russell directly examined whether phagocytosis triggered by receptors
for mannan and antibodies could be modified by TLR signaling (Yates and Russell,
2005). These investigators used silica beads (which are not themselves recognized
by macrophages) coated with mannan or Ig to facilitate phagocytosis through mannose receptors or Fc-receptors, respectively. Upon internalization, phagosome maturation was recorded using dynamic, real time assays: Acidification was measured by
ratiometric imaging of the fluorescein-labeled particles, and phagosome lysosome
fusion was measured using a novel method in which fluorescence resonance energy
transfer between phagosomal and lysosomal markers was recorded. These investigators found that the rate of phagocytosis and phagosome maturation was unaltered
when ligands for TLR2 or TLR4 were additionally incorporated on the beads. The
authors thus conclude that phagocytosis is not affected by co-activation of TLRs.

Using different approaches to defining the role of TLRs in regulating phagocytosis, Blander and Medzhitov have come to the opposite conclusion. Using fluores-
cent bacteria these investigators observed that compared to wild-type macrophages,
macrophages from MyD88$^{-/-}$ or TLR2/TLR4$^{-/-}$ mice internalize bacteria less
efficiently and phagosomal maturation is slower (Blander and Medzhitov, 2004).
Further, these investigators have shown that activation of TLR signaling in a phagosome promotes MHC II antigen presentation of antigens specifically found in that
phagosome; antigens found in non-TLR agonist-containing phagosomes in the same
cell are poorly presented (Blander and Medzhitov 2006). This observation argues in
favor of a specific role for TLR signaling in regulating phagosome fate.

Taken together, the above data show that there is ample reason to believe that
TLR signaling may influence phagocytosis triggered by certain receptors, but that
under other conditions TLR signaling has little or no influence. We have previously
observed that MyD88$^{-/-}$ and TLR2$^{-/-}$ macrophages have no defect in the rate
of binding and internalization of zymosan, suggesting no role for TLR signaling
in enhancing Dectin-1-mediated phagocytosis. There have been no studies to date
exploring the effect of TLR signaling on the maturation fate of Dectin-1-generated
phagosomes.

Dectin-1 triggers phagocytosis by activating tyrosine kinases. As noted earlier,
the cytoplasmic tail of Dectin-1 contains two tyrosines in an "ITAM-like" motif.
Unlike normal ITAMs, only the membrane proximal tyrosine (tyrosine-15) is required for signaling. This has been established by transfection of non-phagocytic
cells with wild-type and mutant forms of Dectin-1 and measuring the ability to
mediate phagocytosis of zymosan particles. Despite the unusual structure of the
"ITAM-like" motif, Dectin-1 signaling results in activation of Src family kinases and
Syk-like regular ITAMs. Inhibitors of Src family kinases block Dectin-1-mediated

phagocytosis in macrophages (Herre et al., 2004), although the particular Src family kinases that participate in Dectin-1-mediated phagocytosis have not been identified. The requirement for Syk is more varied. Syk inhibitors do not block phagocytosis in macrophages, and $Syk^{-/-}$ macrophages internalize zymosan normally (Herre et al., 2004; Underhill et al., 2005). However, Rogers et al. have reported that $Syk^{-/-}$ dendritic cells are deficient in zymosan phagocytosis, suggesting that Syk signaling in these cells might participate in phagocytosis (Rogers et al., 2005).

6 Production of Reactive Oxygen Species

Production of reactive oxygen species (ROS) is coupled to phagocytosis of yeast by myeloid phagocytes, and is thought to be an important mechanism for killing internalized organisms. ROS is produced by the NADPH phagocyte oxidase, a multisubunit enzyme that assembles directly on the phagosomal membrane. Patients with Chronic Granulomatous Disease (CGD) lack specific components of this enzyme due to genetic defects, and are highly susceptible to a host of bacterial and fungal infections (Lehrer and Cline, 1969; Foster et al., 1998). Similarly, mice engineered to mimic these defects are more susceptible to fungal infections than their wild-type counterparts (Aratani et al., 2002a; Aratani et al., 2002b).

Dectin-1 triggers macrophage ROS production, while TLR2 stimulation does not. We measured ROS production by $MyD88^{-/-}$ and $TLR2^{-/-}$ bone marrow-derived macrophages upon stimulation with zymosan and observed normal responses in these cells indicating that TLR signaling does not contribute to ROS production (Gantner et al., 2003). Also, activation of TLR2 or TLR4 with pure agonists failed to trigger a significant ROS response. The first clue that β-glucan recognition was particularly important for zymosan-induced ROS production came from the observation that the soluble β-glucan laminarin blocked the response and that ROS production was enhanced by overexpression of Dectin-1 in the RAW264.7 macrophage cell line (Gantner et al., 2003).

Data demonstrating that Dectin-1 is necessary for zymosan-induced ROS production now come from three laboratories. We have demonstrated that specific reduction of Dectin-1 expression by miRNA in RAW264.7 cells suppresses zymosan-stimulated ROS production (Goodridge et al., 2007). Two groups have shown that the zymosan-induced respiratory burst of macrophages is suppressed in cells from $Dectin-1^{-/-}$ mice (Saijo et al., 2007; Taylor et al., 2007), although serum-opsonization restores the activity (Taylor et al., 2007). We have also demonstrated that Dectin-1 signaling is sufficient to drive ROS production in macrophages: When Dectin-1 is tagged with an extracellular streptavidin-binding protein (SBP) tag, cross linking of the receptor with streptavidin-coated beads specifically triggers ROS production (Underhill et al., 2005).

While it is clear that Dectin-1 is capable of triggering phagocytosis and ROS production, the specific role of Dectin-1 in the net ROS response of macrophages and neutrophils to live fungal pathogens is still being established. We have observed that *C. albicans* yeast (which are recognized by Dectin-1) trigger ROS production from mouse bone marrow-derived macrophages, while filaments (which are not recognized by Dectin-1) do not (Gantner et al., 2005). Further, we observed that soluble β-glucan and blocking Dectin-1 antibodies inhibited macrophage ROS production in response to yeast. Taylor et al. have argued that this apparent role for Dectin-1 in ROS production is largely an effect of the role of Dectin-1 in promoting binding of yeast to macrophages, and that while Dectin-1 may trigger ROS production, other receptors are sufficient to trigger the response in the absence of Dectin-1 (Taylor et al., 2007). On the other end of the spectrum, Saijo et al. have suggested that Dectin-1 is not required at all for ROS responses to *C. albicans* (Saijo et al., 2007). These heterogeneous reports are likely due to a combination of researchers' use of different cells (bone marrow-derived macrophages, thioglycolate-elicited peritoneal macrophages, and alveolar macrophages) and possibly differing methods of measuring ROS production (luminol vs. dihidrorhodamine 123). Dectin-1 has also been implicated in macrophage ROS production in response to *A. fumigatus* (Gersuk et al., 2006) and *P. carinii* (Saijo et al., 2007). In the case of *A. fumigatus*, Dectin-1 appears to play a partial role in the respiratory burst, suggesting that, as for *Candida*, other receptors may additionally recognize the fungus and trigger ROS production. In the case of *P. carinii*, at least for alveolar macrophages, the role for Dectin-1 in triggering ROS appears dominant, since the response is completely lost in Dectin-1$^{-/-}$ cells.

Triggering of ROS production by Dectin-1 requires Src family kinases and Syk. We have demonstrated that ROS production triggered by zymosan in bone marrow-derived macrophages and by specific Dectin-1 cross linking on RAW264.7 cells is inhibited by pharmacological inhibitors of Src and Syk family kinases (Underhill et al., 2005). Further, ROS production in response to zymosan is completely abolished in bone marrow-derived macrophages from Syk$^{-/-}$ mice. Curiously, when we directly measured activation of Syk by tyrosine phosphorylation, we observed that although all cells in a population express Dectin-1, only a subset of these show strong Syk activation (Underhill et al., 2005). Consistent with a requirement for Syk in ROS production, only a subset of the cells (presumably the same cells) produces ROS upon Dectin-1 ligation. We demonstrated that this subset is not a stable, clonable phenotype, but rather each cell is sometimes prepared to activate this pathway and at other times is not. Treatment with specific cytokines could alter the frequency of cells activating Syk downstream of Dectin-1. The ability to active Syk was not simply dependent on cell cycle, as the same observations were made in peritoneal macrophages which do not undergo cell division in culture (Underhill et al., 2005). These observations raise the possibility that cell-to-cell variability in inflammatory response to Dectin-1 activation (or activation of other innate immune receptors) may be an important regulator of the net inflammatory response to infection.

Is there a role for TLR/Dectin-1 collaboration in triggering ROS production? Although TLR signaling triggers little or no ROS production in macrophages on its own, it has long been known that LPS can prime macrophages for an enhanced respiratory burst (Pabst and Johnston, 1980). We have demonstrated that TLR2 activation primes macrophages for an enhanced Dectin-1-stimulated respiratory burst (Gantner et al., 2003). In these cases, TLR signaling must precede phagocytosis and the effect requires new protein synthesis, indicating that TLR signaling up-regulates the cells' capacity to produce ROS. Thus, although there is no evidence for TLR/Dectin-1 signaling cooperativity in triggering ROS production, the TLR-driven transcriptional response enhances ROS production.

7 The Role of TLR2 and Dectin-1 in Production of Inflammatory Mediators

Macrophages and dendritic cells produce a variety of proinflammatory cytokines and chemokines, including TNF-α, IL-6, IL-12, and MIP-2, following exposure to zymosan or live fungi, and both TLRs and Dectin-1 are implicated in their induction. That cytokines and chemokines are produced in responses to TLR2 agonists is well-established, while the role of β-glucan recognition has been less clear.

Wheeler and Fink demonstrated enhanced TNF-α production by macrophages stimulated with *C. albicans* yeast in the presence of the antifungal drug caspofungin, which unmasks β-glucans buried beneath the surface of the fungal cell wall (Wheeler and Fink, 2006). They also observed enhanced TNF-α production in response to "unmasked" *S. cerevisiae* and *C. albicans* mutants that have elevated β-glucan exposure at their surface. Similarly, β-glucan recognition has been implicated in cytokine and chemokine induction by *P. carinii* (Hoffman et al., 1993; Vassallo et al., 2000; Steele et al., 2003). Treatment of a *P. carinii* cell wall isolate with zymolase, which predominantly exhibits β-glucanase activity, significantly compromised its ability to trigger TNF-α release by alveolar macrophages (Vassallo et al., 2000). Furthermore, TNF-α production was suppressed by treatment with soluble β-glucans, but not mannan (Hoffman et al., 1993; Vassallo et al., 2000).

The first evidence for collaboration between TLR2 and Dectin-1 in coordinating inflammatory gene induction came from studies with zymosan. TNF-α and IL-12 induction by zymosan is severely compromised in TLR2$^{-/-}$ and MyD88$^{-/-}$ macrophages, indicating a key role for TLR2 signals in the induction of these proinflammatory cytokines (Gantner et al., 2003). Further, overexpression of Dectin-1 in RAW264.7 macrophages enhances TNF-α and IL-12 p40 production following stimulation with zymosan, but not pure TLR2 agonists, indicating that Dectin-1 specifically enhances these responses (Brown et al., 2003; Gantner et al., 2003). The contribution of Dectin-1 to proinflammatory signaling was confirmed by Brown and colleagues who demonstrated that TNF-α induction by zymosan or *C. albicans* is strongly reduced in macrophages from Dectin-1$^{-/-}$ compared to wild-type macrophages (Taylor et al., 2007). Importantly, TNF-α induction by complement-opsonized zymosan or yeast was also defective in Dectin-1$^{-/-}$ macrophages, despite efficient binding of these particles by complement receptors on the cell surface (Taylor et al., 2007). These data indicate that Dectin-1 signals regulate TNF-α gene induction.

Dectin-1 and TLR2 signals have also been reported to contribute to cytokine induction by *A. fumigatus* conidia (Hohl et al., 2005; Steele et al., 2005;

Gersuk et al., 2006). TNF-α induction by *Aspergillus* germ tubes can be blocked by treatment with a Dectin-1-specific antibody, soluble β-glucan or soluble Dectin-1. TNF-α induction by germ tubes is also suppressed in macrophages from TLR2- or MyD88-deficient mice, and virtually abolished by addition of Dectin-1 antibodies to TLR2- or MyD88-deficient macrophages (Gersuk et al., 2006). Dectin-1 activation has also been implicated in the induction of a variety of other cytokines, chemokines, and growth factors by *A. fumigatus* including MIP-1α, MIP-2, IL-1α, IL-6, G-CSF, and GM-CSF; TLR2 signaling does not appear to be necessary for the induction of these mediators (Steele et al., 2005), although another report suggested MyD88 signals can play a role in the induction of MIP-2 (Hohl et al., 2005). These variations may arise from differing thresholds for activation of each of these cytokines and chemokines, or to different types of macrophages and dendritic cells examined.

A similar role has been described for Dectin-1 in controlling macrophage inflammatory cytokine production in response to *P. carinii*. Steele et al. reported that *P. carinii*-induced MIP-2 production by alveolar macrophages is blocked by an anti-Dectin-1 antibody, and overexpression of Dectin-1 in RAW264.7 macrophages enhanced MIP-2 induction (Steele et al., 2003). However, these investigators did not determine the contribution of TLRs to these responses. In contrast to these findings, Saijo et al. have reported that there is no defect in TNF-α or IL-12 induction in *P. carinii*-stimulated Dectin-1$^{-/-}$ alveolar macrophages, although induction of these cytokines by pure β-glucan was dependent on Dectin-1 (Saijo et al., 2007). The different findings by the two reports may stem from the different cytokines examined, or differences in strains or preparations of *P. carinii*.

Taken together the above data demonstrate that TLR2 and Dectin-1 can collaborate to induce inflammatory gene induction, and that in certain circumstances Dectin-1 signaling may be sufficient to drive these responses. Compared to TLR4, TLR2 is a relatively weak inducer of proinflammatory cytokine production (Hirschfeld et al., 2001). For example, dendritic cells stimulated with TLR2 ligands produce low levels of IL-12 and IFN-γ, thus promoting the development of Th2, rather than Th1, responses (Re and Strominger, 2001). Analysis of the transcriptional responses of macrophages and dendritic cells to fungi has revealed collaboration between TLR2 and Dectin-1 signaling to amplify the TLR2 response and promote the induction of proinflammatory cytokines.

While TLR2-MyD88 signals are sufficient to induce modest proinflammatory cytokine production by macrophages, Dectin-1 signaling alone is not. Boiling zymosan in alkali (depleted zymosan) destroys its ability to trigger TLR signaling but does not affect its recognition by Dectin-1; depleted zymosan is internalized normally, triggers Dectin-1 phosphorylation, and induces robust ROS production, but fails to induce NF-κB activation and cytokine induction by macrophages (Gantner et al., 2003; Underhill et al., 2005). To investigate the ability of Dectin-1 signals to collaborate with TLR2 signals to promote cytokine induction, we stably expressed Dectin-1 in RAW264.7 cells and stimulated them with depleted zymosan and the pure TLR2 agonist Pam₃CSK₄ (Gantner et al., 2003). While treatment with depleted zymosan or Pam₃CSK₄ alone induced little or no IL-12 p40, we observed strong synergy when the two receptors were co-expressed and co-ligated by treating the cells with both agonists. These findings are supported by data from Dectin-1-deficient mice: Dectin-1$^{-/-}$ macrophages show impaired zymosan-induced TNF-α and IL-12 (Taylor et al., 2007). However bone marrow-derived dendritic cells from Dectin-1 deficient mice show little defect in TNF-α and IL-12 induction, although activation of IL-10 is affected (Saijo et al., 2007; Taylor et al., 2007). Macrophages appear to respond more readily to TLR2 stimulation than dendritic cells, and some reports suggest that activation of macrophages by zymosan is more dependent on TLR signaling and does not significantly involve Dectin-1 (Saijo et al., 2007). These findings are likely due to significant variability in the TLR stimulatory activity found in different preparations of zymosan. For TLR-induced cytokines such as TNF-α, the collaborative effect of Dectin-1 activation is most apparent at lower doses of TLR stimulation.

Dendritic cells have also been reported to produce IL-2 and the anti-inflammatory cytokine IL-10 following zymosan stimulation, and Dectin-1 is clearly required (Rogers et al., 2005; Dillon et al., 2006; Goodridge et al., 2007). Zymosan-induced IL-10 production by human monocyte-derived dendritic cells can be blocked by laminarin (Dillon et al., 2006), and IL-10 production by bone marrow-derived dendritic cells from Dectin-1$^{-/-}$ mice is reduced compared to wild-type dendritic cells (Saijo et al., 2007). Reis e Sousa and colleagues reported that stable expression of wild-type, but not truncated, Dectin-1 in a murine B cell hybridoma (LK35.2 cells) was sufficient to enable these cells to produce IL-2 and IL-10 in response to zymosan stimulation, and this response was inhibited by soluble glucan phosphate (Rogers et al., 2005). Expression of Dectin-1 mutants in LK35.2 cells revealed a critical role for the membrane-proximal tyrosine of the ITAM-like motif, but not the membrane-distal tyrosine, in the induction of IL-2 and IL-10, and Dectin-1 signals are probably transduced by Syk because induction of these cytokines is defective in dendritic cells from Syk$^{-/-}$ mice. However, it is not clear from this study whether Dectin-1 signaling is sufficient for the induction of these cytokines or whether endogenous TLR2 expression by the LK35.2 cells contributes to their induction.

TLR signaling is required for zymosan-induced IL-2 production since it is suppressed in dendritic cells from TLR2- or MyD88-deficient mice (Rogers et al., 2005; Goodridge et al., 2007), but the contribution of TLR2-MyD88 signals to the induction of IL-10 by zymosan is more controversial. Several studies have reported normal levels of IL-10 production by bone marrow-derived dendritic cells from MyD88-deficient mice (Rogers et al., 2005; Gross et al., 2006; Saijo et al., 2007). However, we and others have observed reduced zymosan-stimulated IL-10 production by bone marrow-derived dendritic cells from TLR2- and MyD88-deficient mice (Goodridge et al., 2007) and from TLR2-deficient splenic dendritic cells (Dillon et al., 2006).

Production of inflammatory lipid mediators is also a consequence of macrophage activation by zymosan and fungi. For example, zymosan stimulation triggers cPLA$_2$-mediated release of arachidonic acid, which is metabolized to generate eicosanoids including prostaglandins, prostanoids (prostacyclins and thromboxane), and leukotrienes. Arachidonic acid release and eicosanoid production by macrophages is observed within 30 minutes of intraperitoneal injection of mice with zymosan (Lundy et al., 1990). Leukotriene generation is catalyzed by 5-lipoxygenase, while inducible cyclooxygenase (Cox-2) is required for prostaglandin and prostanoid production. TLR2 and Dectin-1 collaborate in triggering Cox-2 synthesis and arachidonic acid release (Suram et al., 2006; Goodridge et al., 2007). Zymosan or *C. albicans*-triggered Cox-2 production and arachidonic acid release is suppressed by soluble β-glucan, and enhanced by overexpression of wild-type but not truncated Dectin-1 in RAW264.7 macrophages (Suram et al., 2006; Goodridge et al., 2007). Furthermore, TLR2 agonists, which induce only very low arachidonic acid release, enhance Dectin-1-triggered arachidonic acid release by particulate β-glucan in peritoneal macrophages (Suram et al., 2006). Zymosan and *C. albicans* trigger Cox-2 synthesis by macrophages from TLR2$^{-/-}$ or MyD88$^{-/-}$ mice, albeit at much lower levels than wild-type macrophages (Suram et al., 2006; Goodridge et al., 2007), and particulate β-glucan triggers robust Cox-2 production and prostaglandin generation (Suram et al., 2006), indicating that Dectin-1 signals are sufficient to induce Cox-2.

8 Stimulation of Transcription Factors by Dectin-1 and TLR2

That TLR2 and Dectin-1 induce production of a host of inflammatory mediators indicates that signaling by these receptors activates transcription factors. NF-κB is a key transcription factor regulating production of many cytokines and chemokines, and TLR-mediated activation of NF-κB is well-established. To assess the collaboration of TLR2 and Dectin-1 signaling in regulating the activation of NF-κB-driven transcription, we transiently transfected HEK293 cells, which do not normally respond to TLR2 ligands, with TLR2 and/or Dectin-1 and measured activity of an ELAM-luciferase reporter. HEK293 cells transfected with TLR2 alone responded poorly to zymosan stimulation, while Dectin-1 transfection alone was not sufficient for induction of ELAM-luciferase reporter activity (Gantner et al., 2003). This is consistent with the finding that β-glucan particles lacking TLR stimulatory activity fail to activate NF-κB in macrophages (Gantner et al., 2003; Underhill 2003). However, co-transfection of HEK293 cells with wild-type Dectin-1, but not signaling-deficient forms of the receptor, enhanced the TLR2 response. Hence Dectin-1 signals appear to collaborate with TLR2 to induce NF-κB activation.

A recent study suggested that Dectin-1 signals can activate NF-κB directly in dendritic cells via the caspase recruitment domain (CARD)-containing adapter CARD9 (Gross et al., 2006) (Figure 4). Bone marrow-derived dendritic cells from CARD9-deficient mice exhibited defective cytokine responses (TNF-α, IL-6, IL-2) to zymosan and *C. albicans*, but not to other TLR ligands, and NF-κB activation was reduced in CARD9$^{-/-}$ cells. The authors also demonstrated that NF-κB activation could be induced by expressing CARD9 along with Bcl10 in HEK293 cells, and that zymosan stimulation enhanced NF-κB activation when Dectin-1 was co-expressed with CARD9 and its CARD domain-interacting partner Bcl10. Furthermore, dendritic cells from mice lacking either Bcl10 or Malt1, which is involved

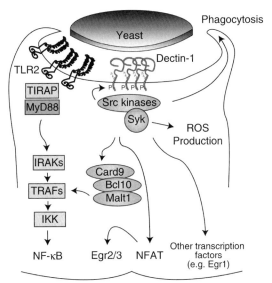

Fig. 4 Signal transduction by TLR2 and Dectin-1. Fungal cell wall particles are recognized by TLRs and Dectin-1 which each signal independently. TLR2 signals to NF-κB via the signaling adaptor molecules TIRAP/Mal and MyD88. These adaptors activate the IKK complex through IRAKs and TRAF. Dectin-1 activates Src and Syk kinases, and triggers phagocytosis and production of reactive oxygen species. In addition, Dectin-1 may activate NF-κB through a signaling complex including CARD9, Bcl10 and MALT1. Dectin-1 also triggers activation of NFAT and other transcription factors. Together, these responses define the net output of inflammatory cytokines and chemokines

in Bcl10-mediated NF-κB activation in lymphocytes, had defective cytokine responses to zymosan. These data suggest that in dendritic cells Dectin-1 can activate NF-κB via CARD9 coupled to Bcl10 and Malt1, although it is unclear whether Dectin 1-CARD9-mediated NF-κB activation is itself sufficient to induce a transcriptional response in the absence of signals from other receptors such as TLRs. Also, it is not yet clear that Dectin-1 is the most relevant CARD9-activating zymosan receptor expressed on dendritic cells. Taylor et al. and Saijo et al. observed minimal defects in zymosan-induced TNF-α and IL-12 induction in dendritic cells from Dectin-1$^{-/-}$ mice, even though macrophage responses were affected (Saijo et al., 2007; Taylor et al., 2007). These data may suggest that another receptor on dendritic cells is key for activating signaling through CARD9.

We recently demonstrated using microarrays that zymosan can trigger a robust transcriptional response in the absence of TLR2 signaling (Goodridge et al., 2007). Among the TLR-independent genes induced in macrophages and dendritic cells by zymosan or *C. albicans* yeast are three members of the Egr family of transcription factors (Egr1, Egr2, and Egr3). Egr gene induction was suppressed in RAW264.7 cells expressing either a Dectin-1 mutant that lacks the intracellular tail

(Dectin-1Δ38) or an miRNA-specific for Dectin-1, demonstrating that Dectin-1 is necessary for Egr induction. We also showed that Dectin-1 signals are sufficient for Egr induction by crosslinking SBP-tagged Dectin-1 with streptavidin beads. Hence, Dectin-1 signals alone are sufficient to induce a transcriptional response.

Furthermore, we demonstrated that Dectin-1 signals, but not TLR2 signals, trigger activation of nuclear factor of activated T cells (NFAT) transcription factors, which are classically associated with adaptive immune responses (TCR, BCR, and FcR ITAM signaling) and not innate antimicrobial responses (Goodridge et al., 2007). Zymosan and depleted zymosan, but not the pure TLR2 agonist Pam_3CSK_4, triggered activity of an NFAT-luciferase reporter in RAW264.7 macrophages expressing wild-type Dectin-1, but not the truncated Dectin-1Δ38 mutant, and we also observed NFAT activation in bone marrow-derived macrophages from NFAT-luciferase reporter transgenic mice. Furthermore, consistent with our previous study describing recognition of *C. albicans* by Dectin-1, we observed NFAT activation in response to exposure to *C. albicans* yeast but not hyphae.

Using the inhibitor cyclosporin A, which blocks NFAT activation by the phosphatase calcineurin, and a specific peptide inhibitor of NFAT activation, 11R-VIVIT, we demonstrated that Dectin-1-triggered Egr2 and Egr3 induction is, at least in part, mediated by NFAT. The role of transcriptional regulation by the Egrs in the antifungal response of myeloid cells is currently unclear. However, NFAT signals also appear to be responsible for the Dectin-1-mediated collaboration with TLR2 signals to promote Cox-2 induction, and consequently prostaglandin E_2 release, by zymosan-stimulated macrophages, as well as the production of IL-2, IL-10, and IL-12 p70 by zymosan-stimulated dendritic cells.

9 TLR2 and Dectin-1 During *In vivo* Fungal Infection

If, as we have discussed above, TLR2 and Dectin-1 collaborate to regulate the inflammatory response of phagocytes to fungi, what is the consequence of this collaboration? This question is best addressed experimentally by examination of *in vivo* mouse models of infection. There are numerous examples to date demonstrating a specific role for TLR2 in immune defense against *Candida* (Bellocchio et al., 2004; Netea et al., 2004a; Villamon et al., 2004), *Aspergillus* (Balloy et al., 2005), *Cryptococcus* (Yauch et al., 2004; Biondo et al., 2005), and *Pneumocystis* (Zhang et al., 2006). The reader is referred to several recent reviews focusing specifically on TLRs and fungal infections (Netea et al., 2004b; Romani, 2004; Netea et al., 2006).

The role of Dectin-1 during *in vivo* infection is less established. To date, three studies have directly explored the contribution of Dectin-1 to *in vivo* infection with pathogenic fungi. Steele et al. demonstrated that inflammatory responses to intratracheal infection with *A. fumigatus* conidia were significantly reduced if a soluble form of Dectin-1 was included during the infection to block β-glucan binding sites. Soluble Dectin-1 reduced cytokine and chemokine production induced by the infection and suppressed recruitment of inflammatory cells to the lung (Steele et al., 2005). Two groups have independently generated Dectin-1-deficient mice in order to evaluate the contribution of Dectin-1 to antifungal responses (Saijo et al., 2007; Taylor et al., 2007). Brown and colleagues found that Dectin-1$^{-/-}$ mice are markedly more susceptible to *C. albicans* infection than wild-type mice, displaying significantly enhanced fungal colonization of the kidneys, stomach, and intestinal tissues (Taylor et al., 2007). Furthermore, inflammatory cell recruitment (neutrophils, monocytes, and eosinophils) and macrophage activation in response to intraperitoneal injection of *C. albicans* were reduced in Dectin-1-deficient mice. In the other study, Iwakura and colleagues observed that Dectin-1-deficient mice are significantly more susceptible to infection with *P. carinii* (Saijo et al., 2007). In contrast to the study by Taylor et al., these investigators found no role for Dectin-1 during infection with *C. albicans*. This difference may be due to the different genetic backgrounds of the subjects used for the knockouts, or to different strains of *C. albicans* used, or to differing methods for preparing the yeast for infection. Nonetheless, the data confirm a role for Dectin-1 during *in vivo* infection with fungi. To date there are no studies specifically examining the in vivo role of Dectin-1 and TLR2 collaboration during infection. These studies will require comparing phenotypes of TLR2$^{-/-}$, Dectin-1$^{-/-}$, and double knockout mice.

10 Concluding Remarks

TLR2 and Dectin-1 both recognize a variety of pathogenic fungi and together coordinate effective innate immune responses. The functional relationships between these receptors offer a useful model for examining how receptor collaboration can help to shape inflammatory responses. Certainly additional receptors participate in recognition of fungi and play important (perhaps even critical) roles in orchestrating effective innate immune responses. In the coming years it will be crucial to expand our understanding of how additional innate immune receptors influence signaling and inflammation triggered by TLRs and Dectin-1.

References

Aratani Y, Kura F, Watanabe H, Akagawa H, Takano Y, Suzuki K, Dinauer MC, Maeda N, Koyama H (2002a) Critical role of myeloperoxidase and nicotinamide adenine dinucleotide phosphate-oxidase in high-burden systemic infection of mice with *Candida albicans*. J Infect Dis 185: 1833–1837

Aratani Y, Kura F, Watanabe H, Akagawa H, Takano Y, Suzuki K, Dinauer MC, Maeda N, Koyama H (2002b) Relative contributions of myeloperoxidase and NADPH-oxidase to the early host defense against pulmonary infections with *Candida albicans* and *Aspergillus fumigatus*. Med Mycol 40: 557–563

Ariizumi K, Shen GL, Shikano S, Xu S, Ritter R, 3rd, Kumamoto T, Edelbaum D, Morita A, Bergstresser PR, Takashima A (2000) Identification of a novel, dendritic cell-associated molecule, Dectin-1, by subtractive cDNA cloning. J Biol Chem 275: 20157–20167

Balloy V, Si-Tahar M, Takeuchi O, Philippe B, Nahori MA, Tanguy M, Huerre M, Akira S, Latge JP, Chignard M (2005) Involvement of Toll-like receptor 2 in experimental invasive pulmonary aspergillosis. Infect Immun 73: 5420–5425

Barrow AD, Trowsdale J (2006) You say ITAM and I say ITIM, let's call the whole thing off: The ambiguity of immunoreceptor signalling. Eur J Immunol 36: 1646–1653

Bellocchio S, Montagnoli C, Bozza S, Gaziano R, Rossi G, Mambula SS, Vecchi A, Mantovani A, Levitz SM, Romani L (2004) The contribution of the Toll-like/IL-1 receptor superfamily to innate and adaptive immunity to fungal pathogens *in vivo*. J Immunol 172: 3059–3069

Biondo C, Midiri A, Messina L, Tomasello F, Garufi G, Catania MR, Bombaci M, Beninati C, Teti G, Mancuso G (2005) MyD88 and TLR2, but not TLR4, are required for host defense against *Cryptococcus neoformans*. Eur J Immunol 35: 870–878

Blander JM, Medzhitov R (2004) Regulation of phagosome maturation by signals from Toll-like receptors. Science 304: 1014–1018

Blander JM, Medzhitov R (2006) Toll-dependent selection of microbial antigens for presentation by dendritic cells. Nature 440: 808–812

Brown GD, Gordon S (2001) Immune recognition. A new receptor for beta-glucans. Nature 413: 36–37

Brown GD, Herre J, Williams DL, Willment JA, Marshall AS, Gordon S (2003) Dectin-1 mediates the biological effects of beta-glucans. J Exp Med 197: 1119–1124

Brown GD, Taylor PR, Reid DM, Willment JA, Williams DL, Martinez-Pomares L, Wong SY, Gordon S (2002) Dectin-1 is a major beta-glucan receptor on macrophages. J Exp Med 196: 407–412

Buchanan KL, Murphy JW (1998) What makes *Cryptococcus neoformans* a pathogen? Emerg Infect Dis 4: 71–83

Calderone RA, Fonzi WA (2001) Virulence factors of *Candida albicans*. Trends Microbiol 9: 327–335

Campos MA, Almeida IC, Takeuchi O, Akira S, Valente EP, Procopio DO, Travassos LR, Smith JA, Golenbock DT, Gazzinelli RT (2001) Activation of Toll-like receptor-2 by glycosylphosphatidylinositol anchors from a protozoan parasite. J Immunol 167: 416–423

Dillon S, Agrawal S, Banerjee K, Letterio J, Denning TL, Oswald-Richter K, Kasprowicz DJ, Kellar K, Pare J, van Dyke T, Ziegler S, Unutmaz D, Pulendran B (2006) Yeast zymosan, a stimulus for TLR2 and Dectin-1, induces regulatory antigen-presenting cells and immunological tolerance. J Clin Invest 116: 916–928

Fodor S, Jakus Z, Mocsai A (2006) ITAM-based signaling beyond the adaptive immune response. Immunol Lett 104: 29–37

Foster CB, Lehrnbecher T, Mol F, Steinberg SM, Venzon DJ, Walsh TJ, Noack D, Rae J, Winkelstein JA, Curnutte JT, Chanock SJ (1998) Host defense molecule polymorphisms influence the risk for immune-mediated complications in chronic granulomatous disease. J Clin Invest 102: 2146–2155

Gantner BN, Simmons RM, Canavera SJ, Akira S, Underhill DM (2003) Collaborative induction of inflammatory responses by Dectin-1 and Toll-like receptor 2. J Exp Med 197: 1107–1117

Gantner BN, Simmons RM, Underhill DM (2005) Dectin-1 mediates macrophage recognition of *Candida albicans* yeast but not filaments. EMBO J 24: 1277–1286

Gersuk GM, Underhill DM, Zhu L, Marr KA (2006) Dectin-1 and TLRs permit macrophages to distinguish between different *Aspergillus fumigatus* cellular states. J Immunol 176: 3717–3724

Giaimis J, Lombard Y, Fonteneau P, Muller CD, Levy R, Makaya-Kumba M, Lazdins J, Poindron P (1993) Both mannose and beta-glucan receptors are involved in phagocytosis of unopsonized, heat-killed *Saccharomyces cerevisiae* by murine macrophages. J Leukoc Biol 54: 564–571

Goodridge H, Simmons R, Underhill DM (2007) Dectin-1 stimulation by *Candida albicans* yeast or zymosan triggers nuclear factor of activated T cells (NFAT) activation in macrophages and dendritic cells. J Immunol (in press)

Gross O, Gewies A, Finger K, Schafer M, Sparwasser T, Peschel C, Forster I, Ruland J (2006) Card9 controls a non-TLR signalling pathway for innate anti-fungal immunity. Nature 442: 651–656

Heinsbroek SE, Taylor PR, Rosas M, Willment JA, Williams DL, Gordon S, Brown GD (2006) Expression of functionally different Dectin-1 isoforms by murine macrophages. J Immunol 176: 5513–5518

Herre J, Marshall AS, Caron E, Edwards AD, Williams DL, Schweighoffer E, Tybulewicz V, Reis e Sousa C, Gordon S, Brown GD (2004) Dectin-1 uses novel mechanisms for yeast phagocytosis in macrophages. Blood 104: 4038–4045

Hirschfeld M, Weis JJ, Toshchakov V, Salkowski CA, Cody MJ, Ward DC, Qureshi N, Michalek SM, Vogel SN (2001) Signaling by Toll-like receptor 2 and 4 agonists results in differential gene expression in murine macrophages. Infect Immun 69: 1477–1482

Hoffman OA, Standing JE, Limper AH (1993) Pneumocystis carinii stimulates tumor necrosis factor-alpha release from alveolar macrophages through a beta-glucan-mediated mechanism. J Immunol 150: 3932–3940

Hohl TM, Van Epps HL, Rivera A, Morgan LA, Chen PL, Feldmesser M, Pamer EG (2005) *Aspergillus fumigatus* triggers inflammatory responses by stage-specific beta-glucan display. PLoS Pathog 1: e30

Hume DA, Ross IL, Himes SR, Sasmono RT, Wells CA, Ravasi T (2002) The mononuclear phagocyte system revisited. J Leukoc Biol 72: 621–627

Janusz MJ, Austen KF, Czop JK (1986) Isolation of soluble yeast beta-glucans that inhibit human monocyte phagocytosis mediated by beta-glucan receptors. J Immunol 137: 3270–3276

Jouault T, Ibata-Ombetta S, Takeuchi O, Trinel PA, Sacchetti P, Lefebvre P, Akira S, Poulain D (2003) *Candida albicans* phospholipomannan is sensed through Toll-like receptors. J Infect Dis 188: 165–172

Kato Y, Adachi Y, Ohno N (2006) Contribution of N-linked oligosaccharides to the expression and functions of beta-glucan receptor, Dectin-1. Biol Pharm Bull 29: 1580–1586

Kollar R, Reinhold BB, Petrakova E, Yeh HJ, Ashwell G, Drgonova J, Kapteyn JC, Klis FM, Cabib E (1997). Architecture of the yeast cell wall. Beta $(1->6)$-glucan interconnects mannoprotein, beta$(1->)$3-glucan, and chitin. J Biol Chem 272: 17762–17775

Lehrer RI, Cline MJ (1969) Leukocyte myeloperoxidase deficiency and disseminated candidiasis: The role of myeloperoxidase in resistance to Candida infection. J Clin Invest 48: 1478–1488

Lemaitre B, Nicolas E, Michaut L, Reichhart JM, Hoffmann JA (1996) The dorsoventral regulatory gene cassette Spätzle/Toll/Cactus controls the potent antifungal response in *Drosophila* adults. Cell 86: 973–983

Lo HJ, Kohler JR, DiDomenico B, Loebenberg D, Cacciapuoti A, Fink GR (1997) Nonfilamentous *C. albicans* mutants are avirulent. Cell 90: 939–949

Lundy SR, Dowling RL, Stevens TM, Kerr JS, Mackin WM, Gans KR (1990) Kinetics of phospholipase A2, arachidonic acid, and eicosanoid appearance in mouse zymosan peritonitis. J Immunol 144: 2671–2677

Marr KA, Patterson T, Denning D (2002) Aspergillosis. Pathogenesis, clinical manifestations, and therapy. Infect Dis Clin North Am 16: 875–894, vi

Medzhitov R, Preston-Hurlburt P, Janeway CA, Jr. (1997) A human homologue of the Drosophila Toll protein signals activation of adaptive immunity. Nature 388: 394–397

Meier A, Kirschning CJ, Nikolaus T, Wagner H, Heesemann J, Ebel F (2003) Toll-like receptor (TLR) 2 and TLR4 are essential for *Aspergillus*-induced activation of murine macrophages. Cell Microbiol 5: 561–570

Netea MG, Sutmuller R, Hermann C, Van der Graaf CA, Van der Meer JW, van Krieken JH, Hartung T, Adema G, Kullberg BJ (2004a) Toll-like receptor 2 suppresses immunity against *Candida albicans* through induction of IL-10 and regulatory T cells. J Immunol 172: 3712–3718

Netea MG, Van der Graaf C, Van der Meer JW, Kullberg BJ (2004b) Recognition of fungal pathogens by Toll-like receptors. Eur J Clin Microbiol Infect Dis 23: 672–676

Netea MG, Van Der Graaf CA, Vonk AG, Verschueren I, Van Der Meer JW, Kullberg BJ (2002) The role of Toll-like receptor (TLR) 2 and TLR4 in the host defense against disseminated candidiasis. J Infect Dis 185: 1483–1489

Netea MG, Van der Meer JW, Kullberg BJ (2006) Role of the dual interaction of fungal pathogens with pattern recognition receptors in the activation and modulation of host defence. Clin Microbiol Infect 12: 404–409

Netea MG, Warris A, Van der Meer JW, Fenton MJ, Verver-Janssen TJ, Jacobs LE, Andresen T, Verweij PE, Kullberg BJ (2003) *Aspergillus fumigatus* evades immune recognition during germination through loss of Toll-like receptor-4-mediated signal transduction. J Infect Dis 188: 320–326

Opitz B, Schroder NW, Spreitzer I, Michelsen KS, Kirschning CJ, Hallatschek W, Zahringer U, Hartung T, Gobel UB, Schumann RR (2001) Toll-like receptor-2 mediates Treponema glycolipid and lipoteichoic acid-induced NF-kappaB translocation. J Biol Chem 276: 22041–22047

Osumi M (1998) The ultrastructure of yeast: Cell wall structure and formation. Micron 29: 207–233

Ozinsky A, Underhill DM, Fontenot JD, Hajjar AM, Smith KD, Wilson CB, Schroeder L, Aderem A (2000) The repertoire for pattern recognition of pathogens by the innate immune system is defined by cooperation between Toll-like receptors. Proc Natl Acad Sci USA 97: 13766–13771

Pabst MJ, Johnston RB, Jr. (1980) Increased production of superoxide anion by macrophages exposed in vitro to muramyl dipeptide or lipopolysaccharide. J Exp Med 151: 101–114

Palma AS, Feizi T, Zhang Y, SToll MS, Lawson AM, Diaz-Rodriguez E, Campanero-Rhodes MA, Costa J, Gordon S, Brown GD, Chai W (2006) Ligands for the beta-glucan receptor, Dectin-1, assigned using "designer" microarrays of oligosaccharide probes (neoglycolipids) generated from glucan polysaccharides. J Biol Chem 281: 5771–5779

Re F, Strominger JL (2001) Toll-like receptor 2 (TLR2) and TLR4 differentially activate human dendritic cells. J Biol Chem 276: 37692–37699

Rogers NC, Slack EC, Edwards AD, Nolte MA, Schulz O, Schweighoffer E, Williams DL, Gordon S, Tybulewicz VL, Brown GD, Reis e Sousa C (2005) Syk-dependent cytokine induction by Dectin-1 reveals a novel pattern recognition pathway for C type lectins. Immunity 22: 507–517

Romani L (2004) Immunity to fungal infections. Nat Rev Immunol 4: 1–23

Saijo S, Fujikado N, Furuta T, Chung SH, Kotaki H, Seki K, Sudo K, Akira S, Adachi Y, Ohno N, Kinjo T, Nakamura K, Kawakami K, Iwakura Y (2007) Dectin-1 is required for host defense against *Pneumocystis carinii* but not against *Candida albicans*. Nat Immunol 8: 39–46

Saville SP, Lazzell AL, Monteagudo C, Lopez-Ribot JL (2003) Engineered control of cell morphology in vivo reveals distinct roles for yeast and filamentous forms of *Candida albicans* during infection. Eukaryot Cell 2: 1053–1060

Steele C, Marrero L, Swain S, Harmsen AG, Zheng M, Brown GD, Gordon S, Shellito JE, Kolls JK (2003) Alveolar macrophage-mediated killing of *Pneumocystis carinii f. sp. muris* involves molecular recognition by the Dectin-1 beta-glucan receptor. J Exp Med 198: 1677–1688

Steele C, Rapaka RR, Metz A, Pop SM, Williams DL, Gordon S, Kolls JK, Brown GD (2005) The beta-glucan receptor Dectin-1 recognizes specific morphologies of *Aspergillus fumigatus*. PLoS Pathog 1: e42

Suram S, Brown GD, Ghosh M, Gordon S, Loper R, Taylor PR, Akira S, Uematsu S, Williams DL, Leslie CC (2006) Regulation of cytosolic phospholipase A2 activation and cyclooxygenase 2 expression in macrophages by the beta-glucan receptor. J Biol Chem 281: 5506–5514

Taylor PR, Brown GD, Reid DM, Willment JA, Martinez-Pomares L, Gordon S, Wong SY (2002) The beta-glucan receptor, Dectin-1, is predominantly expressed on the surface of cells of the monocyte/macrophage and neutrophil lineages. J Immunol 169: 3876–3882

Taylor PR, Martinez-Pomares L, Stacey M, Lin HH, Brown GD, Gordon S (2005) Macrophage receptors and immune recognition. Annu Rev Immunol 23: 901–944

Taylor PR, Tsoni SV, Willment JA, Dennehy KM, Rosas M, Findon H, Haynes K, Steele C, Botto M, Gordon S, Brown GD (2007) Dectin-1 is required for beta-glucan recognition and control of fungal infection. Nat Immunol 8: 31–38

Underhill DM (2003) Macrophage recognition of zymosan particles. J Endotoxin Res 9: 176–180

Underhill DM, Ozinsky A (2002) Phagocytosis of microbes: Complexity in action. Annu Rev Immunol 20: 825–852

Underhill DM, Ozinsky A, Hajjar AM, Stevens A, Wilson CB, Bassetti M, Aderem A (1999a) The Toll-like receptor 2 is recruited to macrophage phagosomes and discriminates between pathogens. Nature 401: 811–815

Underhill DM, Ozinsky A, Smith KD, Aderem A (1999b) Toll-like receptor-2 mediates mycobacteria-induced proinflammatory signaling in macrophages. Proc Natl Acad Sci USA 96: 14459–14463

Underhill DM, Rossnagle E, Lowell CA, Simmons RM (2005) Dectin-1 activates Syk tyrosine kinase in a dynamic subset of macrophages for reactive oxygen production. Blood 106: 2543–2550

Van der Graaf CA, Netea MG, Morre SA, Den Heijer M, Verweij PE, Van der Meer JW, Kullberg BJ (2006) Toll-like receptor 4 Asp299Gly/Thr399Ile polymorphisms are a risk factor for *Candida* bloodstream infection. Eur Cytokine Netw 17: 29–34

Vassallo R, Standing JE, Limper AH (2000) Isolated *Pneumocystis carinii* cell wall glucan provokes lower respiratory tract inflammatory responses. J Immunol 164: 3755–3763

Villamon E, Gozalbo D, Roig P, O'Connor JE, Fradelizi D, Gil ML (2004) Toll-like receptor-2 is essential in murine defenses against *Candida albicans* infections. Microbes Infect 6: 1–7

Wheeler RT, Fink GR (2006) A drug-sensitive genetic network masks fungi from the immune system. PLoS Pathog 2: e35

Willment JA, Gordon S, Brown GD (2001) Characterization of the human beta-glucan receptor and its alternatively spliced isoforms. J Biol Chem 276: 43818–43823

Yadav M, Schorey JS (2006) The beta-glucan receptor Dectin-1 functions together with TLR2 to mediate macrophage activation by mycobacteria. Blood 108: 3168–3175

Yates RM, Russell DG (2005) Phagosome maturation proceeds independently of stimulation of Toll-like receptors 2 and 4. Immunity 23: 409–417

Yauch LE, Mansour MK, Shoham S, Rottman JB, Levitz SM (2004) Involvement of CD14, Toll-like receptors 2 and 4, and MyD88 in the host response to the fungal pathogen *Cryptococcus neoformans in vivo*. Infect Immun 72: 5373–5382

Zhang C, Wang SH, Lasbury ME, Tschang D, Liao CP, Durant PJ, Lee CH (2006) Toll-like receptor 2 mediates alveolar macrophage response to *Pneumocystis murina*. Infect Immun 74: 1857–1864

Heat Shock Proteins and Toll-Like Receptors

Alexzander Asea

Abstract Researchers have only just begun to elucidate the relationship between heat shock proteins (HSP) and Toll-like receptors (TLR). HSP were originally described as an intracellular molecular chaperone of naïve, aberrantly folded, or mutated proteins and primarily implicated as a cytoprotective protein when cells are exposed to stressful stimuli. However, recent studies have ascribed novel functions to the Hsp70 protein depending on its localization: Surface-bound Hsp70 specifically activate natural killer (NK) cells, while Hsp70 released into the extracellular milieu specifically bind to Toll-like receptors (TLR) 2 and 4 on antigen-presenting cells (APC) and exerts immunoregulatory effects, including upregulation of adhesion molecules, co-stimulatory molecule expression, and cytokine and chemokine release—a process known as the chaperokine activity of Hsp70. This chapter discusses the most recent advances in the understanding of heat shock protein (HSP) and TLR interactions in general and highlights recent findings that demonstrate Hsp70 is a ligand for TLR and its biological significance.

Alexzander Asea

Division of Investigative Pathology, Scott & White Memorial Hospital and Clinic and Texas A&M University System Health Science Center College of Medicine, 1901 South 1st Street, Temple, TX 76504, USA

aasea@swmail.sw.org or asea@medicine.tamhsc.edu

S. Bauer, G. Hartmann (eds.), *Toll-Like Receptors (TLRs) and Innate Immunity.*
Handbook of Experimental Pharmacology 183.
© Springer-Verlag Berlin Heidelberg 2008

List of Abbreviations

APC: antigen-presenting cells; *hsp*, heat shock protein gene; HSP, heat shock protein; Hsp70: inducible form of the 70-kilo Dalton heat shock protein; IL: interleukin; IRAK: IL-1 receptor-associated kinase; IFN-γ: interferon-gamma; MyD88: myeloid differentiation factor-88; NK cell: natural killer cell; TLR: Toll-like receptors; TNF: tumor necrosis factor; TRAF-6: TNF-receptor associated factor-6.

1 Introduction

Heat shock proteins (HSP) are highly conserved proteins found in all prokaryotes and eukaryotes. Under normal physiological conditions HSP are expressed at low levels (Craig and Gross, 1991). However, a wide variety of stressful stimul—including environmental (UV radiation, heat shock, heavy metals, and amino acids), pathological (viral, bacterial, parasitic infections or fever, inflammation, malignancy, or autoimmunity), or physiological stimuli (growth factors, cell differentiation, hormonal stimulation, or tissue development)—induces a marked increase in intracellular HSP synthesis (Lindquist, 1986), known as the stress response. Hsp70 is a member of the heat shock protein family, which enables organisms to respond to stress. Under physiological conditions Hsp70 and its cognates play essential roles in modulating protein-protein interaction, participating in the folding, assembling, and translocation of intracellular proteins (Martin, 1997; Nover and Scharf, 1997; Pilon and Schekman, 1999). For this reason, the primary function ascribed to Hsp70 is as intracellular molecular chaperones of naïve, aberrantly folded, or mutated proteins, as well as in cytoprotection, following the kinds of stressful stimuli mentioned above. The focus of this chapter is to discuss the new role of Hsp70 as both chaperone and cytokine—a chaperokine—and to discuss the role of TLR in chaperokine-induced signaling.

Innate immunity is the first line of host defense against infection and malignant transformation and has a profound effect on the establishment of adaptive immunity (Fearon and Locksley, 1996; Medzhitov and Janeway, 1997). Cells of the innate immune system are adorned with recognition structures called pattern recognition receptors (PRRs) (Medzhitov and Janeway, 1997; Medzhitov et al., 1997). PRRs such as Toll-like receptors (TLRs), CD14, β_2-intergrins (CD11/CD18), complement receptors (CR1/CD35), and C-type lectins are expressed either as soluble proteins or plasma membrane-bound proteins that recognize invariant molecular structures called pathogen-associated molecular patterns (PAMPs) (e.g., LPS, peptidoglycan (PGN), unmethylated CpG-DNA, bacterial lipoprotein (BLP), and mannans of yeast) that are shared by numerous pathogens but are not normally expressed on host tissues (Medzhitov and Janeway, 1997). Recent studies on the recognition of microbial PAMPs have highlighted the central role played by one group of PRRs, the Toll-like receptors (TLR), in pathogen recognition and host defense (see review in (Janeway, 1999; Anderson, 2000; Zhang and Ghosh, 2001)).

TLRs are similar in sequence and structure to the *Drosophila* Toll protein, and they share a conserved extracellular leucine-rich region important for ligand binding. Both Toll and TLRs are type 1 transmembrane proteins whose intracellular signaling domains have a Toll/IL-lR homology (TIR) motif (Rock et al., 1998; Kopp and Medzhitov, 1999; Aderem and Ulevitch, 2000). Toll was originally identified as an essential component of dorsal-ventral development in flies and has since been linked to an immune response against fungal infection in adult flies (Lemaitre et al., 1996; Muzio and Mantovani, 2000). The mammalian homologues of Toll also control innate immune responses through conserved signaling pathways in which an adapter protein, MyD88, binds to a receptor TIR-domain through its own TIR motif, while a death domain on its C-terminus recruits IL-lR-associated kinase (IRAK) to the complex. IRAK is then autophosphorylated and released from the complex to bind TNF-receptor associated factor-6 (TRAF6), which can then activate either the NF-κB pathway or the MAP kinase cascade (Kopp and Medzhitov, 1999). The TLR family is a fast growing family whose ligands have not all been identified. The most well-characterized TLRs are TLR2 and TLR4. TLR4 initiates signaling cascades in response to lipopolysaccharide (LPS), the abundant glycolipid of the outer membrane of Gram-negative bacteria, taxol or Hsp60, while TLR2 initiates the signal cascade in response to Gram-positive bacteria, *Mycoplasma, Yeast,* and *Spirochetes*. This chapter will focus on the 70-kDa heat shock protein (Hsp70) as a ligand for TLR.

2 Regulation of the Stress Response

Mammalian cells exhibit a cohort of molecular chaperone proteins, which are induced by a wide variety of stressful stimuli, including: environmental (UV radiation, heat shock, heavy metals, and amino acids); pathological (viral, bacterial, parasitic infections or fever, inflammation, malignancy, or autoimmunity); or physiological stimuli (growth factors, cell differentiation, hormonal stimulation, or tissue development), and which in turn induce a marked increase in intracellular HSP synthesis, known as the stress response. These include "small HSP" typified by Hsp27 and Hsp40, the "intermediate HSP" including Hsp60, Hsp70, Hsp90, and "large HSP," Hsp110 (Lindquist and Craig, 1988; Georgopolis and Welch, 1993). Some of the proteins, including the Hsp70 family, are encoded by more than one gene. In addition, mammalian cells contain 3 HSF family members including HSF1, HSF2, and HSF4 (Rabindran et al., 1991; Wu, 1995; Nakai et al., 1997). No gene corresponding to avian *hsf3* has so far been observed (Nakai and Morimoto, 1993).

Upon sensing stressful stimuli, transcriptional activation of the heat shock response by HSF1 involves trimerization, nuclear localization, and binding to the heat shock elements in HSP promoters (Rabindran et al., 1993; Westwood and Wu, 1993; Zuo et al., 1995). These events involve major unfolding reactions reflected in the hydrodynamic properties of HSF1 (Rabindran et al., 1993; Westwood and Wu, 1993), and HSF1 unfolding is necessary for interactions with other molecules including protein kinases and transcription factors that mediate cross talk with other responses

in the cell (Xie et al., 2002; Soncin et al., 2003). In order to achieve the full transcriptional activation, an additional stress-induced step is required that is dependent
on the activities of upstream tyrosine kinases and results in the hyperphosphoryla-
tion of HSF1 largely on serine residues (Hensold et al., 1990; Price and Calderwood,
1991; Sarge et al., 1993). Hsp90 found in the cytosol has been demonstrated to be
the primary regulator of HSF1. Binding of Hsp90 to HSF1 maintains HSF1 in its
inactive, compacted form in the cell (Zou et al., 1998). The central role of Hsp90 in
this regard is indicated by the fact that HSP90 inhibitors such as geldanomycin can
activate all steps of the stress protein response (Zou et al., 1998). The transcription
factor HSF1 is an unusual Hsp90 client protein in that, while other Hsp90-associated
proteins become destabilized and destroyed by proteolysis by Hsp90 dissociation,
HSF1 is activated and leads to abundant HSP expression (Zou et al., 1998). On the
other hand, HSF1 is repressed by a number of other pathways largely mediated by
phosphorylation, including repression mediated by a double phosphorylation at Serines 307 and 303 by the ERK and GSK3 pathways, and phosphorylation at Serine
363 by protein kinase C (Chu et al., 1996; Klein and Melton, 1996; Knauf et al.,
1996; Chu et al., 1998).

3 Pathophysiological Role of Stress Protein Response

In addition to their functions as molecular chaperones, HSP play a number of roles
in cell and tissue physiology. HSP protect the proteome through their molecular chaperone function, which permits them to recognize damaged proteins, chan-
neling such proteins either into repair/refolding pathways or to proteolysis. For
cell survival these properties of the HSP family permit cells to respond to damage at the source and immediately begin the processes required to resolve the
cellular insult (Kampinga et al., 1994; Kampinga et al., 1995). In addition, HSP
play more generic roles in cell survival and are implicated as inhibitors of pro-
grammed cell death, and block both the intrinsic and extrinsic pathways of caspase-
dependent apoptosis (Beere, 2004). The HSP may thus have been co-opted from
their ancient molecular chaperone roles to play a part in other processes that require cells to negotiate stressful periods. Thus, the molecular chaperone properties of the 70 and 90 kD HSP families have permitted them to play a role in
cell regulation often as stabilizing inhibitory components of transcription factor
or protein kinase complexes (Nollen and Morimoto, 2002). Another feature of
the stress protein response is the power of the gene expression system involved
and the high abundance of HSP expression in stressed cells (Wu, 1995). This appears to have led to a further elaboration of the functions of stress proteins in the
immune system (Srivastava and Amato, 2001; Srivastava, 2002). Dying cells often undergo the stress protein response, leading to lysis and release of HSP into
the extracellular space (Shi and Rock, 2002). Such extracellular HSP appears to
lead to a danger response that can activate the inflammatory response as well as
the innate and adaptive immune response (Asea et al., 2000a; Asea et al., 2002a;
Srivastava, 2002). The proimmune effects of extracellular HSP appear to be coun-
tered by the intracellular stress protein response and both HSF1 and the HSP70

are able to inhibit the expression of proinflammatory cytokines and mediate the extremes of the acute phase response (Cahill et al., 1996; Xie et al., 2003).

4 Dichotomy of HSP Effects

A dichotomy now exists between the effects of HSP based on its relative location and the target cell it binds to and activates. This dichotomy is one of intracellular versus extracellular. The upregulation of intracellular Hsp70 (iHsp72) is generally cytoprotective and induces the cells anti-apoptotic mechanisms (Jaattela et al., 1998), represses gene expression (Tang et al., 2001), modulates cell cycle progression (Hut et al., 2005), and is anti-inflammatory (Housby et al., 1999). On the other hand, the upregulation of extracellular Hsp70 (eHsp72) is generally immunostimulatory and stimulates proinflammatory cytokine synthesis (Asea et al., 2000a; Asea, 2005), augments chemokine synthesis (Lehner et al., 2000; Panjwani et al., 2002), upregulates co-stimulatory molecules (Asea et al., 2002b; Bausero et al., 2005b), and enhances anti-tumor surveillance (Srivastava et al., 1994; Srivastava, 2000; 2005).

5 HSP Release from Cells

The following hypotheses cover concern HSP release from cells.

1. Passive release hypothesis. Gallucci and colleagues initially demonstrated that dendritic cells (DC) are stimulated by endogenous signals received from stressed, viral-infected, or necrosis-induced cells, but not by healthy cells or cells undergoing apoptosis (Gallucci et al., 1999). In a series of elegantly performed experiments, Basu and coworkers later reported that heat shock proteins including gp96, calreticulin, Hsp90, and Hsp72 are released from cells by necrotic but not apoptotic cells (Basu et al., 2000). These authors demonstrated that necrosis induced by freeze thaw, but not apoptosis induced by irradiation, resulted in the release of Hsp into the culture supernatant, respectively (Basu et al., 2000; Basu and Srivastava, 2000; Srivastava and Amato, 2001; Srivastava, 2003). During apoptotic cell death, the contents of the cell are not released into the external milieu but are packaged neatly into apoptotic bodies, which are efficiently scavenged by neighboring professional phagocytes. However, necrotic cell death results in the discharge of intracellular contents into the extracellular milieu thereby liberating heat shock proteins (Srivastava, 2003; Calderwood, 2005). These results make the necrosis hypothesis an attractive explanation for the mechanism by which heat shock proteins are released into the circulation.

   A condition in which necrotic cell death clearly contributes to the release of Hsp72 from cells is after severe trauma. In a study by Pittet and colleagues a significant upregulation in circulating serum Hsp72 can be measured in severely traumatized patients as early as 30 minutes after injury (Pittet et al., 2002). Increased circulating serum Hsp72 has also been measured in patients after coronary artery bypass grafting (Dybdahl et al., 2002; Dybdahl et al., 2004). Importantly, circulating serum Hsp72 has been suggested as a marker of myocardial damage, and reported to have a role in the inflammatory response after acute myocardial infarction (AMI) (Dybdahl et al., 2005). Other conditions in which elevated levels of circulating serum Hsp72 has been demonstrated is in renal disease (Wright et al., 2000), hypertension (Pockley et al., 2002), atherosclerosis (Pockley et al., 2003), aging (Terry et al., 2004), and sickle cell disease (Adewoye et al., 2005). However, in these conditions, although necrosis is proposed as the mechanism of release, conclusive experimental data are still lacking. A more conclusive study was designed in which *in situ* killing of tumor cells using suicide gene transfer to generate death by a nonapoptotic pathway was shown to be associated with high immunogenicity and induction of Hsp (Melcher et al., 1998). The most conclusive reports to demonstrate that necrosis accounts for Hsp release is found following infection with lytic viruses. In a study by Moehler and coworkers, it was demonstrated that parvovirus-mediated cell killing enhances tumor immunogenicity by Hsp72 release and contributes to the antitumor effect of parvoviruses (Moehler et al., 2005). Although these authors did not directly demonstrate that H1-induced cell killing, and its associated Hsp72 release promotes the loading and maturation of antigen-presenting cells, and by extension triggers tumor-specific immune responses, one can speculate that the release of Hsp72 could facilitate priming of T cells specific for viral antigens.

When we take its elements together, we see clearly that the passive release hypothesis seems to be an important mechanism by which Hsp72 is released into the circulation. However, is it the only mechanism? An additional mechanism for Hsp release is now proposed as being of equal importance in the release of Hsp72 into the circulation.

2. Active release hypothesis. The active release hypothesis has been proposed as an additional mechanism to the passive release hypothesis. Three lines of evidence strongly support this hypothesis. First, as early as 1998 Pockley and coworkers demonstrated the presence of soluble Hsp72 and antibodies against Hsp72 in the peripheral circulation of normal individuals (Pockley et al., 1998). Second, Guzhova and colleagues demonstrated that Hsp72 is released by glia cells in the absence of necrotic cell death (Guzhova et al., 2001). Third, and extremely compelling, psychological stress induced by exposure of a Sprague Dawley rat to a cat results in the release of Hsp72 into the circulation (Fleshner et al., 2004). In this study, a rat was put in a glass cage and a cat placed on top of the cage. This form of psychological stress induced a marked increase in circulating Hsp72, as judged by the classical Hsp72 sandwich ELISA. The terrified rat did not run around the cage, thereby negating the possibility that damage to the muscles played a part in increased Hsp72 release. Subsequent studies have demonstrated that Hsp72 is released by B cells (Clayton et al., 2005) and peripheral blood mononuclear cells (Hunter-Lavin et al., 2004) under non necrotic conditions.

Using conditions that would not induce significant cell death, our group showed that IFN-γ and IL-10 induce the active release of constitutively expressed Hsp70 and also designed Hsc70, or Hsp73 from tumors (Barreto et al., 2003). However, these initial studies did not address the mechanism underlying Hsp72 release. Recently, our group (Bausero et al., 2005a; Gastpar et al., 2005) and others (Lancaster and Febbraio, 2005) have begun to elucidate the mechanism of active release of iHsp72 from viable cells. In our study we demonstrated that certain proinflammatory cytokines normally found in high concentrations within inflammatory foci including IFN-γ and IL-10 but not the anti-inflammatory cytokine TGF-β1, mediate the active release of Hsp72. We further showed that whereas some eHsp72 could be found as free Hsp72, a proportion of eHsp72 was released within exosomes (Bausero et al., 2005a). Exosomes are internal vesicles of multivesicular bodies (MVB) released into the extracellular milieu upon fusion of MVB with the cell surface (Raposo et al., 1996; Zitvogel et al., 1998; Zitvogel et al., 1999). In addition to containing Hsp72 (Bausero et al., 2005a; Gastpar et al., 2005), exosomes are highly packed with immunostimulatory mediators including MHC class I and II (Raposo et al., 1996; Zitvogel et al., 1998; Zitvogel et al., 1999) and co-stimulatory molecules (Escola et al., 1998). Additionally, we demonstrated that Hsp72 is released by a nonclassical protein transport pathway and that intact surface membrane lipid rafts are required for efficient stress-induced Hsp72 release (Bausero et al., 2005a; Gastpar et al., 2005). These studies were recently confirmed in B cells (Clayton et al., 2005). Studies by Lancaster and Febbraio recently demonstrated that exosomes provide the major pathway for secretory vesicular release of Hsp72 (Lancaster and Febbraio, 2005). However, using methyl-β-cyclodextrin (the cholesterol depleting agent) to disrupt lipid raft function, these authors were unable to confirm a role for lipid rafts in stress-induced Hsp72 release from human peripheral blood mononuclear cells (Lancaster and Febbraio, 2005). In order to address the cellular location of Hsp72 after stress, a recent study demonstrated that newly synthesized Hsp72 protein localizes within the Golgi region of HeLa cells and also concentrates on the surface of the plasma membrane and in the ruffled zone of migrating cells (Schneider et al., 2002).

Taken together, these studies suggest that the active release hypothesis is an important mechanism by which Hsp72 is released into the circulation. However, studies remain to be performed that conclusively demonstrate that T cell responses are primed in response to active release of Hsp72, especially in the case of psychological stress or exercise.

6 Signaling Events Resulting in Chaperokine-Induced Activities of Hsp70

Although the exact nature of the Hsp70 receptor has not yet been described, studies from the Multhoff laboratory on the expression of Hsp70 on the surface of cells has been well defined. In comparison with immunocompetent cells, malignant tumor cells including biopsies from colorectal, lung, neuronal, and pancreas carcinomas, liver metastases, and leukemic blasts of patients with acute myelogenous leukemia, express high levels of surface-bound Hsp70 (Botzler et al., 1996; Multhoff and Hightower, 1996; Multhoff et al., 1997; Botzler et al., 1998b; Hantschel et al., 2000). The Hsp70 expression on tumors correlates with an increased sensitivity to natural killer (NK)-mediated cytolysis following cytokine stimulation (Botzler et al., 1998a; Multhoff et al., 1999; Multhoff et al., 2001). Indeed, Hsp70-selective NK cell activity was reported to be stimulated in a clinical Phase I trial of patients with advanced, metastasized colorectal and lung carcinoma when treated with Hsp70-peptide TKD plus low-dose IL-2 (Gehrmann et al., 2003).

Our group initially focused on understanding Hsp70 effects on immunocompetent cells as a model for what might occur *in vivo* when immunocompetent cells come into contact with Hsp70 highly expressed by tumors or released from tumors as a consequence of the lytic machinery of the host. Extracellular Hsp70 specifically binds to the surface membrane of distinct cell populations, notably natural killer (NK) cells (Multhoff et al., 1995; Multhoff et al., 1997; Gross et al., 2003), and APC including DC (Reed and Nicchitta, 2000; Asea et al., 2002b; Vabulas et al., 2002a), macrophages, peripheral blood monocytes (Asea et al., 2000a; Sondermann et al., 2000), and B cells (Arnold-Schild et al., 1999). In contrast, T lymphocytes do not appear to specifically bind exogenous Hsp70 (Arnold-Schild et al., 1999).

Following surface binding, exogenous Hsp70 was demonstrated to elicit a rapid intracellular Ca^{2+} flux (Asea et al., 2000a). This is an important signaling step that distinguishes Hsp70- from LPS-induced, signaling since treatment of APC with LPS does not result in intracellular Ca^{2+} flux (McLeish et al., 1989). The possibility that endotoxin contamination might confound our results was addressed by using Polymyxin B and Lipid IVa (LPS inhibitor) which abrogates LPS-induced, but not Hsp70-induced, cytokine expression. Boiling the proteins at 100°C for 1 hour abrogates Hsp70-induced, but not LPS-induced, cytokine expression. We noted that rapid Hsp70-induced intracellular Ca^{2+} flux is followed by the phosphorylation of I-κBα (Asea et al., 2000a). Activation of NF-κB is regulated by its cytoplasmic inhibitor, I-κBα, via phosphorylation at Serine 32 (Ser-32) and 36 (Ser-36) which targets it for degradation by the proteosome and releases NF-κB to migrate to the nucleus and activate the promoter of target genes (Baeuerle and Baltimore, 1988). As early as 30 minutes post exposure to exogenous Hsp70, I-κBα was phosphorylated at Serine 32 (Ser-32) and 36 (Ser-36) resulting in the release and nuclear translocation of NF-κB (Asea et al., 2000a).

Mechanistic studies using the HEK293 model system revealed that Hsp70-induced NF-κB promoter activity is MyD88-dependent, CD14-dependent and is transduced via both TLR2 and TLR4 (Asea et al., 2002b). Our studies show that the presence of both TLR2 and TLR4 synergistically stimulates Hsp70-induced cytokine production (Asea et al., 2002b). Interestingly, we found that the synergistic activation of NF-κB promoter by co-expression of both TLR2 and TLR4 is MyD88-independent, suggesting an alterative pathway by which exogenous Hsp70 stimulates cells of the immune system. As early as 2–4 hours post exposure of APC to exogenous Hsp70, there is significant release of TNF-α, IL-1β, IL-6 and IL-12

(Asea et al., 2000a; Asea et al., 2002b). The human monocytic cell line THP1, transfected with the dominant negative MyD88 plasmid or a combination of both dominant negative TLR2 and TLR4, inhibited a portion of Hsp70-induced IL-6 (Asea et al., 2002b) and IL-1β expression (Asea, 2003). However, only a combination of dominant negative MyD88/TLR2/TLR4 completely inhibited Hsp70-induced IL-6 (Asea et al., 2002b), IL-1β (Asea, 2003), IFN-γ (Asea, 2004), and IL-12 expression. A combination of MyD88-DN and TLR2, or MyD88-DN and TLR4, were not sufficient to completely block Hsp70-induced intracellular IL-12 expression. These results suggest that there is a component of Hsp70-induced cytokine production that is MyD88-independent.

Recent studies seemed to suggest that CD14 is able to enhance HSP-induced cell signaling. This was refuted by data from the group of Delneste who demonstrated that neutralizing antibodies against CD14 does not inhibit the binding of Hsp70 to human APCs (Delneste et al., 2002). The argument that membrane-bound CD14 is a glycosyl phosphatidyl inositol-anchored protein devoid of an intracellular domain seems to support these results.

7 The Endotoxin Question

Pretreatment of cells with $1\,\mu g/ml$ *Rhodopseudomonas spheroids* (RSLP), an LPS inhibitor did not significantly affect Hsp70-induced IL-12 expression, thereby negating the possibility that endotoxin contamination might have resulted in enhanced IL-12 expression. However, heat denaturation at 100°C for 1 hour completely abrogated Hsp70-induced IL-12 expression (data not shown). Pretreatment of cells with RSLP completely inhibited LPS-induced IL-12 expression (data not shown). Controls were cells pretreated with control protein OVA. All Hsp70 preparations were tested for LPS content by *Limulus* amebocyte lysate assay and were found to have no detectable LPS up to the sensitivity limits of the assay (≤ 0.01 endotoxin U/ml). These results were confirmed by independent groups (Ohashi et al., 2000; Vabulas et al., 2001; Vabulas et al., 2002a; Vabulas et al., 2002b; Liu et al., 2003).

In a separate study MacAry and colleagues used physical and functional assays to ensure the "cleanliness" of the Hsp70 protein preparations. Physical assays include adding an additional microdialysis step to remove unbound peptide and other contaminants, passing all Hsp70 protein preparations through polymyxin B column, and only using preparations with less than <1.0 endotoxin units per $20\,\mu g$ of protein. Functional assays include boiling Hsp70 protein preparations at 100°C for 60 minutes, which denatures Hsp70 but not LPS; pretreatment of Hsp70 preparations with protinase K, which inhibits Hsp70-induced, but not LPS induced-cytokine release by APC; addition of soluble CD14 to macrophages, which enhances LPS-induced, but not Hsp70-induced cytokine release; pretreatment of macrophages with BAPTA-AM, an intracellular calcium chelator, which inhibits efficient Hsp70-induced, but not LPS induced-cytokine release; and measurement of intracellular calcium flux, which is only induced by Hsp70, not LPS (Asea et al., 2000b; MacAry et al., 2004). When similar measures were used to control for LPS contamination of rHsp70 preparations, Hsp70 augmented dendritic cell (DC) effector functions and when admixed with specific antigens, triggered autoimmune diseases *in vivo* (Millar et al., 2003), and DC pulsed with peptide-loaded rHsp70 generated potent antigen-specific CTL responses (MacAry et al., 2004). However, mutation of the peptide-binding domain of Hsp70 rendered the mutants incapable of generating antigen-specific CTL responses (MacAry et al., 2004). The most conclusive evidence that LPS contamination cannot account for the functions of HSP was provided by a recent study from the Lehner lab in which they identified stimulating and inhibitory epitopes within microbial Hsp70 that modulate cytokine and chemokine release and the maturation of dendritic cells (Wang et al., 2005). It was demonstrated that Hsp70-derived stimulating peptide (aa407–426), which is devoid of any LPS, is able to elicit stimulating functions comparable to the wild-type Hsp70 (Wang et al., 2005). In addition, it was recently reported that LPS-low Hsp110 activates APC, as judged by enhanced CD86, CD40, MHC class II expression, and TNF-α, IL-6 and IL-12 secretion (Manjili et al., 2005).

Finally, it must be noted that although the most up-to-date techniques to eliminate endotoxin contamination may be used, it is virtually impossible to completely eliminate its possibility. However, all these studies strongly suggest that when special care is taken to control for LPS contamination, clear effects of Hsp70 can be demonstrated.

8 Biological Significance of HSP-TLR Interactions

TLR are innate immune receptors that recognize microbial moieties highly conserved during the evolution of, which are called pathogen-associated molecular patterns (PAMPs) (Takeda et al., 2003). Therefore, an interesting observation is that in addition to HSP's obvious role in the stimulation of innate immunity through TLR, HSP also activate cells of the adaptive immunity, including B cells and T lymphocytes. Initial study by Brelor and coworkers and More et al. independently demonstrated that T lymphocytes potentiate the HSP-induced activation of APCs, as evidenced by an increase of IL-2 and IFN-γ production and proliferation (Breloer et al., 2001; More et al., 2001). In addition, HSP have been shown to directly activate T lymphocytes in a TLR4-independent and TLR2-dependent manner (Zanin-Zhorov et al., 2003; Osterloh et al., 2004). This observation is in agreement with the fact that T lymphocytes can be activated by TLR agonists, mainly microbial moieties (Gelman et al., 2004; Komai-Koma et al., 2004; Caron et al., 2005), in the presence of co-stimuli such as IL-2 or the anti-CD3 antibody. In addition, human Hsp60 has been shown to activate B cells via the recruitment of TLR4 in a LPS-independent manner, resulting in the release of IL-6 and the concomitant up-regulation in expression of plasma membrane activation markers including CD40, CD69, and CD86 (Cohen-Sfady et al., 2005). However, in this study the participation of CD40 in Hsp60-induced B cell activation was not evaluated. Interestingly, both B and T lymphocytes do not express SR, suggesting that HSP-mediated cell activation may occur independently of these molecules. Understanding of the role and the consequences of HSP-mediated T and B cell stimulation on the initiation/development of an antigen-specific immune response remain incomplete.

The role of TLR in Hsp70 signaling in infectious diseases has just begun to be addressed (Aosai et al., 2002; Chen et al., 2002). Aosai and colleagues recently demonstrated that *Toxoplasma gondii*-derived Hsp70 (TgHsp70) functions as a B cell mitogen (Aosai et al., 2002). These authors demonstrated that B cells but not CD4$^+$ or CD8$^+$ T lymphocytes respond to TgHsp70. In addition, C3H/HeN mice, but not C3H/HeJ mice, that carry a point mutation in the TLR4 gene activated TgHsp70 (Aosai et al., 2002). Taken together these results suggest an important role for Hsp70-based proteins signaling through TLR in controlling infectious diseases.

Recent studies of patients undergoing cardiopulmonary bypass using coronary artery bypass grafting (CABG) suggest a role for TLR in Hsp70-induced inflammatory response (Dybdahl et al., 2002). Elevated levels of Hsp70 were detected in the plasma of patients referred for elective CABG, and the expression of TLR2 and TLR4 on monocytes was enhanced one day post surgery, suggesting that extracellular Hsp70 may act as an endogenous ligand for TLR4 and this may account for the enhanced inflammatory response seen after CABG (Dybdahl et al., 2002).

Our findings (Asea et al., 2002b) and those of others (Vabulas et al., 2002a) demonstrate that the chaperokine activity of Hsp70 is transduced via Toll/IL-1 receptor signal transduction pathways and helps to identify Hsp70 as an endogenous natural adjuvant. In addition, these studies now pave the way for the development of highly effective pharmacological or molecular tools that will either upregulate or suppress Hsp70-induced functions. If the hypothesis is correct, in conditions where Hsp70-induced effects are desirable, including cancer, therapeutic protocols should be aimed at enhancing Hsp70 release, since this would in turn enhance tumor immunogenicity and host antitumor responses. On the other hand, in disorders where Hsp70-induced effects are undesirable including CABG, arthritis, and arteriosclerosis, downregulating Hsp70-induced effects would be beneficial to the host survival.

Acknowledgements The author thanks Edwina Asea, Edith Kabingu, Rajani Mallick, Rahilya Napoli, Elizabeth Palaima, Fred Powell and Preethi Rao for expert technical assistance, and Drs. Maria A. Bausero, Vadiraja Bhat, Nagaraja Mallappa, Nirmal Singh, and Hongying Zheng for helpful discussions. This work was supported in part by the National Institute of Health grant RO1CA91889 and Institutional support from the Department of Pathology Scott & White Memorial Hospital and Clinic, the Texas A&M University System Health Science Center College of Medicine, the Central Texas Veterans Health Administration, and an Endowment from the Cain Foundation.

References

Aderem A, Ulevitch RJ (2000) Toll-like receptors in the induction of the innate immune response. Nature 406: 782–787

Adewoye AH, Klings ES Farber HW, Palaima E, Bausero MA, McMahon L, Odhiambo A, Surinder S, Yoder M, Steinberg MH, Asea A (2005) Sickle cell vaso-occlusive crisis induces the release of circulating serum heat shock protein-70. Am J Hematol 78: 240–242

Anderson KV (2000) Toll signaling pathways in the innate immune response. Curr Opin Immunol 12: 13–19

Aosai F, Chen M, Kang HK, Mun HS, Norose K, Piao LX, Kobayashi M, Takeuchi O, Akira S, Yano A (2002) *Toxoplasma gondii*-derived heat shock protein HSP70 functions as a B cell mitogen. Cell Stress Chaperones 7: 357–364

Arnold-Schild D, Hanau D, Spehner D, Schmid C, Rammensee HG, de la Salle H, Schild H (1999) Receptor-mediated endocytosis of heat shock proteins by professional antigen-presenting cells. J Immunol 162: 3757–3760

Asea A (2003) Chaperokine-induced signal transduction pathways. Exerc Immunol Rev 9: 25–33

Asea A (2005) Stress proteins and initiation of immune response: chaperokine activity of hsp72. Exerc Immunol Rev 11: 34–45

Asea A, Kraeft SK, Kurt-Jones EA, Stevenson MA, Chen LB, Finberg RW, Koo GC, Calderwood SK (2000a) HSP70 stimulates cytokine production through a CD14-dependent pathway, demonstrating its dual role as a chaperone and cytokine. Nat Med 6: 435–442

Asea A, Kraeft SK, Kurt-Jones EA, Stevenson MA, Chen LB, Finberg RW, Koo GC, Calderwood SK (2000b) HSP70 stimulates cytokine production through a CD14-dependent pathway, demonstrating its dual role as a chaperone and cytokine. Nat Med 6: 435–442

Asea A, Rehli M, Kabingu E, Boch JA, Bare O, Auron PE, Stevenson MA, Calderwood SK (2002a) Novel signal transduction pathway utilized by extracellular HSP70: Role of Toll-like receptor (TLR) 2 and TLR4. J Biol Chem 277: 15028–15034

Asea A, Rehli M, Kabingu E, Boch JA, Bare O, Auron PE, Stevenson MA, Calderwood SK (2002b) Novel signal transduction pathway utilized by extracellular HSP70: Role of Toll-like receptor (TLR) 2 and TLR4. J Biol Chem 277: 15028–15034

Baeuerle PA, Baltimore D (1988) I kappa B: A specific inhibitor of the NF-kappa B transcription factor. Science 242: 540–546

Barreto A, Gonzalez JM, Kabingu E, Asea A, Fiorentino S (2003) Stress-induced release of HSC70 from human tumors. Cell Immunol 222: 97–104

Basu S, Binder RJ, Suto R, Anderson KM, Srivastava PK (2000) Necrotic but not apoptotic cell death releases heat shock proteins, which deliver a partial maturation signal to dendritic cells and activate the NF-kappa B pathway. Int Immunol 12: 1539–1546

Basu S, Srivastava PK (2000) Heat shock proteins: The fountainhead of innate and adaptive immune responses. Cell Stress Chaperones 5: 443–451

Bausero MA, Gastpar R, Multhoff G, Asea A (2005a) Alternative mechanism by which IFN-{gamma} enhances tumor recognition: Active release of heat shock protein 72. J Immunol 175: 2900–2912

Bausero MA, Gastpar R, Multhoff G, Asea A (2005b) Alternative mechanism by which IFN-gamma enhances tumor recognition: Active release of heat shock protein 72. J Immunol 175: 2900–2912

Beere HM (2004) 'The stress of dying': The role of heat shock proteins in the regulation of apoptosis. J Cell Sci 117: 2641–2651

Botzler C, Issels R, Multhoff G (1996) Heat-shock protein 72 cell-surface expression on human lung carcinoma cells in associated with an increased sensitivity to lysis mediated by adherent natural killer cells. Cancer Immunol Immunother 43: 226–230

Botzler C, Li G, Issels RD, Multhoff G (1998a) Definition of extracellular localized epitopes of Hsp70 involved in an NK immune response. Cell Stress Chaperones 3: 6–11

Botzler C, Schmidt J, Luz A, Jennen L, Issels R, Multhoff G (1998b) Differential Hsp70 plasma-membrane expression on primary human tumors and metastases in mice with severe combined immunodeficiency. Int J Cancer 77: 942–948

Breloer M, Dorner B, More SH, Roderian T, Fleischer B, von Bonin A (2001) Heat shock proteins as "danger signals": Eukaryotic Hsp60 enhances and accelerates antigen-specific IFN-gamma production in T cells. Eur J Immunol 31: 2051–2059

Cahill CM, Waterman WR, Auron PE, Calderwood SK (1996) Transcriptional repression of the prointerleukin1B gene by heat shock factor 1. J Biol Chem 271: 24874–24879

Calderwood SK (2005) Chaperones and slow death—A recipe for tumor immunotherapy. Trends Biotechnol 23: 57–59

Caron G, Duluc D, Fremaux I, Jeannin P, David C, Gascan H, Delneste Y (2005) Direct stimulation of human T cells via TLR5 and TLR7/8: Flagellin and R-848 up-regulate proliferation and IFN-gamma production by memory CD4 + T cells. J Immunol 175: 1551–1557

Chen M, Aosai F, Norose K, Mun HS, Takeuchi O, Akira S, Yano A (2002) Involvement of MyD88 in host defense and the down-regulation of anti-heat shock protein 70 autoantibody formation by MyD88 in *Toxoplasma gondii*-infected mice. J Parasitol 88: 1017–1019

Chu B, Soncin F, Price BD, Stevenson MA, Calderwood SK (1996) Sequential phosphorylation by mitogen–activated protein kinase and glycogen synthase kinase 3 represses transcriptional activation by heat shock factor-1. J Biol Chem 271: 30847–30857

Chu B, Zhong R, Soncin F, Stevenson MA, Calderwood SK (1998) Transcriptional activity of heat shock factor 1 at 37°C is repressed through phosphorylation on two distinct serine residues by glycogen synthase kinase 3 and protein kinase C a and Cz. J Biol Chem. 273: 18640–18646

Clayton A, Turkes A, Navabi H, Mason MD, Tabi Z (2005) Induction of heat shock proteins in B-cell exosomes. J Cell Sci 118: 3631–3638

Cohen-Sfady M, Nussbaum G, Pevsner-Fischer M, Mor F, Carmi P, Zanin-Zhorov A, Lider O, Cohen IR (2005) Heat shock protein 60 activates B cells via the TLR4-MyD88 pathway. J Immunol 175: 3594–3602

Craig EA, Gross CA (1991) Is hsp70 the cellular thermometer? Trends Biochem Sci 16: 135–140

Delneste Y, Magistrelli G, Gauchat J, Haeuw J, Aubry J, Nakamura K, Kawakami-Honda N, Goetsch L, Sawamura T, Bonnefoy J, Jeannin P (2002) Involvement of LOX-1 in dendritic cell-mediated antigen cross-presentation. Immunity 17: 353–362

Dybdahl B, Slordahl SA, Waage A, Kierulf P, Espevik T, Sundan A (2005) Myocardial ischaemia and the inflammatory response: Release of heat shock protein 70 after myocardial infarction. Heart 91: 299–304

Dybdahl B, Wahba A, Haaverstad R, Kirkeby-Garstad I, Kierulf P, Espevik T, Sundan A (2004) On-pump versus off-pump coronary artery bypass grafting: More heat-shock protein 70 is released after on-pump surgery. Eur J Cardiothorac Surg 25: 985–992

Dybdahl B, Wahba A, Lien E, Flo TH, Waage A, Qureshi N, Sellevold OF, Espevik T, Sundan A (2002) Inflammatory response after open heart surgery: Release of heat-shock protein 70 and signaling through Toll-like receptor-4. Circulation 105: 685–690

Escola JM, Kleijmeer MJ, Stoorvogel W, Griffith JM, Yoshie O, Geuze HJ (1998) Selective enrichment of tetraspan proteins on the internal vesicles of multivesicular endosomes and on exosomes secreted by human B-lymphocytes. J Biol Chem 273: 20121–20127

Fearon DT, Locksley RM (1996) The instructive role of innate immunity in the acquired immune response. Science 272: 50–53

Fleshner M, Campisi J, Amiri L, Diamond DM (2004) Cat exposure induces both intra- and extra-cellular Hsp72: The role of adrenal hormones. Psychoneuroendocrinol 29: 1142–1152

Gallucci S, Lolkema M, Matzinger P (1999) Natural adjuvants: Endogenous activators of dendritic cells. Nat Med 5: 1249–1255

Gastpar R, Gehrmann M, Bausero MA, Asea A, Gross C, Schroeder JA, Multhoff G (2005) Heat shock protein 70 surface-positive tumor exosomes stimulate migratory and cytolytic activity of natural killer cells. Cancer Res 65: 5238–5247

Gehrmann M, Schmetzer H, Eissner G, Haferlach T, Hiddemann W, Multhoff G (2003) Membrane-bound heat shock protein 70 (Hsp70) in acute myeloid leukemia: A tumor specific recognition structure for the cytolytic activity of autologous NK cells. Haematolog 88: 474–476

Gelman AE, Zhang J, Choi Y, Turka LA (2004) Toll-like receptor ligands directly promote activated CD4 + T cell survival. J Immunol 172: 6065–6073

Georgopolis C, Welch WJ (1993) Role of the major heat shock proteins as molecular chaperones. Ann Rev Cell Biol 9: 601–634

Gross C, Hansch D, Gastpar R, Multhoff G (2003) Interaction of heat shock protein 70 peptide with NK cells involves the NK receptor CD94. Biol Chem 384: 267–279

Guzhova I, Kislyakova K, Moskaliova O, Fridlanskaya I, Tytell M, Cheetham M, Margulis B (2001) *In vitro* studies show that Hsp70 can be released by glia and that exogenous Hsp70 can enhance neuronal stress tolerance. Brain Res 914: 66–73

Hantschel M, Pfister K, Jordan A, Scholz R, Andreesen R, Schmitz G, Schmetzer H, Hiddemann W, Multhoff G (2000) Hsp70 plasma membrane expression on primary tumor biopsy material and bone marrow of leukemic patients. Cell Stress Chaperones 5: 438–442

He H, Soncin F, Grammatikakis N, Li Y, Siganou A, Gong J, Brown SA, Kingston RE, Calderwood SK (2003) Elevated expression of heat shock factor 2a stimulates HSF1-induced transcription during stress. J Biol Chem 278: 35465–35475

Hensold JO, Hunt CR, Calderwood SK, Houseman DE, Kingston RE (1990) DNA binding of heat shock factor to the heat shock element is insufficient for transcriptional activation in murine erythroleukemia cells. Mol Cell Biol 10: 1600–1608

Housby JN, Cahill CM, Chu B, Prevelige R, Bickford K, Stevenson MA, Calderwood SK (1999) Non-steroidal anti-inflammatory drugs inhibit the expression of cytokines and induce HSP70 in human monocytes. Cytokine 11: 347–358

Hunter-Lavin C, Davies EL, Bacelar MM, Marshall MJ, Andrew SM, Williams JH (2004) Hsp70 release from peripheral blood mononuclear cells. Biochem Biophys Res Commun 324: 511–517

Hut HM, Kampinga HH, Sibon OC (2005) Hsp70 protects mitotic cells against heat-induced centrosome damage and division abnormalities. Mol Biol Cell 16: 3776–3785

Jaattela M, Wissing D, Kokholm K, Kallunki T, Egeblad M (1998) Hsp70 exerts its anti-apoptotic function downstream of caspase-3-like proteases. EMBO J 17: 6124–6134

Janeway CAJ (1999) Lipoproteins tale their toll on the host. Curr Biol 9, R879–R882

Kampinga HH, Brunsting JF, Stege GJ, Burgman PW, Konings AW (1995) Thermal protein denaturation and protein aggregation in cells made thermotolerant by various chemicals: Role of heat shock proteins. Exp Cell Res 219: 536–546

Kampinga HH, Brunsting JF, Stege GJ, Konings AW, Landry J (1994) Cells overexpressing Hsp27 show accelerated recovery from heat-induced nuclear protein aggregation. Biochem Biophys Res Commun 204: 1170–1177

Klein PS, Melton DA (1996) A molecular mechanism for the effect of lithium on development. Proc Natl Acad Sci USA 93: 8455–8459

Knauf U, Newton EM, Kyriakis J, Kingston RE (1996) Repression of heat shock factor 1 activity at control temperature by phosphorylation. Genes Dev 10: 2782–2793

Komai-Koma M, Jones L, Ogg GS, Xu D, Liew FY (2004) TLR2 is expressed on activated T cells as a costimulatory receptor. Proc Natl Acad Sci USA 101: 3029–3034

Kopp EB, Medzhitov R (1999) The Toll-receptor family and control of innate immunity. Curr Opin Immunol 11: 13–18

Lancaster GI, Febbraio MA (2005) Exosome-dependent trafficking of HSP70: A novel secretory pathway for cellular stress proteins. J Biol Chem 280: 23349–23355

Lehner T, Bergmeier LA, Wang Y, Tao L, Sing M, Spallek R, van der Zee R (2000) Heat shock proteins generate beta-chemokines which function as innate adjuvants enhancing adaptive immunity. Eur J Immunol 30: 594–603

Lemaitre B, Nicolas E, Michaut L, Reichhart JM, Hoffmann JA (1996) The dorsoventral regulatory gene cassette Spätzle/Toll/Cactus controls the potent antifungal response in *Drosophila* adults. Cell 86: 973–983

Lindquist S (1986) The heat-shock response. Ann Rev Biochem 55: 1151–1191

Lindquist S, Craig EA (1988) The heat shock proteins. Ann Rev Genet 22: 631–637

Liu B, Dai J, Zheng H, Stoilova D, Sun S, Li Z (2003) Cell surface expression of an endoplasmic reticulum resident heat shock protein gp96 triggers MyD88-dependent systemic autoimmune diseases. Proc Natl Acad Sci USA 100: 15824–15829

MacAry PA, Javid B, Floto RA, Smith KG, Oehlmann W, Singh M, Lehner PJ (2004) HSP70 peptide binding mutants separate antigen delivery from dendritic cell stimulation. Immunity 20: 95–106

Manjili MH, Park J, Facciponte G, Subjeck JR (2005) HSP110 induces "danger signals" upon interaction with antigen presenting cells and mouse mammary carcinoma. Immunobiol 210: 295–303

McLeish KR, Dean WL, Wellhausen SR, Stelzer GT (1989) Role of intracellular calcium in priming of human peripheral blood monocytes by bacterial lipopolysaccharide. Inflammation 13: 681–692

Medzhitov R, Janeway CAJ (1997) Innate immunity: Impact on the adaptive immune response. Curr Opin Immunol 9: 4–9

Medzhitov R, Preston-Hurlburt P, Janeway CA, Jr (1997) A human homologue of the *Drosophila* Toll protein signals activation of adaptive immunity. Nature 388: 394–397

Melcher A, Todryk S, Hardwick N, Ford M, Jacobson M, Vile RG (1998) Tumor immunogenicity is determined by the mechanism of cell death via induction of heat shock protein expression. Nat Med 4: 581–587

Millar DG, Garza KM, Odermatt B, Elford AR, Ono N, Li Z, Ohashi PS (2003) Hsp70 promotes antigen-presenting cell function and converts T-cell tolerance to autoimmunity *in vivo*. Nat Med 9: 1469–1476

Moehler MH, Zeidler M, Wilsberg V, Cornelis JJ, Woelfel T, Rommelaere J, Galle PR, Heike M (2005) Parvovirus H-1-induced tumor cell death enhances human immune response *in vitro* via increased phagocytosis, maturation, and cross-presentation by dendritic cells. Hum Gene Ther 16: 996–1005

More SH, Breloer M, von Bonin A (2001) Eukaryotic heat shock proteins as molecular links in innate and adaptive immune responses: Hsp60-mediated activation of cytotoxic T cells. Int Immunol 13: 1121–1127

Multhoff G, Botzler C, Jennen L, Schmidt J, Ellwart J, Issels R (1997) Heat shock protein 72 on tumor cells: A recognition structure for natural killer cells. J Immunol 158: 4341–4350

Multhoff G, Botzler C, Wiesnet M, Eissner G, Issels R (1995) CD3-large granular lymphocytes recognize a heat-inducible immunogenic determinant associated with the 72-kD heat shock protein on human sarcoma cells. Blood 86: 1374–1382

Multhoff G, Hightower LE (1996) Cell surface expression of heat shock proteins and the immune response. Cell Stress Chaperones 1: 167–176

Multhoff G, Mizzen L, Winchester CC, Milner CM, Wenk S, Eissner G, Kampinga HH, Laumbacher B, Johnson J (1999) Heat shock protein 70 (Hsp70) stimulates proliferation and cytolytic activity of natural killer cells. Exp Hematol 27: 1627–1636

Multhoff G, Pfister K, Gehrmann M, Hantschel M, Gross C, Hafner M, Hiddemann W (2001) A 14-mer Hsp70 peptide stimulates natural killer (NK) cell activity. Cell Stress Chaperones 6: 337–344

Muzio M, Mantovani A (2000) Toll-like receptors. Microbes Infect 2: 251–255

Nakai A, Morimoto RI (1993) Characterization of a novel chicken heat shock transcription factor, HSF3 suggests a new regulatory factor. Mol Cell Biol 13: 1983–1997

Nakai A, Tanabe M, Kawazoe Y, Inazawa J, Morimoto RI, Nagata K (1997) HSF4, a new member of the human heat shock factor family which lacks properties of a transcriptional activator. Mol Cell Biol 17: 469–481

Nollen EA, Morimoto RI (2002) Chaperoning signaling pathways: Molecular chaperones as stress-sensing 'heat shock' proteins. J Cell Sci 115: 2809–2816

Ohashi K, Burkart V, Flohe S, Kolb H (2000) Cutting edge: Heat shock protein 60 is a putative endogenous ligand of the Toll-like receptor-4 complex. J Immunol 164: 558–561

Osterloh A, Meier-Stiegen F, Veit A, Fleischer B, von Bonin A, Breloer M (2004) Lipopolysaccharide-free heat shock protein 60 activates T cells. J of Biol Chem 279: 47906–47911

Panjwani NN, Popova L, Srivastava PK (2002) Heat shock proteins gp96 and hsp70 activate the release of nitric oxide by APCs. J Immunol 168: 2997–3003

Pittet JF, Lee H, Morabito D, Howard MB, Welch WJ, Mackersie RC (2002) Serum levels of Hsp 72 measured early after trauma correlate with survival. J Trauma 52: 611–617 (see discussion p. 617)

Pockley AG, De Faire U, Kiessling R, Lemne C, Thulin T, Frostegard J (2002) Circulating heat shock protein and heat shock protein antibody levels in established hypertension. J Hypertens 20: 1815–1820

Pockley AG, Georgiades A, Thulin T, de Faire U, Frostegard J (2003) Serum heat shock protein 70 levels predict the development of atherosclerosis in subjects with established hypertension. Hypertension 42: 235–238

Pockley AG, Shepherd J, Corton JM (1998) Detection of heat shock protein 70 (Hsp70) and anti-Hsp70 antibodies in the serum of normal individuals. Immunol Invest 27: 367–377

Price BD, Calderwood SK (1991) Calcium is essential for multistep activation of the heat shock factor in permeabilized cells. Mol Cell Biol 11: 3365–3368

Rabindran SK, Gioorgi G, Clos J, Wu C (1991) Molecular cloning and expression of a human heat shock factor, HSF1. Proc Natl Acad Sci (USA) 88: 6906–6910

Rabindran SK, Haroun RI, Clos J, Wisniewski J, Wu C (1993) Regulation of heat shock factor trimer formation: Role of a conserved leucine zipper. Science 259: 230–234

Raposo G, Nijman HW, Stoorvogel W, Liejendekker R, Harding CV, Melief CJ, Geuze HJ (1996) B lymphocytes secrete antigen-presenting vesicles. J Exp Med 183: 1161–1172

Reed RC, Nicchitta CV (2000) Chaperone-mediated cross-priming: A hitchhiker's guide to vesicle transport (review). Int J Mol Med 6: 259–264

Rock FL, Hardiman G, Timans JC, Kastelein RA, Bazan JF (1998) A family of human receptors structurally related to *Drosophila* Toll. Proc Natl Acad Sci USA 95: 588–593

Sarge KD, Murphy SP, Morimoto RI (1993) Activation of heat shock gene transcription by heat shock factor 1 involves oligomerization, acquisition of DNA-binding activity, and nuclear localization and can occur in the absence of stress. Mol Cell Biol 13: 1392–1407

Schneider EM, Niess AM, Lorenz I, Northoff H, Fehrenbach E (2002) Inducible hsp70 expression analysis after heat and physical exercise: Transcriptional, protein expression, and subcellular localization. Ann NY Acad Sci 973: 8–12

Shi Y, Rock KL (2002) Cell death releases endogenous adjuvants that selectively enhance immune surveillance of particulate antigens. Eur J Immunol 32: 155–162

Soncin F, Zhang X, Chu B, Wang X, Asea A, Ann Stevenson M, Sacks DB, Calderwood SK (2003) Transcriptional activity and DNA binding of heat shock factor-1 involve phosphorylation on threonine 142 by CK2. Biochem Biophys Res Commun 303: 700–706

Sondermann H, Becker T, Mayhew M, Wieland F, Hartl FU (2000) Characterization of a receptor for heat shock protein 70 on macrophages and monocytes. Biol Chem 381: 1165–1174

Srivastava P (2002) Interaction of heat shock proteins with peptides and antigen presenting cells: Chaperoning of the innate and adaptive immune responses. Annu Rev Immunol 20: 395–425

Srivastava PK (2000) Heat shock protein-based novel immunotherapies. Drug News Perspect 13: 517–522

Srivastava PK (2003) Hypothesis: Controlled necrosis as a tool for immunotherapy of human cancer. Canc Immun 3: 4

Srivastava PK (2005) Immunotherapy for human cancer using heat shock protein-Peptide complexes. Curr Oncol Rep 7: 104–108

Srivastava PK, Amato RJ (2001) Heat shock proteins: the 'Swiss Army Knife' vaccines against cancers and infectious agents. Vaccine 19: 2590–2597

Srivastava PK, Udono H, Blachere NE, Li Z (1994) Heat shock proteins transfer peptides during antigen processing and CTL priming. Immunogenet 39: 93–98

Takeda K, Kaisho T, Akira S (2003) Toll-like receptors. Annu Rev Immunol 21: 335–376

Tang D, Xie Y, Zhao M, Stevenson MA, Calderwood SK (2001) Repression of the HSP70B promoter by NFIL6, Ku70, and MAPK involves three complementary mechanisms. Biochem Biophys Res Commun 280: 280–285

Terry DF, McCormick M, Andersen S, Pennington J, Schoenhofen E, Palaima E, Bausero M, Ogawa K, Perls T, Asea A (2004) Cardiovascular disease delay in centenarian offspring: Role of heat shock proteins. Ann NY Acad Sci 1019: 502–505

Vabulas RM, Ahmad-Nejad P, da Costa C, Miethke T, Kirschning CJ, Hacker H, Wagner H (2001) Endocytosed HSP60s use Toll-like receptor 2 (TLR2) and TLR4 to activate the Toll/interleukin-1 receptor signaling pathway in innate immune cells. J Biol Chem 276: 31332–31339

Vabulas RM, Ahmad-Nejad P, Ghose S, Kirschning CJ, Issels RD, Wagner H (2002a) HSP70 as endogenous stimulus of the Toll/interleukin-1 receptor signal pathway. J Biol Chem 277: 15107–15112

Vabulas RM, Braedel S, Hilf N, Singh-Jasuja H, Herter S, Ahmad-Nejad P, Kirschning CJ, Da Costa C, Rammensee HG, Wagner H, Schild H (2002b) The endoplasmic reticulum-resident heat shock protein Gp96 activates dendritic cells via the Toll-like receptor 2/4 pathway. J Biol Chem 277: 20847–20853

Wang Y, Whittall T, McGowan E, Younson J, Kelly C, Bergmeier LA, Singh M, Lehner T (2005) Identification of stimulating and inhibitory epitopes within the heat shock protein 70 molecule that modulate cytokine production and maturation of dendritic cells. J Immunol 174: 3306–3316

Westwood T, Wu C (1993) Activation of *Drosophila* heat shock factor: Conformational changes associated with monomer-to-trimer transition. Mol Cell Biol 13: 3481–3486

Wright BH, Corton JM, El-Nahas AM, Wood RF Pockley AG (2000) Elevated levels of circulating heat shock protein 70 (Hsp70) in peripheral and renal vascular disease. Heart Vessels 15: 18–22

Wu C (1995) Heat shock transcription factors: structure and regulation. Ann Rev Cell Dev Biol 11: 441–469

Xie Y, Chen C, Stevenson MA, Auron PE, Calderwood SK (2002) Heat shock factor 1 represses transcription of the IL-1b gene through physical interaction with nuclear factor of interleukin 6. J Biol Chem. 277: 11802–11810

Xie Y, Zhong R, Chen C, Calderwood SK (2003) Heat Shock factor 1 contains two functional domains that mediate transcriptional repression of the c-fos and c-fms genes. J Biol Chem 278: 4687–4698

Zanin-Zhorov A, Nussbaum G, Franitza S, Cohen IR, Lider O (2003) T cells respond to heat shock protein 60 via TLR2: Activation of adhesion and inhibition of chemokine receptors. Faseb J 17: 1567–1569

Zhang G, Ghosh S (2001) Toll-like receptor-mediated NF-kB activation: A phylogenetically conserved paradigm in innate immunity. J Clin. Invest 107: 13–19

Zitvogel L, Fernandez N, Lozier A, Wolfers J, Regnault A, Raposo G, Amigorena S (1999) Dendritic cells or their exosomes are effective biotherapies of cancer. Eur J Cancer 35 Suppl 3, S36–38

Zitvogel L, Regnault A, Lozier A, Wolfers J, Flament C, Tenza D, Ricciardi-Castagnoli P, Raposo G, Amigorena S (1998) Eradication of established murine tumors using a novel cell-free vaccine: Dendritic cell-derived exosomes. Nat Med 4: 594–600

Zou J, Guo Y, Guettouche T, Smith DF, Voellmy R (1998) Repression of heat shock transcription factor HSF1 activation by HSP90 (HSP90 complex) that forms a stress-sensitive complex with HSF1. Cell 94: 471–480

Zuo J, Rungger D, Voellmy R (1995) Activation of the DNA-binding form of human heat shock factor 1 may involve the transition from an intramolecular to an intermolecular triple-stranded coiled-coil structure. Mol Cell Biol 15: 4319–4330

Nucleic Acid Recognition Receptors in Autoimmunity

Anne Krug

Abstract Recent studies in mouse models of systemic autoimmune diseases have drawn attention to the involvement of Toll-like receptors (TLRs) in the generation of autoreactive immune responses. The endosomally localized TLRs7 and 9 are activated by autoimmune complexes containing self DNA and RNA in B lymphocytes and dendritic cells. These endogenous TLR ligands act as autoadjuvants providing a stimulatory signal together with the autoantigen and thus contribute to break peripheral tolerance against self antigens in systemic lupus erythematosus (SLE), for example. *In vivo* studies in SLE mouse models demonstrate an essential role for

Anne Krug

II. Medizinische Klinik, Klinkum Rechts der Isar, Technische Universität München, Trogerstr. 32,
D-81675 München, Germany
anne.krug@lrz.tum.de

S. Bauer, G. Hartmann (eds.), *Toll-Like Receptors (TLRs) and Innate Immunity.*
Handbook of Experimental Pharmacology 183.

TLR7 in the generation of RNA-containing antinuclear antibodies and deposition of pathogenic immune complexes in the kidney. TLR9, however, appears to have immunostimulatory as well as regulatory functions in SLE mouse models. Type I Interferon, which is produced by plasmacytoid dendritic cells in response to auto-immune complexes containing RNA and DNA recognized by TLR7 and 9 acts as a potent amplifier of the autoimmune response. TLR-independent recognition of self nucleic acids by cytosolic RNA and DNA sensors may also play a role in the gener-ation of autoimmune responses. Defects in protective mechanisms, which normally prevent immunostimulation by self nucleic acids in healthy individuals, promote the development of autoimmune diseases. For example, defects in nucleases that clear nucleic acids derived from apoptotic material, changes in the level and localization of TLR expression, defects in negative regulators of TLR signaling, or changes in the posttranscriptional modification of mammalian DNA and RNA may contribute to autoreactive responses. A better understanding of the exact function of differ-ent nucleic acid recognition receptors in the development of systemic autoimmunity will allow targeting of these innate immune receptors for the therapy of patients with systemic autoimmune diseases.

1 Function of Nucleic Acid Recognition Receptors in the Generation of Autoimmune Responses

Evidence for the critical role of nucleic acid recognition in the generation of au-toimmune responses is provided by the finding that humans and mice lacking functional nucleases, which digest excess DNA and RNA molecules in extracel-lular and intracellular compartments, develop inflammatory disorders and autoim-mune diseases such as, for example, systemic lupus erythematosus (SLE), chronic polyarthritis, myocarditis, and noninfectious encephalitis syndromes (Crow et al., 2006a; Crow et al., 2006b; Kawane et al., 2003; Kawane et al., 2006; Morita et al., 2004; Napirei et al., 2000; Shin et al., 2005; Shin et al., 2004; Yasutomo et al., 2001; Yoshida et al., 2005). In addition, several other defects in the clear-ance of apoptotic material have been shown to predispose to the development of SLE (Alarcon-Riquelme, 2005). These studies suggest that excess self nucleic acids and associated proteins trigger unwanted innate immune responses, which may then promote the generation of adaptive immunity against self antigens.

1.1 Recognition of Foreign and Self Nucleic Acids by Toll-Like Receptors

TLR3, 7, 8, and 9 have been shown to recognize nucleic acids within specific early endosomes (De Bouteiller et al., 2005; Heil et al., 2003; Latz et al., 2004; Nishiya et al., 2005). TLR3 has been reported to recognize viral or synthetic double-stranded (ds) RNA (Alexopoulou et al., 2001). Intracellular delivery of dsRNA is either achieved by uptake of virally infected apoptotic cells by dendritic cells (DC) and macrophages (Schulz et al., 2005) or by binding of free extracellular dsRNA to CD14 expressed on the surface of myeloid cells, which transports the RNA to the TLR3-containing intracellular compartment (Lee et al., 2006). TLR3 is also expressed in non-immune cell types such as vascular endothelial cells, epithelial cells (Tissari et al., 2005) and glomerular mesangial cells (Patole et al., 2005a). TLR3 signaling via adaptor molecule TRIF leads to IRF3-dependent IFN-β production and expression of NF-κB target genes (Akira et al., 2006). Triggering of TLR3 signaling by mammalian mRNA has also been reported (Kariko et al., 2004), however no *in vivo* evidence has been provided for an involvement of TLR3 in the generation of autoimmune responses against self nucleic acids.

Instead, it has been suggested that TLR3 triggering by viral RNA plays a role in the development of glomerulonephritis during viral infections such as hepatitis C, for example (Patole et al., 2005a; Pawar et al., 2006).

TLR7 and 8 recognize synthetic imidazoquinoline compounds (imiquimod, resiquimod), which are currently used for the external treatment of HPV-associated genital warts and skin cancer (Hemmi et al., 2002). The natural ligand of TLR7 and TLR8 is single-stranded (ss)RNA containing uridine-rich sequences as has been demonstrated using isolated Influenza virus RNA, which are synthetic oligonucleotides derived from viral RNA sequences or Poly U-RNA (Diebold et al., 2004; Heil et al., 2004). More recently several groups have provided evidence that specific nuclear RNAs, the U-RNAs, which are part of small nuclear ribonucleoprotein (snRNP) particles in the spliceosome, can activate B cells and DCs via TLR7 and TLR8 (Lau et al., 2005; Savarese et al., 2006; Vollmer et al., 2005). U-RNAs form stem-loop structures containing uridine-rich ds and ssRNA sequences. U1snRNP particles and the Smith (Sm)-antigen contained within U1snRNP are major autoantigens in SLE patients, which is most likely due to their TLR7-activating capacity. TLR7 is expressed on human and murine plasmacytoid and myeloid DCs as well as B cells, whereas TLR8 appears to be functional mainly in human myeloid DCs and monocytes/macrophages (Akira et al., 2006; Jarrossay et al., 2001; Kadowaki et al., 2001; Krug et al., 2001). Interestingly TLR8 has also been shown to be specifically expressed in human CD4+regulatory T cells (Peng et al., 2005). TLR9 has been identified as the receptor for bacterial and viral DNA containing unmethylated CpG dinucleotides within specific hexamer sequence motifs. The study by Leadbetter et al., showed for the first time that TLR9 in B lymphocytes can also be triggered by mammalian DNA within chromatin-containing autoimmune complexes occurring in SLE (Leadbetter et al., 2002). Defects in DNA methylation in SLE patients (Richardson et al., 1990) or preferential release of DNA containing hypomethylated CpG motifs (Sano and Morimoto, 1982) from mitochondrial DNA or CpG-islands during apoptotic cell death may lead to TLR9 activation by mammalian DNA within immune complexes in SLE patients (Marshak-Rothstein, 2006). Expression of TLR9 is restricted to plasmacytoid DCs and B cells in the human system, whereas in mice myeloid DCs and macrophages also express TLR9 (Jarrossay et al., 2001; Kadowaki et al., 2001; Krug et al., 2001).

Nucleic acid recognition pathways

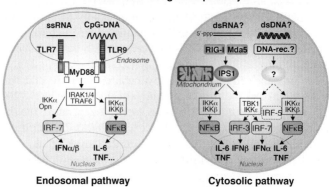

Endosomal pathway   Cytosolic pathway

Fig. 1 Nucleic acid recognition receptors and signaling pathways. Exogenous and endogenous nucleic acids (derived from bacteria/viruses and apoptotic material) can trigger the endosomal TLRs 7, 8, and 9 (left), which signal exclusively via MyD88, inducing proliferation and cytokine release in B cells, type I IFN and proinflammatory cytokine production in plasmacytoid DCs, as well as maturation and cytokine release in conventional DCs. The cytosolic pathway of nucleic acid recognition (right) involves the binding of RNA from replicating viruses to RIG-I and mda5, which signal via the essential signaling adapter IPS-1 located in the mitochondrial membrane. Viral RNA (and possibly also host RNA under specific circumstances) can trigger this pathway in many cell types including nonimmune cells. Type I IFN and inflammatory cytokine expression are induced via IRF3/7 and NF-kB activation. The existence of a similar pathway for cytosolic DNA recognition has been proposed

Interaction of TLR7, 8, and 9 with their respective ligands and initiation of signal transduction occurs within the early endosomal compartment and requires an acidic pH milieu. TLR7, 8, and 9 share a common signaling pathway (reviewed recently in (Akira 2006)), which is entirely dependent on the TIR domain-containing adaptor MyD88. MyD88 associates with TRAF6 and IRAK1/4 leading to the activation of the TAK1 complex, which subsequently activates the IKK-complex (NEMO, IKK-α, IKK-β), leading to expression of NFκB target genes. In addition the MAP kinase cascade (JNK, p38) is activated leading to the expression of AP-1 target genes. In addition to this signaling pathway, which is required for the induction of proinflammatory cytokine production by most members of the TLR family, engagement of TLR7 and 9 directly triggers IFN-α production in plasmacytoid DC via a supramolecular complex formed between MyD88, TRAF6, IRAK4, IRAK1, and IRF7, leading to phosphorylation and nuclear translocation of IRF7 (Honda et al., 2004; Kawai et al., 2004). IRF7 is constitutively expressed in plasmacytoid DC (Kerkmann et al., 2003) and induces transcription of IFN-α and IFN-β genes upon triggering of TLR7 and TLR9 (see Figure 1).

1.2 Cytosolic Sensors of Microbial RNA and DNA

Two cytosolic receptors, the caspase recruitment domain (CARD)-containing RNA helicases RIG-I (retinoic acid inducible gene I) and mda5 (melanoma differentiation antigen 5), have been identified as sensors of viral RNA generated in the cytoplasm of cells infected with RNA viruses (e.g., Influenza virus, VSV, NDV, Sendai virus) during viral replication (Kato et al., 2006; Yoneyama et al., 2005; Yoneyama et al., 2004). RIG-I specifically recognizes RNA containing a triphosphate group at the 5′ end generated by polymerases of specific RNA viruses. Addition of a 7-methyl-guanosine cap, which occurs posttranscriptionally in mammalian cells, abrogates RIG-I activation (Hornung et al., 2006; Pichlmair et al., 2006). It is therefore un-likely that self RNA could activate the RIG-I pathway, but it cannot be excluded that this may occur under specific circumstances, for example, when excess RNA is not properly degraded by nucleases or mitochondrial RNA is released. Synthetic Poly I:C RNA and EMCV RNA are specifically recognized by Mda5; however, a spe-cific RNA-sequence or structure activating Mda5 has not been identified yet (Gitlin et al., 2006; Kato et al., 2006). The cytosolic RNA helicases bind their RNA lig-ands and are then recruited to the signaling adaptor IPS-1, which is localized within the mitochondrial membrane (Kawai et al., 2005; Meylan et al., 2005; Seth et al., 2005; Xu et al., 2005). A signaling complex containing TBK1/IKKε is assembled there leading to direct activation of IRF3 and also IRF7, which trigger type I IFN expression. In addition, NF-κ B is activated in an IPS-1-dependent manner via a signaling pathway which has not been fully elucidated yet. In contrast to the TLRs which are expressed in specific immune cell types, these cytosolic RNA receptors are expressed ubiquitously also in non-immune cells (see Figure 1).

In addition to the cytosolic RNA helicases the existence of a cytosolic DNA sen-sor is postulated by several groups that have shown activation of IPS-1-independent, TBK1/IKKε-mediated activation of IRF3 and NFκB by viral, bacterial, or mam-malian DNA transfected intracellularly using cationic liposomes (see Figure 1; Ishii et al., 2006; Ishii et al., 2001; Stetson and Medzhitov, 2006). The same pathway ap-pears to be triggered by DNA viruses and intracellular bacteria. DNA within apop-totic material that is picked up by macrophages may potentially trigger this pathway, especially when there is a defect in DNA degradation or an overload with apoptotic material (Kawane et al., 2003; Kawane et al., 2006; Okabe et al., 2005; Yoshida et al., 2005). Therefore non-TLR nucleic acid recognition receptors may also be involved in the generation of inflammation and autoimmunity.

1.3 Direct Activation of B Cells by Nuclear Antigens via BCR and TLR Engagement

Since TLRs recognizing nucleic acids are sequestered within the endosomal com-partment self nucleic acids must be delivered into endosomes in order to trigger immune responses via TLRs. This can achieved in B cells by two mechanisms: First, autoreactive B cells which are quite frequent in healthy individuals (5–20%) and even more abundant in SLE patients (25–50%) due to defects in B cell tolerance checkpoints (Yurasov et al., 2005) can directly bind autoantigens released from dy-ing cells via their specific B cell receptor (BCR). Nuclear autoantigens containing nucleic acids can trigger the endosomal TLR 7 and 9 after they have been internalized by BCR-mediated endocytosis. By simultaneous engagement of BCR and TLR the autoantigen acts as an autoadjuvant and boosts the proliferation and differentiation of autoreactive B cells into plasma cells producing class switched IgG2a and IgG2b antibodies against nuclear antigens which are pathogenic. This has been shown formally *in vitro* by using BCR-transgenic B cells reacting directly with chromatin (Fields et al., 2006; Viglianti et al., 2003). A second possibility for delivery of nuclear antigens to the endosomal compartment for engagement of TLR7 and TLR9 is the binding and internalization of autoimmune complexes containing autologous IgG2a by rheumatoid factor specific B cells, which occur in high frequency in several autoimmune disorders. Studies by Ann Marshak-Rothstein's group have proven this point by making use of the AM14-BCR-transgenic mouse. AM14 B cells which express a BCR recognizing autologous IgG2a proliferate in response to autoimmune complexes formed with chromatin and monoclonal antibodies of IgG2a isotype against histone or DNA in a TLR9-dependent manner (Leadbetter et al., 2002). Correspondingly immune complexes formed with snRNP and monoclonal antibodies against the Sm protein or against RNA induced TLR7-dependent proliferation in AM14 B cells (Lau et al., 2005).

It has been known for a long time that viral and bacterial infections can trigger the initial manifestation of autoimmune diseases and can cause disease flares later on. In addition to the fact that during infections more autoantigens are released due to the death of infected host cells, infection may directly or indirectly promote activation of autoreactive B cells. Simultaneously engagement of TLRs by microbial ligands and BCR by autoantigen may lower the threshold for activation of autoreactive B cells. This has been shown recently *in vitro* and *in vivo* by Ding et al., who used anti-snRNP BCR-transgenic mice (Ding et al., 2006). Infection with viruses such as EBV may lead to the expansion of autoreactive B cell clones, which produce cross reactive antibodies against viral antigen and autoantigens (for example, the EBNA1 protein of EBV and the Sm-antigen) (McClain et al., 2005). Autoreactive B cell activation is also supported indirectly by cytokines released from infected dendritic cells and by autoreactive T helper cells. Specific Th cells recognizing self antigens can be activated by infected DCs which present autoantigens derived from dying infected cells together with microbial antigens (Banchereau and Pascual, 2006).

1.4 TLR-Mediated Activation of Dendritic Cells by Internalized Autoimmune Complexes

DCs serve a dual role in the immune system: They are essential for maintaining tolerance against self antigens and at the same time are critically involved in the initiation of effective immune responses against invading pathogens. In the absence of endogenous danger signals or infectious agents, immature DCs constantly pick up autoantigens in the form of apoptotic material and migrate to the draining lymph node, where autoantigens are presented to naïve autoreactive T cells in the absence of co-stimulation or inflammatory cytokines. Thus, autoreactive T cells are rendered anergic or are even deleted. A second mechanism for maintaining peripheral tolerance is the induction and support of regulatory T cells by dendritic cells. The generation of an effective innate and adaptive immune response against pathogens requires activation of DCs via pattern recognition receptors to induce expression of co-stimulatory molecules, MHC I and II as well as proinflammatory cytokines and chemokines. It is very likely that inappropriate activation of DCs by endogenous ligands of pattern recognition receptors is critically involved in the generation of autoimmune responses.

Most studies performed with DCs have found that myeloid as well as plasmacytoid DCs can be stimulated by nuclear antigens via TLR7 and TLR9 only when the DNA- or RNA-containing antigens are delivered intracellularly into the endosomal compartment. This can be achieved artificially by encapsulation in cationic liposomes or more physiologically by formation of immune complexes with autoimmune sera from lupus patients or with monoclonal anti-nucleosome or anti-Sm antibodies and the corresponding nuclear antigens. Early studies by Lars Ronnblom's group showed that apoptotic or necrotic material incubated with IgG from the serum of SLE patients is a potent inducer of IFN-α in plasmacytoid DCs. Type I IFN induction required the presence of SLE-IgG and the presence of nucleic acids (Bave et al., 2000; Bave et al., 2001; Lovgren et al., 2004). It was subsequently shown by confocal microscopy that DNA-containing immune complexes isolated from the serum of SLE patients bound to Fcγ RIIa/CD32a on the cell surface and then colocalized with TLR9 in acidic lysosomes in the 293 cell line transfected with CD32 and TLR9. Blocking the Fcγ RIIa/CD32a in human plasmacytoid DC with a monoclonal antibody or inhibition of endosomal acidification by bafilomycin abrogated the response to SLE-immune complexes (Bave et al., 2003; Means et al., 2005), suggesting that both the Fc receptor and TLR9 are required for activation of plasmacytoid DCs. Using TLR9-deficient and Fcγ R-deficient mice, Boule et al. showed that induction of TNF-α by chromatin-containing immune complexes in murine myeloid DC required the expression of TLR9 and Fcγ RIII. Interestingly, expression of BAFF, which is an important B cell survival factor produced by DCs, was induced independently of TLR9 (Boule et al., 2004).

More recently it has been shown that human and murine plasmacytoid and myeloid DCs are activated by defined immune complexes formed by isolated U1snRNP and SLE-IgG or monoclonal anti-Sm antibody to produce type I IFN, proinflammatory cytokines and to upregulate co-stimulatory molecules. We and others could show that DC activation by these immune complexes or by isolated U1snRNA in complex with cationic liposomes was largely mediated by TLR7 and independent of TLR3 (Savarese et al., 2006; Vollmer et al., 2005). However as has been shown by Boule et al., for TLR9 some residual DC activation (for example, upregulation of co-stimulatory molecules) was also observed in the absence of TLR7 (Boule et al., 2004; Savarese et al., 2006). Intravenous injection of U1snRNP complexes also triggered a largely TLR7-dependent cytokine response *in vivo* (unpublished data).

Taken together, these *in vitro* studies demonstrate that in contrast to autoreactive B cells, which can be directly activated by nuclear antigens, the presence of autoantibodies and the formation of autoimmune complexes is a prerequisite for TLR-mediated activation of DCs by nuclear antigens. Consequently TLR-mediated DC activation may be more important for amplification of the autoimmune response via cytokine release and activation of autoreactive T cells, than for the initiation of autoreactivity. It is possible however that TLR engagement in DCs as professional APCs is involved in the priming of autoreactive Th cells and cytotoxic T cells when apoptotic material is internalized in the context of a viral or bacterial infection, which triggers endosomal TLR7 and 9 (see Figure 2 for a model of

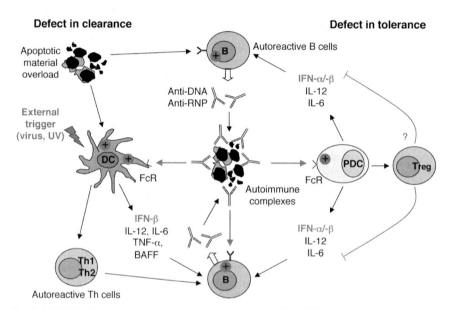

Fig. 2 Model for the generation of autoimmune responses in SLE. SLE patients and mice suffering from SLE-like disease have defects in the clearance of apoptotic cells, leading to accumulation of apoptotic material at sites of high cell turnover rates. Autoreactive B cells, which are abundant in SLE, can directly recognize nuclear antigens via their BCR and produce autoantibodies. Dendritic cells and other antigen-presenting cells pick up excess apoptotic material and present self antigens. Apoptotic material and nucleosomes themselves trigger TLR-independent DC activation. But autoantigens could also be presented in the context of a viral infection or other danger signals leading to the expression of co-stimulatory molecules, MHC class II, and cytokines by DCs, thus overcoming the threshhold for activation of autoreactive Th cells which further promote differentiation of B cells to autoantibody-producing plasma cells. Antinuclear antibodies bind to apoptotic material and form highly immunostimulatory immune complexes, which are internalized via the BCR into B cells and via Fc receptors into DCs. B cells are thus triggered via TLRs (TLR7 and 9) to produce more autoantibodies. Autoimmune complexes also trigger the activation of conventional and plasmacytoid DCs via TLR 7 and 9 ligation. Plasmacytoid DC produce large amounts of type I IFN, which together with other cytokines, promotes autoantibody production, myeloid DC differentiation, and T cell activation. Activated plasmacytoid DC can also support the generation of regulatory T cells which block immune responses against self antigens by interacting with effector T cells, DCs, and B cells. However, IL-6 released by activated DCs can reverse suppressor function of regulatory T cells

the generation of autoimmune responses in SLE). It has been shown in a recent study that DCs can also be directly activated by isolated nucleosomes in the absence of anti-nucleosome antibodies in a TLR-independent fashion (Decker et al., 2005; Ronnefarth et al., 2006). This TLR-independent pathway may be identical with the previously mentioned cytosolic DNA recognition pathway, which has not been exactly defined yet.

1.5 Type I Interferon—Amplifier of Autoimmune Responses?

As has been described in detail above, type I IFN production is induced effectively in plasmacytoid DCs in response to endogenous ligands of TLR7 and TLR9. In fact, plasmacytoid DC have been shown to be the major source of type I IFN in human SLE (Vallin et al., 1999). Early clinical studies have found elevated IFN-α levels in the serum of most patients with active SLE (Shi et al., 1987). More recently peripheral blood leucocytes of SLE patients have been shown to express type I IFNs and IFN-induced genes. This "IFN-signature" of gene expression correlated with disease activity (Baechler et al., 2003; Bennett et al., 2003). Treatment of patients with recombinant IFN-α (for hepatitis C, for example) leads to the production of antinuclear antibodies and, occasionally, SLE-like symptoms. Studies in the NZB x NZW SLE mouse model (Mathian et al., 2005; Santiago-Raber et al., 2003) and the observed correlation between trisomy of the type I IFN cluster on human chromosome 9 and SLE-like autoimmune syndromes (Zhuang et al., 2006) also indicate that type I IFNs and the interferon-producing plasmacytoid DCs may play an important role in SLE pathogenesis (Banchereau and Pascual, 2006).

Type I IFNs present in the blood of SLE patients promote autoantigen presentation by dendritic cells by supporting the differentiation of peripheral blood monocytes to DCs and inducing the expression of co-stimulatory molecules, MHC class I and class II, TAP (transporter associated with antigen processing) proteins and inflammatory cytokines in DCs, which supports expansion and activation of autoreactive Th1 cells and cytotoxic T cells. Type I IFNs promote survival and cytotoxic activity of CD8+T cells and NK cells, but also enhance the sensitivity of target cells for cytotoxicity. In addition, type I IFNs act directly on B cells to promote differentiation to plasma cells and the production of autoantibodies with pathogenic IgG2a and IgG2b isotype. Autoreactive B cell activation by U1snRNP immune complexes is amplified by the upregulation of TLR7 and MyD88 in response to type I IFN. Type I IFN receptors signaling also leads to the upregulation of IRF7 in plasmacytoid DCs and other cell types, which further upregulates IFN-α/-β release in response to endogenous TLR ligands. Thus, type I IFNs are critical for the amplification for systemic autoimmune responses in SLE, but also in other autoimmune disorders, such as Sjögren's syndrome, scleroderma, diabetes, psoriasis, and rare noninfectious encephalitis syndromes.

1.6 Role of Nucleic Acid Recognition Receptors for Organ Damage in Autoimmune Diseases

It has been shown quite convincingly that TLRs are critically involved in the initiation and amplification of immune response to self antigens. How does this relate to the development of organ damage in autoimmune diseases? Taking the example of SLE, the deposition of autoimmune complexes containing nuclear antigens and pathogenic antinuclear antibodies of the IgG2a and IgG2b isotype in glomular capillaries of the kidney leads to the activation of the complement system as well as activation of tissue resident macrophages and dendritic cells via the FcγRIV, which preferentially binds class-switched IgG2a and IgG2b antibodies. Thus, an inflammatory immune response is generated locally in the kidney; inflammatory cytokines and chemokines such as MCP-1 are produced, which further recruit immune cells including dendritic cells, macrophages, and activated T lymphocytes. The current hypothesis is that endogenous TLR ligands within deposited autoimmune complexes may participate in the activation of tissue resident and recruited hematopoetic inflammatory cells in the kidney during lupus nephritis. Direct activation of renal mesangial cells by nucleic acid recognition receptors leading to proliferation and inflammation may also occur (Patole et al., 2005a).

2 Opposing Roles of TLR7 and 9 in Mouse Models of SLE

Several recent reports provide evidence for an essential role of TLR7 in the generation of autoimmune disease in mouse models of SLE. The *yaa* (y chromosome autoimmune accelerator) mutation confers susceptibility to the development of SLE in several autoimmune-prone mouse strains. It was found by two groups that the *yaa* mutation results from a duplication and translocation to the y-chromosome of a cluster of x-linked genes, which contains TLR7 (Pisitkun et al., 2006; Subramanian et al., 2006). This leads to higher expression of TLR7 and increased TLR7 responsiveness in *yaa* mice. Backcrossing of mice carrying the *yaa* mutation to FcγRIIb-deficient mice, which have a defect in peripheral tolerance, leads to a severe aggravation of the SLE-like disease in this mouse strain, one which otherwise shows only mild disease activity. This is associated with a shift in the autoantibody repertoire from mainly anti-DNA antibodies to antinucleolar antibodies (Pisitkun et al., 2006). Similarly the *yaa* mutation exacerbates SLE-like disease in autoimmune-prone B6.NZM-*sle1* mice. The *sle1* mice carrying the *yaa* mutation produce higher titers of anti-snRNP IgG develop more severe renal disease and die earlier than those without the *yaa* mutation (Subramanian et al., 2006). These studies suggest that overexpression of TLR7 leads to an amplification of the anti-snRNP autoantibody response, which is associated with more severe SLE-like disease. However other x-linked genes translocated in the *yaa* mutation could be involved as well. Interestingly, it has been shown that females—in which SLE occurs nine times more frequently than in males—show an increased responsiveness to TLR7 ligands with regard to type I IFN production in plasmacytoid DC (Berghofer et al., 2006). There is also a strong correlation in SLE patients between expression of type I IFN and IFN-induced genes, anti-snRNP antibodies, and disease activity (Kirou et al., 2005).

By generating knock-in mice, which express the 564 autoantibody that recognizes RNA (as well as ssDNA and nucleosomes) on the C57Bl/6 background and crossing these mice with TLR7-deficient mice, Berland et al. were able to demonstrate that autoantibody production and immune complex deposition in the kidney was TLR7-dependent (Berland et al., 2006). In line with this finding the paper by Christensen et al. shows that autoantibodies against RNA-containing autoantigens are not produced in the absence of TLR7 in the spontaneous SLE model of the MRL/Mp$^{lpr/lpr}$ mouse strain (Christensen et al., 2006). Despite similar levels of anti-DNA antibodies, TLR7-deficient MRL/Mp$^{lpr/lpr}$ mice developed less severe renal disease than TLR7-expressing MRL/Mp$^{lpr/lpr}$ mice. We have found that anti-snRNP antibody production and glomerulonephritis severity are also significantly reduced in the absence of TLR7 in an inducible model of SLE in the C57BL/6 mouse strain (unpublished data). These studies suggest that the generation of antibodies against RNA-containing autoantigens specifically requires that RNA-autoantigens exert their autoadjuvant activity via activation of TLR7 in B cells and other antigen-presenting cells. Therefore, the adaptive autoimmune response is shaped by the innate immune activation by endogenous TLR ligands.

The situation is more complicated however with regard to the role of TLR9 for SLE development *in vivo*. The dramatic decrease in anti-dsDNA antibody production observed by Christensen et al. in TLR9-deficient MRL/Mp$^{lpr/lpr}$ mice (measured by Hep2 and *Chritidia luciliae* kinetoplast staining) (Christensen et al., 2006) could not be confirmed by other studies in the MRL/Mp$^{lpr/lpr}$, C57BL/6$^{lpr/lpr}$ and the *Ali5* model of SLE (measured by ELISA) (Lartigue et al., 2006; Wu and Peng, 2006; Yu et al., 2006). The different studies agree however that TLR9-deficient mice have more severe renal disease and higher mortality compared to WT mice. In some of the models studied this disease exacerbation in the absence of TLR9 was associated with an increase in the titer of RNA-reactive autoantibodies and in the percentage of mice producing these antibodies. These results are surprising because they contradict previous *in vitro* results, which showed TLR9-dependent B cell and DC activation by chromatin-containing immune complexes. In the FcγRIIb-deficient mouse model of SLE in which mainly anti-DNA and anti-nucleosome antibodies are produced, MyD88-deficiency protects against class-switching to pathogenic IgG2a and IgG2b anti-DNA autoantibodies. In FcγRIIb-deficient mice expressing an anti-nucleosome VDJ heavy chain knock in (56R), MyD88 and TLR9 are required for the production of class-switched pathogenic IgG2a and IgG2b subclasses of anti-nucleosome antibodies, but not for the production of IgM or IgG1 antinucleosome antibodies (Ehlers et al., 2006). The study goes on to show that the loss of IgG2a and IgG2b autoantibodies in TLR9-deficient mice is a B cell intrinsic defect. Therefore, the protective effect of TLR9 in the MRL/Mp$^{lpr/lpr}$, C57BL/6$^{lpr/lpr}$, and the *Ali5* models of SLE may be explained by tolerogenic effects of TLR9 activation in cells other than B cells.

The different results obtained in TLR9$^{-/-}$ and TLR7$^{-/-}$ MRL/Mp$^{lpr/lpr}$ mice (Christensen et al., 2006) were not expected, since TLR7 and TLR9 have largely overlapping expression patterns and signaling pathways. However, there may be differences in signaling downstream of TLR7 and TLR9 that have not been identified yet. For example, stimulation of plasmacytoid DCs by autoimmune complexes via TLR9 can promote regulatory T cell development that has not been reported for TLR7 activation in this cell type (Moseman et al., 2004). In contrast to TLR9, TLR7 expression is upregulated by type I IFN in B cells and DCs (Berkeredjian-Ding et al., 2005; Lau et al., 2005; Savarese et al., 2006; Vollmer et al., 2005). This amplification of the immune response to RNP-containing autoimmune complexes, which does not occur for TLR9-activating autoantigens, may make RNA-reactive autoantibodies more pathogenic. In the absence of TLR9, when TLR9-dependent regulatory factors are missing, the expansion of RNA-reactive autoantibodies leads to the development of more severe SLE disease in this specific mouse model. The specific function of TLR7 and TLR9 in human SLE is not clear yet. No association between TLR9 polymorphisms and SLE susceptibility has been found so far (De Jager et al., 2006; Hur et al., 2005). Polymorphisms of the TLR7 gene have not been studied.

3 TLR Signaling Pathways as Targets for Pharmacological Intervention

It is becoming clear now that antimalarial drugs, such as hydroxychloroquine, which have been used for several decades to treat SLE patients with reasonable efficacy, may actually target TLR7 and TLR9 signaling by blocking endosomal acidification. Chloroquine and bafilomycin have been shown to abrogate the response of B lymphocytes and dendritic cells to synthetic ligands of TLR7, 8, and 9 as well as DNA- or RNA-containing autoimmune complexes (Leadbetter et al., 2002; Vollmer et al., 2005). There has been one report showing that chloroquine and quinacrin can also directly interfere with binding of CpG-DNA to TLR9 *in vitro*, thus acting as TLR9-antagonists (Rutz et al., 2004).

Specific oligodesoxynucleotide sequences have been found that do not activate immune cells but rather inhibit the response to exogenous and endogenous ligands of TLR7 and 9 by acting as competitive antagonists. Inhibitory sequence motifs have been identified that specifically block either TLR7 or TLR9 activation or both at the same time. *In vitro* these inhibitory oligonucleotides block activation of TLR9 and/or TLR7 by nucleic acid-containing autoimmune complexes in B cells and plasmacytoid DC (Barrat et al., 2005; Lau et al., 2005; Leadbetter et al., 2002). Treatment of mice with inhibitory oligodesoxynucleotides, which interfere with both TLR9 and TLR7 activation, ameliorate SLE disease and prolong survival in the spontaneous SLE mouse models of the MRL/Mp$^{lpr/lpr}$ and NZB × NZW strains (Dong et al., 2005; Patole et al., 2005b). The effect of specific TLR7 or TLR9 blockade on SLE activity in mice has not been investigated yet. The impressive results of these preclinical studies provide evidence that TLR7 and possibly also TLR9 are attractive targets for pharmacological intervention in SLE. Other signaling molecules downstream from both TLR7 and 9 could also be targets for inhibitors, such as, for example, IRAK1/4 for specific kinase inhibitors. Other approaches aim at preventing amplification of the systemic autoimmune response by inhibiting type I IFN production by plasmacytoid DCs in response to autoimmune complexes. For example monoclonal antibodies have been developed which specifically inhibit only the type I IFN response of plasmacytoid DCs (Blasius et al., 2004; Dzionek et al., 2001).

4 TLRs and Regulation of Autoimmunity

4.1 Negative Regulation of TLR Signaling

Several molecules have been identified which specifically interfere with TLR signaling and may thus be involved in dampening innate immune responses not only to pathogens but also to self antigens. These regulation mechanisms are critical for preventing inappropriate inflammatory responses and may be defective in autoimmune diseases. They include soluble decoy TLRs, intracellular negative regulators of MyD88 signaling (e.g., IRAKM, SOCS1, NOD2, PI3Kinase, TOLLIP, A20), membrane-bound regulator proteins (e.g., ST2, SIGIRR, TRAILR, RP105), degradation of TLRs (e.g., TRIAD3A) and TLR-induced apoptosis (reviewed by Liew et al., 2005). SOCS1-deficient mice develop a severe multiorgan inflammatory disease suggesting that SOCS1 is an essential regulator of autoimmune response and inflammation. SOCS1 inhibits TLR4 and TLR9 signaling directly by interacting with IRAK1 and additionally inhibits type I IFN signaling by interfering with STAT1 phosphorylation. IRAKM-deficient mice show enhanced production of inflammatory cytokines in response to TLR4 and TLR9 ligands as well as bacterial infection, but do not develop autoimmunity or inflammation spontaneously. IRAKM interferes with the formation of IRAK1-TRAF6 complexes and may therefore inhibit signaling in responses to LPS and IL-1, but possibly also to type I IFN induction by TLR7 and 9 ligands in plasmacytoid DC, which is IRAK1-dependent. A20 blocks the MyD88-dependent and -independent signaling pathway by deubiquitylating TRAF6. A20-deficieny therefore enhances the response to several TLR ligands (TLR2, 3, 4, 9). Elevated levels of soluble ST2 are found in the serum of patients with SLE and other autoimmune and inflammatory conditions. The mechanism of action of sST2 has not been entirely clarified yet, however. The intracellular TIR-domain of SIGIRR inhibits TLR signaling by interfering with the recruitment of receptor-proximal signaling components to TLRs. In the absence of SIGIRR, dendritic cells showed enhanced inflammatory cytokine response to TLR4 and TLR9 ligands. SIGIRR-deficient mice suffer from more severe dextran sodium sulfate induced colitis than wild-type mice. None of the described negative regulators of TLR signaling have been studied in the context of systemic autoimmune diseases relevant for human diseases such as SLE. The association of a higher susceptibility to autoimmune disease with defects in the regulation of TLR signaling would provide further evidence for the important role of TLRs in the pathogenesis of systemic autoimmune diseases.

4.2 Influence of TLRs on Suppression of Systemic Autoimmunity by Regulatory T Cells

Aside from the adjuvant effect of endogenous TLR ligands mediated by direct activation of dendritic cells and B cells, TLR ligation may also break peripheral tolerance to self antigens by abrogating the suppression of immune responses by regulatory T cells (Mudd et al., 2006). Foxp3+ CD4+ CD25+ regulatory T cells, which are produced in the thymus ("natural Treg") or develop from naïve antigen-specific Th cells, are critically involved in maintaining tolerance to self antigens. Foxp3 has been identified as a critical regulator of CD4+ CD25+ Treg development and function (Fontenot et al., 2003). Foxp3-mutant scurfy mice and neonatal mice depleted of Foxp3-expressing Treg cells develop a lethal multiorgan autoimmune syndrome (Brunkow et al., 2001; Lahl et al., 2007). Adoptive transfer of Treg cells has been used successfully for the prevention and treatment of several autoimmune disorders in mouse models (Suri-Payer and Fritzsching, 2006). *In vitro* Treg cells act directly on effector T cells to suppress their proliferation and differentiation. On the other hand, *in vivo* immunosuppression by Treg cells is also mediated by downmodulation of dendritic cell function by inducing the expression of inhibitory cytokines (TGF-β, IL-10) and cell surface molecules which block effector T cells development and function.

Pasare and Medzhitov have shown that TLR triggering by microbial ligands blocks the suppressive function of Treg cells and therefore allows the generation of an effective adaptive immune response to pathogens (Pasare and Medzhitov, 2003). This inhibition of suppressor function was dependent on TLR-induced IL-6 production by antigen-presenting cells. It has been shown, however, that TLR ligands can also directly act on effector T cells and regulatory T cells (Caron et al., 2005; Peng et al., 2005). TLR ligation in effector T cells may confer resistance to Treg cell-mediated suppression, whereas TLR ligation in Treg cells may directly block their suppressive function. Human Treg cells have been shown to express TLR1, 2, 3, 4, 5, 6, 7, and 8 but not TLR9 (Caramalho et al., 2003). Peng et al. showed in a recent publication that TLR8 triggering in Treg cells abrogated their inhibitory action on effector T cells (Peng et al., 2005). Considering the critical role of TLR7 (and possibly TLR8 in humans) for the generation of autoimmune responses in SLE, we propose that inhibition of Treg cell suppressor function, either directly by interaction with endogenous TLR7/8 ligands or indirectly via TLR7/8-mediated activation of DCs and B cells, also contributes to development of SLE disease.

Coming back to the surprising finding that in contrast to TLR7, TLR9 has protective effects in a spontaneous mouse model of SLE, it should be mentioned that TLR9 ligands might also induce tolerance instead of immune activation. For example, intravenous injection of CpG together with a model antigen leads to tolerance induction (in contrast to subcutaneous injection) (Wingender et al., 2006). It has also been reported that intravenous CpG injection induces the production of tolerogenic indolamindioxygenase (IDO) in a specialized subpopulation of plasmacytoid DC (Mellor et al., 2005). Human plasmacytoid DC activated by TLR9 ligand CpG have also been shown to induce the generation of Treg cells *in vitro* (Moseman et al., 2004). Therefore TLR9 may have immunostimulatory as well as regulatory functions and its exact role in SLE remains to be determined.

5 Protective Mechanisms Preventing Autoimmune Activation by Self Nucleic Acids

Several mechanisms exist that can prevent activation of immune cells by self nucleic acids. Localization of nucleic acid recognition receptors in defined intracellular compartments (such as the endosomal compartment for TLR3, 7, 8, 9) provides a barrier for the recognition of self nucleic acids. We and others have seen that activation of these receptors by chromatin or RNA-containing autoantigen requires sufficient intracellular delivery by liposomes or uptake of immune complexes via Fc receptors or the BCR (Lau et al., 2005; Means et al., 2005; Savarese et al., 2006). Forced expression of TLR9 on the cell surface, for example, can overcome this barrier and enables recognition of free extracellular self-DNA (Barton et al., 2006).

Another important protective mechanism is the rapid clearance of apoptotic material and degradation of excess nucleic acids by nucleases. Severe autoimmune disorders develop in mice and humans with defects in these enzymes. Mice lacking the extracellular nuclease DNAseI spontaneously develop SLE-like disease (Napirei et al., 2000) and mutations in the DNAseI gene have been found in two Japanese patients with SLE (Yasutomo et al., 2001). In Korean SLE patients DNAseI polymorphisms correlated with anti-DNA and anti-RNP antibody levels (Shin et al., 2004). DNAseII, which is localized in the phagosomal compartment of macrophages, is responsible for the digestion of DNA from apoptotic cells and nuclei expelled from erythroid progenitor cells, which are engulfed by macrophages (Kawane et al., 2003; Yoshida et al., 2005). DNAseII-deficient mice die *in utero* due to development of lethal anemia, which is due to a strong induction of type I IFN and IFN-responsive genes in macrophages, which interferes with hematopoesis (Yoshida et al., 2005). TLR9 was not responsible for type I IFN induction in DNAseII-deficient cells, suggesting the involvement of a different intracellular DNA-sensor (Okabe et al., 2005). DNAseII$^{-/-}$ mice with defective type I IFN signaling develop a chronic polyarthritis syndrome associated with the overexpression of TNF-α in macrophages (Kawane et al., 2006). Genetic studies have found a higher risk for renal disease in SLE patients with single nucleotide polymorphisms in the DNAse

II gene (Shin et al., 2005). DNAseIII (Trex1)-deficient mice develop inflammatory myocarditis and die prematurely from heart failure (Morita et al., 2004). The mechanism of protection from inflammation by Trex1 is not clear yet. However, two recent reports describe four mutations in patients with a rare non-infectious encephalitis syndrome (Aicardi–Goutieres syndrome), one of which affects the Trex1 gene (Crow et al., 2006a). The other three mutations were located to another nuclease, the RNAseH2 (Crow et al., 2006b). Aicardi–Goutieres syndrome is associated with elevated type I IFN levels and lymphocyte numbers in the cerebrospinal fluid, and IFN-α appears to play a critical role for the pathogenesis of this disease (Akwa et al., 1998; Goutieres, 2005; Lebon et al., 1988). Some patients with AGS also have skin lesions similar to those of SLE patients (De Laet et al., 2005). Most likely, a so-far unidentified nucleic acid recognition receptor (possibly RIG-I or mda5) is triggered by undigested intracellular RNA and mediates type I IFN induction in this disease. However, TLR7 or 8 in plasmacytoid DCs, which can be recruited to the brain, could also be involved (Pashenkov et al., 2002). These reports emphasize the importance of nucleases to prevent autoimmunity due to recognition of self nucleic acids.

Recent data also support the paradigm that pattern recognition receptors that have evolved to recognize pathogens are able to distinguish between self and foreign nucleic acids, which provides another mechanism of protection against immune stimulation by self nucleic acids. For example, RNA transcribed in mammalian cells is subject to posttranscriptional modification. Incorporation of 2′O-methylated nucleotides, pseudouridines, and 2-thiouridines, or the addition of 7-methyl-guoanosine caps, can prevent activation of TLR7/8 or RIG-I by self RNA (Hornung et al., 2006; Kariko et al., 2005; Pichlmair et al., 2006; Savarese et al., 2006). However, as an exception to this rule we have found that U1snRNA, for example, stimulates TLR7 despite the presence of several modifications when transfected into mammalian cells (Savarese et al., 2006). Similarly, methylation of mammalian DNA cannot entirely prevent activation of TLR9 by self DNA, because hypomethylated CpG islands and mitochondrial DNA can be released which trigger immune responses. It can be envisioned that defects in methylation and other modifications of nucleic acids or preferential release of unmodified DNA and RNA sequences during apoptotic or necrotic cell death contribute to SLE susceptibility.

6 Concluding Remarks

From the studies discussed in this review it is becoming clear that exogenous and endogenous ligands of nucleic acid receptors may have important functions in the pathogenesis of autoimmune diseases such as SLE. Convincing studies in SLE mouse models point to a specific role of TLR7 in the generation of autoimmunity, which may be applicable to a subgroup of patients with SLE. It is not clear at present how the different cell populations expressing TLR7 (DCs, B cells, Treg cells) contribute to disease development. It also remains to be investigated which exact role TLR9 plays in SLE and if tolerance or autoimmune activation dominates the response to endogenous TLR9 ligands. The question as to how autoimmunity is initiated and which innate immune receptors and cell types are involved in these early events remain to be answered at present. Addressing these questions experimentally will advance the development of therapeutics targeting nucleic acid recognition pathways for the treatment of systemic autoimmune diseases.

References

Akira S, Uematsu S, Takeuchi O (2006) Pathogen recognition and innate immunity. Cell 124: 783–801

Akwa Y, Hassett DE, Eloranta ML, Sandberg K, Masliah E, Powell H, Whitton JL, Bloom FE, Campbell IL (1998) Transgenic expression of IFN-alpha in the central nervous system of mice protects against lethal neurotropic viral infection but induces inflammation and neurodegeneration. J Immunol 161: 5016–526

Alarcon-Riquelme ME (2005) The genetics of systemic lupus erythematosus. J Autoimmun 25 Suppl: 46–48

Alexopoulou L, Holt AC, Medzhitov R, Flavell RA (2001) Recognition of double-stranded RNA and activation of NF-kappaB by Toll- like receptor 3. Nature 413: 732–738

Baechler EC, Batliwalla FM, Karypis G, Gaffney PM, Ortmann WA, Espe KJ, Shark KB, Grande WJ, Hughes KM, Kapur V, Gregersen PK, Behrens TW (2003) Interferon-inducible gene expression signature in peripheral blood cells of patients with severe lupus. Proc Natl Acad Sci USA 100: 2610–2615

Banchereau J, Pascual V (2006) Type I interferon in systemic lupus erythematosus and other autoimmune diseases. Immunity 25: 383–392

Barrat FJ, Meeker T, Gregorio J, Chan JH, Uematsu S, Akira S, Chang B, Duramad O, Coffman RL (2005) Nucleic acids of mammalian origin can act as endogenous ligands for Toll-like receptors and may promote systemic lupus erythematosus. J Exp Med 202: 1131–1139

Barton GM, Kagan JC, Medzhitov R (2006) Intracellular localization of Toll-like receptor 9 prevents recognition of self DNA but facilitates access to viral DNA. Nat Immunol 7: 49–56

Bave U, Alm GV, Ronnblom L (2000) The combination of apoptotic U937 cells and lupus IgG is a potent IFN-alpha inducer. J Immunol 165: 3519–3526

Bave U, Magnusson M, Eloranta ML, Perers A, Alm GV, Ronnblom L (2003) Fc gamma RIIa is expressed on natural IFN-alpha-producing cells (plasmacytoid dendritic cells) and is required for the IFN-alpha production induced by apoptotic cells combined with lupus IgG. J Immunol 171: 3296–3302

Bave U, Vallin H, Alm GV, Ronnblom L (2001) Activation of natural interferon-alpha producing cells by apoptotic U937 cells combined with lupus IgG and its regulation by cytokines. J Autoimmun 17: 71–80

Bennett L, Palucka AK, Arce E, Cantrell V, Borvak J, Banchereau J, Pascual V (2003) Interferon and granulopoiesis signatures in systemic lupus erythematosus blood. J Exp Med 197: 711–723

Berghofer B, Frommer T, Haley G, Fink L, Bein G, Hackstein H (2006) TLR7 ligands induce higher IFN-alpha production in females. J Immunol 177: 2088–2096

Berkeredjian-Ding IB, Wagner M, Hornung V, Giese T, Schnurr M, Endres S, Hartmann G (2005) Plasmacytoid dendritic cells control TLR7 sensitivity of naive B cells via type I IFN. J Immunol 174: 4043–4050

Berland R, Fernandez L, Kari E, Han JH, Lomakin I, Akira S, Wortis HH, Kearney JF, Ucci AA, Imanishi-Kari T (2006) Toll-like Receptor 7-dependent loss of B cell tolerance in pathogenic autoantibody knockin mice. Immunity 25: 429–440

Blasius A, Vermi W, Krug A, Facchetti F, Cella M, Colonna M (2004) A cell-surface molecule selectively expressed on murine natural interferon-producing cells that blocks secretion of interferon-alpha. Blood 103: 4201–4206

Boule MW, Broughton C, Mackay F, Akira S, Marshak-Rothstein A, Rifkin IR (2004) Toll-like receptor 9-dependent and -independent dendritic cell activation by chromatin-immunoglobulin G complexes. J Exp Med 199: 1631–1640

Brunkow ME, Jeffery EW, Hjerrild KA, Paeper B, Clark LB, Yasayko SA, Wilkinson JE, Galas D, Ziegler SF, Ramsdell F (2001) Disruption of a new forkhead/winged-helix protein, Scurfin, results in the fatal lymphoproliferative disorder of the scurfy mouse. Nat Genet 27: 68–73

Caramalho I, Lopes-Carvalho T, Ostler D, Zelenay S, Haury M, Demengeot J (2003) Regulatory T cells selectively express Toll-like receptors and are activated by lipopolysaccharide. J Exp Med 197: 403–411

Caron G, Duluc D, Fremaux I, Jeannin P, David C, Gascan H, Delneste Y (2005) Direct stimulation of human T cells via TLR5 and TLR7/8: Flagellin and R-848 up-regulate proliferation and IFN-gamma production by memory CD4+T cells. J Immunol 175: 1551–1557

Christensen SR, Shupe J, Nickerson K, Kashgarian M, Flavell RA, Shlomchik MJ (2006) Toll-like receptor 7 and TLR9 dictate autoantibody specificity and have opposing inflammatory and regulatory roles in a murine model of lupus. Immunity 25: 417–428

Crow YJ, Hayward BE, Parmar R, Robins P, Leitch A, Ali M, Black DN, van Bokhoven H, Brunner HG, Hamel BC, Corry PC, Cowan FM, Frints SG, Klepper J, Livingston JH, Lynch SA, Massey RF, Meritet JF, Michaud JL, Ponsot G, Voit T, Lebon P, Bonthron DT, Jackson AP, Barnes DE, Lindahl T (2006a) Mutations in the gene encoding the 3'-5' DNA exonuclease TREX1 cause Aicardi–Goutieres syndrome at the AGS1 locus. Nat Genet 38: 917–920

Crow YJ, Leitch A, Hayward BE, Garner A, Parmar R, Griffith E, Ali M, Semple C, Aicardi J, Babul-Hirji R, Baumann C, Baxter P, Bertini E, Chandler KE, Chitayat D, Cau D, Dery C, Fazzi E, Goizet C, King MD, Klepper J, Lacombe D, Lanzi G, Lyall H, Martinez-Frias ML, Mathieu M, McKeown C, Monier A, Oade Y, Quarrell OW, Rittey CD, Rogers RC, Sanchis A, Stephenson JB, Tacke U, Till M, Tolmie JL, Tomlin P, Voit T, Weschke B, Woods CG, Lebon P, Bonthron DT, Ponting CP, Jackson AP (2006b) Mutations in genes encoding ribonuclease H2 subunits cause Aicardi–Goutieres syndrome and mimic congenital viral brain infection. Nat Genet 38: 910–916

De Bouteiller O, Merck E, Hasan UA, Hubac S, Benguigui B, Trinchieri G, Bates EE, Caux C (2005) Recognition of double-stranded RNA by human Toll-like receptor 3 and downstream receptor signaling requires multimerization and an acidic pH. J Biol Chem 280: 3813–3845

De Jager PL, Richardson A, Vyse TJ, Rioux JD (2006) Genetic variation in Toll-like receptor 9 and susceptibility to systemic lupus erythematosus. Arthritis Rheum 54: 1279–1282

De Laet C, Goyens P, Christophe C, Ferster A, Mascart F, Dan B (2005) Phenotypic overlap between infantile systemic lupus erythematosus and Aicardi–Goutieres syndrome. Neuropediatrics 36: 399–402

Decker P, Singh-Jasuja H, Haager S, Kotter I, Rammensee HG (2005) Nucleosome, the main autoantigen in systemic lupus erythematosus, induces direct dendritic cell activation via a MyD88-independent pathway: Consequences on inflammation. J Immunol 174: 3326–3334

Diebold SS, Kaisho T, Hemmi H, Akira S, Reis ESC (2004) Innate antiviral responses by means of TLR7-mediated recognition of single-stranded RNA. Science 303: 1529–1531

Ding C, Wang L, Al-Ghawi H, Marroquin J, Mamula M, Yan J (2006) Toll-like receptor engagement stimulates anti-snRNP autoreactive B cells for activation. Eur J Immunol 36: 2013–2024

Dong L, Ito S, Ishii KJ, Klinman DM (2005) Suppressive oligodeoxynucleotides delay the onset of glomerulonephritis and prolong survival in lupus-prone NZB × NZW mice. Arthritis Rheum 52: 651–658

Dzionek A, Sohma Y, Nagafune J, Cella M, Colonna M, Facchetti F, Gunther G, Johnston I, Lanzavecchia A, Nagasaka T, Okada T, Vermi W, Winkels G, Yamamoto T, Zysk M, Yamaguchi Y, Schmitz J (2001) BDCA-2, a novel plasmacytoid dendritic cell-specific type II C-type lectin, mediates antigen capture and is a potent inhibitor of interferon alpha/beta induction. J Exp Med 194: 1823–1834

Ehlers M, Fukuyama H, McGaha TL, Aderem A, Ravetch JV (2006) TLR9/MyD88 signaling is required for class switching to pathogenic IgG2a and 2b autoantibodies in SLE. J Exp Med 203: 553–561

Fields ML, Metzgar MH, Hondowicz BD, Kang SA, Alexander ST, Hazard KD, Hsu AC, Du YZ, Prak EL, Monestier M, Erikson J (2006) Exogenous and endogenous TLR ligands activate anti-chromatin and polyreactive B cells. J Immunol 176: 6491–6502

Fontenot JD, Gavin MA, Rudensky AY (2003) Foxp3 programs the development and function of CD4+ CD25+ regulatory T cells. Nat Immunol 4: 330–336

Gitlin L, Barchet W, Gilfillan S, Cella M, Beutler B, Flavell RA, Diamond MS, Colonna M (2006) Essential role of mda-5 in type I IFN responses to polyriboinosinic:polyribocytidylic acid and encephalomyocarditis picornavirus. Proc Natl Acad Sci USA 103: 8459–8464

Goutieres F (2005) Aicardi–Goutieres syndrome. Brain Dev 27: 201–206

Heil F, Ahmad-Nejad P, Hemmi H, Hochrein H, Ampenberger F, Gellert T, Dietrich H, Lipford G, Takeda K, Akira S, Wagner H, Bauer S (2003) The Toll-like receptor 7 (TLR7)-specific stimulus loxoribine uncovers a strong relationship within the TLR7, 8 and 9 subfamily. Eur J Immunol 33: 2987–2997

Heil F, Hemmi H, Hochrein H, Ampenberger F, Kirschning C, Akira S, Lipford G, Wagner H, Bauer S (2004) Species-specific recognition of single-stranded RNA via Toll-like receptor 7 and 8. Science 303: 1526–1529

Hemmi H, Kaisho T, Takeuchi O, Sato S, Sanjo H, Hoshino K, Horiuchi T, Tomizawa H, Takeda K, Akira S (2002) Small anti-viral compounds activate immune cells via the TLR7 MyD88-dependent signaling pathway. Nat Immunol 3: 196–200

Honda K, Yanai H, Mizutani T, Negishi H, Shimada N, Suzuki N, Ohba Y, Takaoka A, Yeh WC, Taniguchi T (2004) Role of a transductional-transcriptional processor complex involving MyD88 and IRF-7 in Toll-like receptor signaling. Proc Natl Acad Sci USA 101: 15416–15421

Hornung V, Ellegast J, Kim S, Brzozka K, Jung A, Kato H, Poeck H, Akira S, Conzelmann KK, Schlee M, Endres S, Hartmann G (2006) 5′-triphosphate RNA is the ligand for RIG-I. Science 314: 994–997

Hur JW, Shin HD, Park BL, Kim LH, Kim SY, Bae SC (2005) Association study of Toll-like receptor 9 gene polymorphism in Korean patients with systemic lupus erythematosus. Tissue Antigens 65: 266–270

Ishii KJ, Coban C, Kato H, Takahashi K, Torii Y, Takeshita F, Ludwig H, Sutter G, Suzuki K, Hemmi H, Sato S, Yamamoto M, Uematsu S, Kawai T, Takeuchi O, Akira S (2006) A Toll-like receptor-independent antiviral response induced by double-stranded B-form DNA. Nat Immunol 7: 40–48

Ishii KJ, Suzuki K, Coban C, Takeshita F, Itoh Y, Matoba H, Kohn LD, Klinman DM (2001) Genomic DNA released by dying cells induces the maturation of APCs. J Immunol 167: 2602–2607

Jarrossay D, Napolitani G, Colonna M, Sallusto F, Lanzavecchia A (2001) Specialization and complementarity in microbial molecule recognition by human myeloid and plasmacytoid dendritic cells. Eur J Immunol 31: 3388–3393

Kadowaki N, Ho S, Antonenko S, Malefyt RW, Kastelein RA, Bazan F, Liu YJ (2001) Subsets of human dendritic cell precursors express different Toll-like receptors and respond to different microbial antigens. J Exp Med 194: 863–869

Kariko K, Buckstein M, Ni H, Weissman D (2005) Suppression of RNA recognition by Toll-like receptors: The impact of nucleoside modification and the evolutionary origin of RNA. Immunity 23: 165–175

Kariko K, Ni H, Capodici J, Lamphier M, Weissman D (2004) mRNA is an endogenous ligand for Toll-like receptor 3. J Biol Chem 279: 12542–12550

Kato H, Takeuchi O, Sato S, Yoneyama M, Yamamoto M, Matsui K, Uematsu S, Jung A, Kawai T, Ishii KJ, Yamaguchi O, Otsu K, Tsujimura T, Koh CS, Reis e Sousa C, Matsuura Y, Fujita T, Akira S (2006) Differential roles of mda5 and RIG-I helicases in the recognition of RNA viruses. Nature 441: 101–105

Kawai T, Sato S, Ishii KJ, Coban C, Hemmi H, Yamamoto M, Terai K, Matsuda M, Inoue J, Uematsu S, Takeuchi O, Akira S (2004) Interferon-alpha induction through Toll-like receptors involves a direct interaction of IRF7 with MyD88 and TRAF6. Nat Immunol 5: 1061–1068

Kawai T, Takahashi K, Sato S, Coban C, Kumar H, Kato H, Ishii KJ, Takeuchi O, Akira S (2005) IPS-1, an adaptor triggering RIG-I- and Mda5-mediated type I interferon induction. Nat Immunol 6: 981–988

Kawane K, Fukuyama H, Yoshida H, Nagase H, Ohsawa Y, Uchiyama Y, Okada K, Iida T, Nagata S (2003) Impaired thymic development in mouse embryos deficient in apoptotic DNA degradation. Nat Immunol 4: 138–144

Kawane K, Ohtani M, Miwa K, Kizawa T, Kanbara Y, Yoshioka Y, Yoshikawa H, Nagata S (2006) Chronic polyarthritis caused by mammalian DNA that escapes from degradation in macrophages. Nature 443: 998–1002

Kerkmann M, Rothenfusser S, Hornung V, Towarowski A, Wagner M, Sarris A, Giese T, Endres S, Hartmann G (2003) Activation with CpG-A and CpG-B oligonucleotides reveals two distinct regulatory pathways of type I IFN synthesis in human plasmacytoid dendritic cells. J Immunol 170: 4465–4474

Kirou KA, Lee C, George S, Louca K, Peterson MG, Crow MK (2005) Activation of the interferon-alpha pathway identifies a subgroup of systemic lupus erythematosus patients with distinct serologic features and active disease. Arthritis Rheum 52: 1491–1503

Krug A, Towarowski A, Britsch S, Rothenfusser S, Hornung V, Bals R, Giese T, Engelmann H, Endres S, Krieg AM, Hartmann G (2001) Toll-like receptor expression reveals CpG DNA as a unique microbial stimulus for plasmacytoid dendritic cells which synergizes with CD40 ligand to induce high amounts of IL-12. Eur J Immunol 31: 3026–3037

Lahl K, Loddenkemper C, Drouin C, Freyer J, Arnason J, Eberl G, Hamann A, Wagner H, Huehn J, Sparwasser T (2007) Selective depletion of Foxp3+ regulatory T cells induces a scurfy-like disease. J Exp Med 204: 57–63

Lartigue A, Courville P, Auquit I, Francois A, Arnoult C, Tron F, Gilbert D, Musette P (2006) Role of TLR9 in anti-nucleosome and anti-DNA antibody production in lpr mutation-induced murine lupus. J Immunol 177: 1349–1354

Latz E, Schoenemeyer A, Visintin A, Fitzgerald KA, Monks BG, Knetter CF, Lien E, Nilsen NJ, Espevik T, Golenbock DT (2004) TLR9 signals after translocating from the ER to CpG DNA in the lysosome. Nat Immunol 5: 190–198

Lau CM, Broughton C, Tabor AS, Akira S, Flavell RA, Mamula MJ, Christensen SR, Shlomchik MJ, Viglianti GA, Rifkin IR, Marshak-Rothstein A (2005) RNA-associated autoantigens activate B cells by combined B cell antigen receptor/Toll-like receptor 7 engagement. J Exp Med 202: 1171–1177

Leadbetter EA, Rifkin IR, Hohlbaum AM, Beaudette BC, Shlomchik MJ, Marshak-Rothstein A (2002) Chromatin-IgG complexes activate B cells by dual engagement of IgM and Toll-like receptors. Nature 416: 603–607

Lebon P, Badoual J, Ponsot G, Goutieres F, Hemeury-Cukier F, Aicardi J (1988) Intrathecal synthesis of interferon-alpha in infants with progressive familial encephalopathy. J Neurol Sci 84: 201–208

Lee HK, Dunzendorfer S, Soldau K, Tobias PS (2006) Double-stranded RNA-mediated TLR3 activation is enhanced by CD14. Immunity 24: 153–163

Liew FY, Xu D, Brint EK, O'Neill LA (2005) Negative regulation of toll-like receptor-mediated immune responses. Nat Rev Immunol 5: 446–458

Lovgren T, Eloranta ML, Bave U, Alm GV, Ronnblom L (2004) Induction of interferon-alpha production in plasmacytoid dendritic cells by immune complexes containing nucleic acid released by necrotic or late apoptotic cells and lupus IgG. Arthritis Rheum 50: 1861–1872

Marshak-Rothstein A (2006) Toll-like receptors in systemic autoimmune disease. Nat Rev Immunol 6: 823–835

Mathian A, Weinberg A, Gallegos M, Banchereau J, Koutouzov S (2005) IFN-alpha induces early lethal lupus in preautoimmune (New Zealand Black × New Zealand White) F1 but not in BALB/c mice. J Immunol 174: 2499–2506

McClain MT, Heinlen LD, Dennis GJ, Roebuck J, Harley JB, James JA (2005) Early events in lupus humoral autoimmunity suggest initiation through molecular mimicry. Nat Med 11: 85–89

Means TK, Latz E, Hayashi F, Murali MR, Golenbock DT, Luster AD (2005) Human lupus autoantibody-DNA complexes activate DCs through cooperation of CD32 and TLR9. J Clin Invest 115: 407–417

Mellor AL, Baban B, Chandler PR, Manlapat A, Kahler DJ, Munn DH (2005) Cutting edge: CpG oligonucleotides induce splenic CD19+ dendritic cells to acquire potent indoleamine 2,3-dioxygenase-dependent T cell regulatory functions via IFN type 1 signaling. J Immunol 175: 5601–5605

Meylan E, Curran J, Hofmann K, Moradpour D, Binder M, Bartenschlager R, Tschopp J (2005) Cardif is an adaptor protein in the RIG-I antiviral pathway and is targeted by hepatitis C virus. Nature 437: 1167–1172

Morita M, Stamp G, Robins P, Dulic A, Rosewell I, Hrivnak G, Daly G, Lindahl T, Barnes DE (2004) Gene-targeted mice lacking the Trex1 (DNase III) $3'- > 5'$ DNA exonuclease develop inflammatory myocarditis. Mol Cell Biol 24: 6719–6727

Moseman EA, Liang X, Dawson AJ, Panoskaltsis-Mortari A, Krieg AM, Liu YJ, Blazar BR, Chen W (2004) Human plasmacytoid dendritic cells activated by CpG oligodeoxynucleotides induce the generation of CD4+ CD25+ regulatory T cells. J Immunol 173: 4433–4442

Mudd PA, Teague BN, Farris AD (2006) Regulatory T cells and systemic lupus erythematosus. Scand J Immunol 64: 211–218

Napirei M, Karsunky H, Zevnik B, Stephan H, Mannherz HG, Moroy T (2000) Features of systemic lupus erythematosus in Dnase-1-deficient mice. Nat Genet 25: 177–181

Nishiya T, Kajita E, Miwa S, Defranco AL (2005) TLR3 and TLR7 are targeted to the same intracellular compartments by distinct regulatory elements. J Biol Chem 280: 37107–37117

Okabe Y, Kawane K, Akira S, Taniguchi T, Nagata S (2005) Toll-like receptor-independent gene induction program activated by mammalian DNA escaped from apoptotic DNA degradation. J Exp Med 202: 1333–1339

Pasare C, Medzhitov R (2003) Toll pathway-dependent blockade of CD4+ CD25+ T cell-mediated suppression by dendritic cells. Science 299: 1033–1036

Pashenkov M, Teleshova N, Kouwenhoven M, Smirnova T, Jin YP, Kostulas V, Huang YM, Pinegin B, Boiko A, Link H (2002) Recruitment of dendritic cells to the cerebrospinal fluid in bacterial neuroinfections. J Neuroimmunol 122: 106–116

Patole PS, Grone HJ, Segerer S, Ciubar R, Belemezova E, Henger A, Kretzler M, Schlondorff D, Anders HJ (2005a) Viral double-stranded RNA aggravates lupus nephritis through Toll-like receptor 3 on glomerular mesangial cells and antigen-presenting cells. J Am Soc Nephrol 16: 1326–1338

Patole PS, Zecher D, Pawar RD, Grone HJ, Schlondorff D, Anders HJ (2005b) G-rich DNA suppresses systemic lupus. J Am Soc Nephrol 16: 3273–3280

Pawar RD, Patole PS, Wornle M, Anders HJ (2006) Microbial nucleic acids pay a Toll in kidney disease. Am J Physiol Renal Physiol 291: F509–516

Peng G, Guo Z, Kiniwa Y, Voo KS, Peng W, Fu T, Wang DY, Li Y, Wang HY, Wang RF (2005) Toll-like receptor 8-mediated reversal of CD4+ regulatory T cell function. Science 309: 1380–1384

Pichlmair A, Schulz O, Tan CP, Naslund TI, Liljestrom P, Weber F, Reis ESC (2006) RIG-I-mediated antiviral responses to single-stranded RNA bearing $5'$ phosphates. Science 314: 997–1001

Pisitkun P, Deane JA, Difilippantonio MJ, Tarasenko T, Satterthwaite AB, Bolland S (2006) Autoreactive B cell responses to RNA-related antigens due to TLR7 gene duplication. Science 312: 1669–1672

Richardson B, Scheinbart L, Strahler J, Gross L, Hanash S, Johnson M (1990) Evidence for impaired T cell DNA methylation in systemic lupus erythematosus and rheumatoid arthritis. Arthritis Rheum 33: 1665–1673

Ronnefarth VM, Erbacher AI, Lamkemeyer T, Madlung J, Nordheim A, Rammensee HG, Decker P (2006) TLR2/TLR4-independent neutrophil activation and recruitment upon endocytosis of nucleosomes reveals a new pathway of innate immunity in systemic lupus erythematosus. J Immunol 177: 7740–7749

Rutz M, Metzger J, Gellert T, Luppa P, Lipford GB, Wagner H, Bauer S (2004) Toll-like receptor 9 binds single-stranded CpG-DNA in a sequence- and pH-dependent manner. Eur J Immunol 34: 2541–2550

Sano H, Morimoto C (1982) DNA isolated from DNA/anti-DNA antibody immune complexes in systemic lupus erythematosus is rich in guanine-cytosine content. J Immunol 128: 1341–1345

Santiago-Raber ML, Baccala R, Haraldsson KM, Choubey D, Stewart TA, Kono DH, Theofilopoulos AN (2003) Type-I interferon receptor deficiency reduces lupus-like disease in NZB mice. J Exp Med 197: 777–788

Savarese E, Chae OW, Trowitzsch S, Weber G, Kastner B, Akira S, Wagner H, Schmid RM, Bauer S, Krug A (2006) U1 small nuclear ribonucleoprotein immune complexes induce Type I interferon in plasmacytoid dendritic cells through TLR7. Blood 107: 3229–3234

Schulz O, Diebold SS, Chen M, Naslund TI, Nolte MA, Alexopoulou L, Azuma YT, Flavell RA, Liljestrom P, Reis e Sousa C (2005) Toll-like receptor 3 promotes cross-priming to virus-infected cells. Nature 433: 887–892

Seth RB, Sun L, Ea CK, Chen ZJ (2005) Identification and characterization of MAVS, a mitochondrial antiviral signaling protein that activates NF-kappaB and IRF 3. Cell 122: 669–682

Shi SN, Feng SF, Wen YM, He LF, Huang YX (1987) Serum interferon in systemic lupus erythematosus. Br J Dermatol 117: 155–159

Shin HD, Park BL, Cheong HS, Lee HS, Jun JB, Bae SC (2005) DNase II polymorphisms associated with risk of renal disorder among systemic lupus erythematosus patients. J Hum Genet 50: 107–111

Shin HD, Park BL, Kim LH, Lee HS, Kim TY, Bae SC (2004) Common DNase I polymorphism associated with autoantibody production among systemic lupus erythematosus patients. Hum Mol Genet 13: 2343–2350

Stetson DB, Medzhitov R (2006) Recognition of cytosolic DNA activates an IRF3-dependent innate immune response. Immunity 24: 93–103

Subramanian S, Tus K, Li QZ, Wang A, Tian XH, Zhou J, Liang C, Bartov G, McDaniel LD, Zhou XJ, Schultz RA, Wakeland EK (2006) A TLR7 translocation accelerates systemic autoimmunity in murine lupus. Proc Natl Acad Sci USA 103: 9970–9975

Suri-Payer E, Fritzsching B (2006) Regulatory T cells in experimental autoimmune disease. Springer Semin Immunopathol 28: 3–16

Tissari J, Siren J, Meri S, Julkunen I, Matikainen S (2005) IFN-alpha enhances TLR3-mediated antiviral cytokine expression in human endothelial and epithelial cells by up-regulating TLR3 expression. J Immunol 174: 4289–4294

Vallin H, Blomberg S, Alm GV, Cederblad B, Ronnblom L (1999) Patients with systemic lupus erythematosus (SLE) have a circulating inducer of interferon-alpha (IFN-alpha) production acting on leucocytes resembling immature dendritic cells. Clin Exp Immunol 115: 196–202

Viglianti GA, Lau CM, Hanley TM, Miko BA, Shlomchik MJ, Marshak-Rothstein A (2003) Activation of autoreactive B cells by CpG dsDNA. Immunity 19: 837–847

Vollmer J, Tluk S, Schmitz C, Hamm S, Jurk M, Forsbach A, Akira S, Kelly KM, Reeves WH, Bauer S, Krieg AM (2005) Immune stimulation mediated by autoantigen binding sites within small nuclear RNAs involves Toll-like receptors 7 and 8. J Exp Med 202: 1575–1585

Wingender G, Garbi N, Schumak B, Jungerkes F, Endl E, von Bubnoff D, Steitz J, Striegler J, Moldenhauer G, Tuting T, Heit A, Huster KM, Takikawa O, Akira S, Busch DH, Wagner H, Hammerling GJ, Knolle PA, Limmer A (2006) Systemic application of CpG-rich DNA suppresses adaptive T cell immunity via induction of IDO. Eur J Immunol 36: 12–20

Wu X, Peng SL (2006) Toll-like receptor 9 signaling protects against murine lupus. Arthritis Rheum 54: 336–42

Xu LG, Wang YY, Han KJ, Li LY, Zhai Z, Shu HB (2005) VISA is an adapter protein required for virus-triggered IFN-beta signaling. Mol Cell 19: 727–740

Yasutomo K, Horiuchi T, Kagami S, Tsukamoto H, Hashimura C, Urushihara M, Kuroda Y (2001) Mutation of DNASE1 in people with systemic lupus erythematosus. Nat Genet 28: 313–314

Yoneyama M, Kikuchi M, Matsumoto K, Imaizumi T, Miyagishi M, Taira K, Foy E, Loo YM, Gale M, Jr., Akira S, Yonehara S, Kato A, Fujita T (2005) Shared and unique functions of the DExD/H-box helicases RIG-I, MDA5, and LGP2 in antiviral innate immunity. J Immunol 175: 2851–2858

Yoneyama M, Kikuchi M, Natsukawa T, Shinobu N, Imaizumi T, Miyagishi M, Taira K, Akira S, Fujita T (2004) The RNA helicase RIG-I has an essential function in double-stranded RNA-induced innate antiviral responses. Nat Immunol 5: 730–737

Yoshida H, Okabe Y, Kawane K, Fukuyama H, Nagata S (2005) Lethal anemia caused by interferon-beta produced in mouse embryos carrying undigested DNA. Nat Immunol 6: 49–56

Yu P, Wellmann U, Kunder S, Quintanilla-Martinez L, Jennen L, Dear N, Amann K, Bauer S, Winkler TH, Wagner H (2006) Toll-like receptor 9–independent aggravation of glomerulonephritis in a novel model of SLE. Int Immunol 18: 1211–1219

Yurasov S, Wardemann H, Hammersen J, Tsuiji M, Meffre E, Pascual V, Nussenzweig MC (2005) Defective B cell tolerance checkpoints in systemic lupus erythematosus. J Exp Med 201: 703–711

Zhuang H, Kosboth M, Lee P, Rice A, Driscoll DJ, Zori R, Narain S, Lyons R, Satoh M, Sobel E, Reeves WH (2006) Lupus-like disease and high interferon levels corresponding to trisomy of the Type I interferon cluster on chromosome 9p. Arthritis Rheum 54: 1573–1579

Dendritic Cell Subsets and Toll-Like Receptors

Hubertus Hochrein(✉) and Meredith O'Keeffe

Abstract Toll-like receptors exist as highly conserved pathogen sensors through-out the animal kingdom and they represent a key family of molecules bridging the ancient innate and adaptive immune systems. The first molecules of adaptive immunity appeared in the cartilaginous fishes and, with these, major histocompatibility proteins and cells expressing these molecules, and thus, by definition, the advent of antigen-presenting cells and the "professional" antigen-presenting cells, the dendritic cells. Dendritic cells themselves are highly specialized subsets of cells with the major roles of antigen presentation and stimulation of lymphocytes. The dendritic cell functions of inducing immunity are regulated by their own activation status, which is governed by their encounter with pathogen-associated molecular patterns that signal through pattern recognition receptors, including Toll-like receptors, expressed at the surface and within the cytoplasm and endosomal membranes of dendritic cells. Thus although dendritic cells play a crucial role in the induction of adaptive immunity, the adaptive response is itself initiated at the level of ancient

Hubertus Hochrein

Bavarian Nordic GmbH, Fraunhoferstrasse 13, D-82152 Martinsried, Germany

hubertus.hochrein@bavarian-nordic.com

S. Bauer, G. Hartmann (eds.), *Toll-Like Receptors (TLRs) and Innate Immunity.*
Handbook of Experimental Pharmacology 183.

receptors of the innate immune system. A further degree in the complexity of dendritic cell activation is established by the fact that not all dendritic cells are equal. Dendritic cells exist as multiple subsets that vary in location, function, and phenotype. Distinct dendritic cell subsets display great variation in the type of Toll-like receptors expressed and consequently variation in the type of pathogens sensed and the subsequent type of immune responses initiated.

1 Mouse Dendritic Cells

Within all species studied, dendritic cells (DC) are rare cells present in blood, skin, and all lymphoid organs. In the spleen, for example, they account for only about 1% of total splenocytes. Yet it is clear that these rare cells are crucial for normal immune responses. Mice depleted of DC display defective immune responses to viral (Ciavarra et al., 2006), parasitic (Jung et al., 2002; Liu et al., 2006a) and bacterial infections (Jung et al., 2002).

The most extensive studies of DC subtypes have been carried out in the mouse system. It is clear that within every mouse lymphoid organ and blood there are two distinct categories of DC: conventional (c)DC and plasmacytoid (p)DC. The same scenario exists in other mammalian species, including in humans and rats, although the further separation of these DC categories into subsets that are paralleled across species barriers is not straightforward. The following sections provide an overview of mouse DC subsets, with a comparison to human and rat DC subsets in Section 3.

1.1 Conventional Dendritic Cells

Within mouse lymphoid organs the cDC can be recognized by the expression of high levels of CD11c and MHC II (Shortman and Liu, 2002). The cDC conform to the historical, functional, and morphological definition of a DC, that is, a veiled cell that has the unique ability to stimulate a naïve T cell into cycle (Steinman 1991). Further separation of the cDC into subsets depends upon the organ in question and these subsets are discussed below.

1.1.1 Spleen

The DC of spleen are present at an abundance of 1% of total splenocytes. Of these, approximately 80% are cDC and the remaining 20% are pDC (these numbers are somewhat skewed to higher pDC numbers in 129sv mice Asselin-Paturel et al., 2003). The separation of spleen cDC into functionally distinct subsets is possible by the separation of CD11c^{hi}MHC II$^+$ cells based on the expression of CD4 and the

Table 1 Differential expression of selected molecules on the cell surface of spleen cDC subsets

	CD4⁻CD8⁻	CD4⁺CD8⁻	CD4⁻CD8⁺
CD1d[1]	+/−	+/−	++
CD5[1]	+	++	+/−
CD11b[2]	++	++	+/−
CD22[1]	+	++	+/−
CD24[2]	+	+	+++
CD36[3]	+/−	+/−	++
CD49f[2]	+	+	+++
CD72[1]	+	+	−
CD81[1]	+	+/−	++
CD103[1]	−	−	++
CD205[2]	+	+	+++
F4/80[2]	++	++	+/−
Sirp-α[4]	++	++	+/−

[1](Edwards et al., 2003a), [2](Vremec et al., 2000),
[3](Belz et al., 2002), [4](Lahoud et al., 2006)

CD8αα homodimer (Vremec et al., 2000). Numerous other cell surface molecules are also differentially expressed between the three subsets (summarized in Table 1).

CD8⁺ Spleen DC

The CD8⁺CD4⁻ subset, about 25% of total spleen cDC, resides in the T cell areas of spleen and is the shortest lived of the spleen cDC subtypes with a turnover rate of about three days (Kamath et al., 2000). The CD8⁺ cDC, unlike other cDC of spleen, absolutely require Interferon response factor 8 (IRF8, also known as ISCBP) for development and normal function (Tamura et al., 2005).

The CD8⁺ DC are important *in vivo* due to their ability to secrete extremely high levels of the pro-inflammatory cytokine IL-12p70 upon activation, lending these cells with a Th-1-inducing profile (Maldonado-Lopez et al., 1999). The CD8⁺ cDC also express other cytokines upon activation including IL-6, TNF-α, and low levels of chemokines including Mip-1α and β and RANTES (Proietto et al., 2004). Under some circumstances the CD8α⁺ DC also produce type I IFN (Hochrein et al., 2001).

The CD8⁺ cDC in all organs are unique amongst the cDC as they have the exquisite ability to constitutively present exogenous cell-associated or soluble proteins very efficiently in the context of MHC I (den Haan et al., 2000; Pooley et al., 2001; Schnorrer et al., 2006). This process is known as "cross-presentation" and it is thought to be important in the context of CD8 T cell priming in viral infections and in tumour surveillance and maintenance of peripheral tolerance (for recent reviews see Cresswell et al., 2005; Groothuis and Neefjes, 2005; Shen and Rock, 2006). Amongst the splenic DC, the CD8⁺ cells are the primary cells that induce CTL immunity to lytic and nonlytic viruses and intracellular bacteria (Belz et al., 2004a;

Belz et al., 2005). Although noninfection of the CD8$^+$ cDC has not been proven in all cases, their enhanced ability to cross-present and cross-prime probably plays a major role in this ability to prime CTL.

CD4$^+$ Spleen DC

The CD4$^+$CD8$^-$ cDC of mouse spleen comprise about 50% of spleen cDC and are located in non-T cell zones of the spleen. They require IRF4 and IRF2 for development and normal function (Ichikawa et al., 2004; Tamura et al., 2005). The CD4$^+$ cDC stand out as the cDC population that produces the highest levels of inflammatory-type chemokines: Mip-3α, Mip-3β, RANTES (Proietto et al., 2004). Quite high levels of these chemokines are produced by the CD4$^+$cDC, even in the resting state. The functional significance of this is not yet understood.

When compared to the CD8$^+$ cDC, the cross-presentation capacity of CD4$^+$ cDC in the steady state is poor. However, the CD4$^+$ cDC display a high capacity to stimulate CD4$^+$ and CD8$^+$ T cells in "direct" presentation assays. In fact the CD4$^+$ cDC, together with the CD4$^-$CD8$^-$ cDC are the most potent presenters of MHC II-antigen complexes to CD4$^+$ T cells (den Haan and Bevan, 2002; Pooley et al., 2001). Contrary to CD8$^+$ cDC, the CD4$^+$ cDC and CD4$^-$CD8$^-$ cDC have been shown to induce TH2 responses by responder T cells (Hammad et al., 2004; Maldonado-Lopez et al., 1999).

CD4$^-$CD8$^-$ Spleen DC

DC in mouse spleen that lack both CD4 and CD8 expression comprise about 20–25% of spleen cDC and closely resemble the CD4$^+$ DC in function. Similarly, they also produce high levels of Mip-3α, Mip-3β and RANTES, although the levels produced in the steady state are considerably lower than those produced by the CD4$^+$ cDC. The CD4$^-$CD8$^-$ cDC are also poor at cross-presenting exogenous antigen, although they are as efficient as CD4$^+$ cDC in direct MHC I and MHC II presentation (Schnorrer et al., 2006). It was earlier believed that the CD4$^-$CD8$^-$ cDC produced quite high levels of IFN-γ. However, the recent identification of the immediate cDC precursor in spleen has revealed that the IFN-γ activity is derived from a small population of Sirpα^- DC precursors within the CD4$^-$CD8$^-$ subset (Vremec et al., 2007).

Studies examining the BrdU incorporation of cDC subsets indicated that the CD4$^-$CD8$^-$ cDC are not the precursors of either CD4$^+$ or CD8$^+$ cDC, although the microarray data now available does suggest that at least the majority of cells that are identified as CD4$^-$CD8$^-$ DC are extremely closely related to the CD4$^+$ cDC (Edwards et al., 2003a; Lahoud et al., 2006). However, it remains true that the CD4$^-$CD8$^-$ cDC are not as heavily reduced in numbers as the CD4$^+$ cDC in an

IRF4, IRF2 (Tamura et al., 2005), or NF-κ B p50 knockout mouse (O'Keeffe et al., 2005). Moreover, mice treated with fms-like tyrosine kinase 3 ligand (Flt3-L) have a large increase in CD4$^-$CD8$^-$ and CD8$^+$ cDC but not CD4$^+$ cDC, and, in contrast, the CD4$^+$ cDC are preferentially increased in a mouse treated with pegylated GM-CSF (O'Keeffe et al., 2002b).

A caveat to these studies is that they were carried out before the identification of the CD4$^-$CD8$^-$ Sirpα$^-$ precursor subset. Given the identification of contaminating cells within the CD4$^-$CD8$^-$ cDC population, the concept of CD4$^-$CD8$^-$ cDC as a distinct cell type and not as a direct precursor of the CD4$^+$ cDC needs to be reinvestigated.

It should be noted here that both spleen CD8$^-$ cDC subsets can, under certain circumstances, cross-present antigen at least as well as CD8$^+$ cDC. den Haan and Bevan (2002) have shown that ovalbumin/Ig complexes are efficiently cross-presented to CTL by CD8$^-$ cDC. The key here is signaling and or intracellular rerouting of antigen via the FcR-γ. Thus, the context of antigen with additional activatory ligands, if in an immune complex, or additionally if seen together with Toll-like receptor (TLR) ligands (Maurer et al., 2002), may endow all cDC, at least in spleen, with the ability to cross-present antigens.

1.1.2 Thymic cDC

As in the spleen, the primary separation of DC in mouse thymus can be made by the distinction between pDC and cDC, with the pDC:cDC ratio approximately 1:3 in C57BL/6 mice.

Most thymic DC are located in the medulla or at the cortico-medullary junction. The thymic cDC all stain positively for low levels of CD8αβ, contributed by "uptake" from thymocytes (Vremec et al., 2000) and thus it is difficult to cleanly separate the cells based on CD8α expression alone. All thymic cDC are also CD205$^+$, regardless of the CD8 expression (Kamath et al., 2002). However, CD8α^{hi} cells also are negative for the expression of Sirpα, and thus cells can be separated as CD8α^{hi}Sirpα$^-$ and CD8α^{lo}Sirpα$^+$ subsets (Lahoud et al., 2006).

Their location in the thymic medulla suggests that the cDC would not play a major role in positive selection, this role being carried out predominantly by cortical epithelial cells. However, the cDC are purported to play a role in negative selection in the medulla (reviewed in Wu and Shortman, 2005), and in the medullary positive selection of regulatory T cells (Watanabe et al., 2005; Wu and Shortman, 2005).

It is clear that unseparated thymic cDC have a high capacity to directly present antigen to CD4$^+$ T cells (Wilson et al., 2003). Whether the CD8α^{hi} DC are capable of cross-presenting antigen, akin to the spleen cDC, has not been reported. As in the spleen, the CD8α^{hi} cDC are the most proficient producers of IL-12p70 (Hochrein et al., 2001), although at levels about 50% that of the spleen cells. The effects on thymocyte selection upon cDC activation in the thymus have not been examined.

1.1.3 Lymph Node cDC

All lymph nodes (LN) contain the two major classes of DC, pDC, and cDC, although their subsets of cDC are not identical. All lymph nodes appear to contain the "resident" CD8$^+$ and CD8$^-$ cDC, but they also contain heterogeneous populations of migratory DC. The nature of these migratory cDC differs between organ- and skin-draining lymph nodes and also possibly differs depending on the location of the lymph node.

The CD11c^{hi}MHC II$^+$ cells of the subcutaneous LN can be divided into four main categories—those which have one of the following phenotypes: CD8α^{hi} CD205$^+$MHC II^{int}Sirpα^-; CD8$\alpha^{-/lo}$MHC II^{hi}CD205^{hi}; CD8α^-CD205^{int}MHC II^{hi}; and CD8α^-CD205$^-$MHC II^{int}. The CD8$\alpha^{-/lo}$CD205^{hi} cells are the skin-derived Langerhans cells, cDC that have migrated from the epidermis, dermal-derived DC are the CD8$^-$CD205^{int} cells. The separation between the Langerhans, dermal-derived DC, and the CD205$^-$ cDC is quite arbitrary, particularly if the CD205 staining is suboptimal. The recent inclusion of Sirpα as a marker to separate CD8$^+$ and CD8$^-$ cDC may be extremely useful in discerning the subcutaneous LN subsets further. Recent studies by Lahoud et al. (2006) show a biphasic distribution of Sirpα expression by those cells thought to contain the dermal cDC subset, with half of these cells bearing the phenotype Sirpα^{hi} and the other half Sirpα^{lo}. The functional significance of this, and potential relevance to their origin, is yet to be investigated.

The CD8$^-$CD205$^-$ cDC of LN also contain a low number of CD4$^+$ cDC. However, the CD4 marker is not reliable to distinguish LN cDC subsets since Henri et al., (2001) have shown that DC derived from CD4-deficient bone marrow (BM) cells acquire CD4 expression in the LN, presumably due to pick-up from CD4$^+$ T cells.

Lymph Node CD8$^+$ cDC

As with the spleen and thymus, lymph node CD8^{hi} cDC are the major producers of IL-12p70, although they produce considerably less of this cytokine than their spleen counterparts (Hochrein et al., 2001). It is tempting to speculate that the IL-12p70 producing LN CD8$^+$ cDC constitutes only one compartment of the LN CD8$^+$ cDC, perhaps only that which is involved in immunity and not tolerance. Indeed, it is clear that the CD8$^+$ cDC of the LN are extremely important in both arms of the adaptive immune system. Studies by the Belz, Heath, and Carbone groups have shown that CD8$^+$ DC of lymph nodes, whether they be skin- or tissue-draining are, like spleen CD8$^+$ cDC, major players in the induction of CD8$^+$ T cell immunity to viral infection via intranasal, footpad, or subcutaneous routes (Allan et al., 2003; Belz et al., 2004a; Belz et al., 2004b; Belz et al., 2005; Smith et al., 2003).

On the other hand, the CD8$^+$ cDC of lymph node are also thought to be essential for the maintenance of peripheral tolerance to tissue antigens. In the transgenic mouse model of Belz et al., (2002) peptides derived from proteins expressed under the rat insulin promoter in the pancreas were presented by CD8$^+$ cDC in the pancreatic draining lymph node, in a process termed cross-tolerance.

Clearly the potent ability of the LN CD8$^+$ cDC to cross-present antigen and to subsequently cross-prime and cross-tolerize CTL is of upmost importance in the adaptive immune system. However, it is likely that the signals to the CD8$^+$ cDC that tip the balance from tolerance to immunity are induced via innate receptors such as TLR.

Langerhans and Dermal-Derived Dendritic Cells

The CD8$^{-/lo}$CD205^{hi} Langerhans and CD8$^-$CD205^{int} dermal-derived DC within the subcutaneous LN are long-lived, with a half-life of 9–10 days (Kamath et al., 2002). The Langerhans cells, originating from the skin, are radio-resistant and can be recognized histologically by the presence of intracellular Birbeck granules within the cytoplasm. A marker of Langerhans cells expressed on the surface and within the Birbeck granules is the C-type lectin Langerin. Recent elegant studies by Kissenpfennig et al. (2005) indicate that the Langerhans cells and dermal-derived DC traffic to, and reside in, nonoverlapping areas of the LN paracortex. Moreover, skin painting with TRITC and the ability to clearly distinguish Langerhans cells by EGFP expression, revealed as previously suggested (Kamath et al., 2002), that the dermal DC traffic to LN with much faster kinetics than the Langerhans cells. Dermal DC reaching the LN peaked at two days whilst it took four days for Langerhans cells to reach peak numbers in the LN.

The skin-derived dendritic cells within the LN are the only cDC thus far described that have an activated phenotype in the steady state. These cells in LN express at least a log-fold higher of MHC II and co-stimulation markers than other cDC. When resident within the epidermis and dermis the Langerhans and dermal DC, with a much less activated phenotype, continually acquire antigen. Upon extravasation into the LN (which, under steady state conditions, continues only at a slow "trickle"), they are activated, leaving these cells with the "frozen" antigen-carrying phenotype that they acquired in the skin, since once activated they are unable to further process LN-borne antigen (Wilson et al., 2003). The level of activation of Langerhans cells upon entering the LN is similar whether in steady state or inflammatory conditions. Thus, in the skin-draining LN the Langerhans act as "snapshots" of the local skin environment. The precise role of Langerhans cells in T cell stimulation in skin-draining LN remains rather controversial, with opposing views regarding their ability to cross-present and/or directly present antigen to T cells (Allan et al., 2003; Iezzi et al., 2006; Kissenpfennig and Malissen, 2006; Le et al., 2006).

It is currently a prominent view that Langerhans and dermal DC act as couriers in ferrying antigen from cutaneous locations to other DC for presentation in the draining LN. However, it is still possible that any of the following—the nature of the antigen or, for example, whether the DC themselves are infected by a virus, or the type of pattern recognition stimulus received by the Langerhans cell or dermal DC in the epidermis—may influence the subsequent T cell presentation and the nature of the DC directly involved. It is also clear that different researchers use a variety of established techniques to isolate Langerhans cells that may hamper the correlation of results. They are variously purified from LN or called from skin explants using CCL21 (Saeki et al., 1999) and/or several days' culture (Ortner et al., 1996) or isolated directly from the epidermis using trypsin (Schuler and Steinman, 1985) or generated *in vitro* from CD34$^+$ precursors using TGFβ (Geissmann et al., 1998; Strobl et al., 1997). The isolation of Langerhans cell preparations, probably also containing dermal DC, from subcutaneous LN has been undertaken at various time points after infections or skin sensitization. Given the finding that peak numbers of Langerhans cells do not reach the lymph node until four days after TRITC skin painting, whereas dermal DC take only two days (Kissenpfennig et al., 2005), the need for multiple-day kinetic studies to accurately examine the function of different skin-derived DC subsets seems necessary. Recent studies have also shown that the expression of Langerin is not confined to Langerhans cells but it is also expressed by CD8$^+$ cDC of lymphoid organs (Kissenpfennig et al., 2005) and thus functions previously attributed to Langerin$^+$ cells could in fact be attributable to the CD8$^+$ cDC.

A feature of Langerhans cells is high expression of CD1a. Hunger et al., (2004) have shown that Langerhans cells can efficiently present microbial lipopeptides but this CD1a-mediated lipopeptide presentation remains to be proven *in vivo*. In addition, the role of Langerhans cells per se in "supervision" of skin resident T cells or their interaction with memory CD8 T cells that home to the skin after viral infection (Liu et al., 2006b) remains to be elucidated.

Migrating DC from Non-Skin-Draining Lymph Nodes

LN that drain non-skin tissues also contain a heterogeneous population of cells with a phenotype resembling the dermal DC of subcutaneous LN. These CD8$^-$CD205^{int} DC are en masse termed "migratory DC," the majority of which are thought to derive from the drained tissue. Within the mediastinal LN draining the lungs this population of migratory DC contains a subset of F4/80$^+$CD11b$^-$ DC that, along with the LN resident CD8$^+$ cDC, have been shown to be potent stimulators of CTL after intranasal viral infection (Belz et al., 2004b). DC with a similar phenotype were also shown to be present in renal and hepatic LN, but no functional assays were carried out. Skin-draining LN and the mesenteric LN did not appear to contain DC with this F4/80$^+$ CD11b$^-$ phenotype. Within the gastric LN CD8$^-$ and CD8$^+$ cDC, both subsets probably CD205$^+$ (although cell scarcity restricted phenotypic analyses, and only microscopic analysis of CD205 was possible) can present stomach tissue antigen to specific T cells (Scheinecker et al., 2002). Whether the probable CD8$^-$CD205$^+$ cDC population capable of this is also F4/80$^+$ was not investigated.

Another group has recently published the identification of DC that express high levels of the integrin CD103, also expressed on spleen CD8$^+$ cDC (Edwards et al., 2003a) that are found in the lung epithelia and arteriolar wall (Sung et al., 2006). These cDC also express Langerin and are CD11b$^{-/lo}$. Whether these DC express DEC205 or F4/80 was not examined in this study. However, it is tempting to speculate that these CD103$^+$ cells may indeed be the tissue form of the CD8$^-$F4/80$^+$CD11b$^-$CD205^{int} cells identified by Belz et al. (2004). In addition, given the Langerin$^+$ phenotype and the production of IL-12 in response to TLR3 ligands, perhaps these cells are the non-lymphoid tissue equivalents of CD8$^+$ cDC.

It has recently been shown that within the muscular layer of the intestine (not including the lamina propria and submucosa) exists an extensive network of cDC with the phenotype CD11c$^+$CD205$^+$Langerin$^+$ (Flores-Langarica et al., 2005). These novel cDC take up anti-CD205/ovalbumin conjugates *in vivo*, and when then admixed with OT-I and OT-II T cells *in vitro*, can present ovalbumin peptides in the context of both MHC I and MHC II. These DC also respond with cell surface upregulation of co-stimulation markers (CD80, CD86) in response to orally administered pathogens. It has not yet been investigated whether these DC traffic to mesenteric LN. Like the newly identified lung epithelial DC, the cells migrating to mesenteric LN from the intestine are CD103$^+$ (Salazar-Gonzalez et al., 2006). Whether the cells of the muscularis layer described by Flores-Langarica et al. (2005) are actually those thought to arise from the lamina propria is not clear nor has the expression of CD103 been examined. The study of Worbs et al. (2006) has shown that removal of mesenteric LN ablates oral tolerance, and that CD103$^+$ DC migrating in a CCR7-dependent manner from the intestine are probably the essential players. The CCR7-dependent migration of lamina propria CD205$^+$CD11b$^+$/CD11b$^-$ DC subsets to mesenteric LN has also been shown by Jang et al. (2006). With the additional information of Chung et al., (2005) that CD8$^-$CD11b$^+$ cDC are the cells responsible for tolerance to gastrointestinally induced antigen, it is strikingly clear that at least one other subset of DC exists in the mouse that is capable of efficient cross-presentation in the absence of exogenous stimulus. Whether the different intestinal cell populations mentioned above are one and the same requires further investigation, as does their relationship to the mediastinal cross-priming cells described by Belz et al., (2004) and the lung epithelial cells described by Sung et al. (2006).

1.1.4 cDC of Other Organs

The liver has notoriously been a difficult organ from which to directly purify DC due to the difficulty of separating DC from autofluorescent and fragile Kupffer cells. Lian et al. (2003) have described a gentle PBS perfusion method that allowed the isolation and identification of two subsets of cDC in murine liver. These cDC have the phenotype CD11c$^+$CD11b$^+$ and CD11c$^+$CD11b$^-$. Both populations lack CD205 expression and are biphasic for MHC II expression, with both containing a clearly MHC II^{hi} population and a MHC II$^{lo/-}$ population. Both subsets appear capable of allogeneic T cell stimulation and in the low-level production of IL-12p40, IL-6 and TNF-α. Further investigation into these liver DC subsets, including the separation based on MHC II expression, may help to shed further light into the DC subsets and their differential functions within mouse liver.

Recently, the kidney has also been shown to contain multiple cDC subsets (Soos et al., 2006). All appear to be CD11b$^+$F4/80^{lo} and could be separated into at least two subsets based on the expression of CX3CR1.

1.1.5 Immature cDC of Blood and Bone Marrow

The blood of mice contains very few cells that display the level of CD11c and MHC II of organ DC. In a steady state mouse we have previously found a variable low number of these DC, numbering only up to about 1000 in the total blood obtained from a mouse (O'Keeffe et al., 2003). BM likewise contains very few CD11c^{hi}MHC II$^+$ DC. The low numbers of these cDC found in the blood, and BM has precluded their detailed study but we have seen that they are CD4$^-$CD8$^-$ and mainly CD11b$^+$ (O'Keeffe et al., 2003, and unpublished observations).

Instead both blood (O'Keeffe et al., 2003) and BM (unpublished observations) contains a population of CD11c^{int}MHC II$^{lo/-}$ CD11b$^+$CD4$^-$CD8$^-$ cells that up-regulate MHC II and co-stimulation markers after overnight culture and maturation is further enhanced with GM-CSF or, additionally, TNFα.

1.2 Plasmacytoid DC

Plasmacytoid DC (pDC) defy the classical definition of a DC since in the steady state they completely lack any cytoplasmic protrusions or veils and lack the ability to stimulate naïve T cells into cycle. However, upon activation by viruses, TLR7, 8, or 9 ligands (discussed below) they rapidly acquire the morphological and phenotypical characteristics of a cDC together of course with their trade mark high type I IFN production. There is no doubt that these cells have a major function in innate immune responses with their exceptional ability to produce rapid, high levels of type I IFN upon activation. Several recent reviews have described pDC development and functional properties known to date (Barchet et al., 2005b; Barchet et al., 2005a; Fuchsberger et al., 2005; Liu, 2005; Naik et al., 2005a; Soumelis and Liu 2006).

It remains though, from the studies of numerous groups, that the ability of pDC to stimulate naïve Tcells into cycle is still somewhat under a cloud—yes they can—but the majority opinion would be that relative to the cDC populations they are not very good at it. This lack of potent stimulatory activity has raised the argument that pDC should not be inducted into the DC "family" at all.

Several recent reports cite pDC as capable and necessary of maintaining tolerance (Abe et al., 2005a; de Heer et al., 2004; Ochando et al., 2006). Indeed the study of Ochando et al., (2006) elegantly portrayed the pDC as an essential cell type in the induction of tolerance to allogeneic cardiac transplants via the induction of alloantigen-specific regulatory T cells (T-regs). Perhaps the interaction of pDC with T-regs is of general and major importance given the observation that pDC, at least from BM, prolong hematopoietic stem cell engraftment (Fugier-Vivier et al., 2005).

The pDC of mice display, fortunately to date, nowhere near the subset complexity of the cDC. The pDC in all organs have the phenotype $CD11c^{int}MHC\ II^{lo}CD11b^-$ $CD205^-$. In mouse blood the pDC are $CD4^-CD8^-$ but in all other organs the pDC exist in each of the following four phenotypes $CD4^-CD8^-$, $CD4^-CD8^+$, $CD4^+$ $CD8^-$, $CD4^+CD8^+$.

The expression of CD4 is clearly a differentiation marker, with $CD4^-$ pDC differentiating into $CD4^+$ pDC. Although $CD4^+$ and $CD4^-$ pDC also display different functional attributes, possibly due to differences in the expression of pattern recognition receptors during development. The expression of $CD8\alpha$ on steady state pDC has no known function but it is clearly upregulated to high levels on all pDC subsets with activation (O'Keeffe et al., 2002a).

Another marker differentially expressed on pDC is Ly49Q. In Balb/c mice it has been reported that Ly49Q is expressed on essentially all peripheral pDC outside of the BM. In BM Ly49Q divides pDC into 2 functionally distinct cell populations with $Ly49Q^-$ cells less responsive to Influenza virus and producers of lower levels of IL-6 and $TNF\alpha$ in response to CpG stimulation (Kamogawa-Schifter et al., 2005). Using a different mAb and in C57BL/6 mice, Omatsu et al. (2005) showed that whilst the majority of $Ly49Q^-$ cells exist in C57BL/6 BM, significant numbers also exist in lymphoid organs outside of the BM. The $Ly49Q^-$ and $Ly49Q^+$ pDC also differed in their cytokine responses to CpG and Sendai virus (Omatsu et al., 2005). Both studies showed that Ly49Q is a differentiation marker of pDC, $Ly49Q^-$ cells are also $CD4^-$ and that they develop into $Ly49Q^+CD4^+$ pDC.

Although detailed studies on the functional attributes of pDC from different anatomical locations is still in its infancy, there is some indication that different tissue locations lend different functional attributes to pDC. The pDC of BM respond to HSV-1 in a TLR9-dependent and independent manner (Hochrein et al., 2004). Only the TLR9 dependent response is detectable in spleen pDC (Hochrein et al., 2004; Krug et al., 2004b). Whether environmental factors influence the function of the same pDC subsets or whether distinct pDC subsets exist in different environments is not yet clear.

2 Relationship of Mouse DC Subsets to Human DC

The logistical and ethical constraints limiting access to human tissues have meant a strong mouse bias in defining and characterising *ex vivo* isolated DC subsets. Many surface markers used to define functionally distinct mouse DC are not expressed on human DC, and thus correlations between the species have proven difficult. For instance, the $CD8\alpha$ molecule is not expressed on any human DC population and conversely, all human DC express CD4. Thus, the majority of studies working with freshly isolated human cDC define only pDC and cDC populations, without further subdivision. The exception here is the differentiation of human skin cDC into Langerhans cells and dermal-derived DC.

Although the phenotypes of mouse and human pDC are not identical, they share many surface molecules such as CD45RA, CD45RB and CD68. Moreover, they express a similar pattern of intracellular TLR (see Section 5) that endows both human and mouse pDC with the ability to respond to similar pathogens. Morphologically, the human and mouse cells are very similar, they are similarly found in blood, throughout lymphoid organs, and inflamed tissue, and they share the same capacity to produce very high levels of type I IFN.

The Hart group has published extensive surface phenotype data that will further the characterization of human DC subsets. These researchers have identified five DC subsets in human blood (MacDonald et al., 2002) and tonsils (Summers et al., 2001), four cDC subsets that differ in surface phenotype and the pDC, and they have characterized the DC subsets' T cell allostimulatory potential. However, other functional information on each of the subsets is lacking. The commercial availability of the antibodies BDCA-1 and -3 for human cDC isolation has assisted in standardizing the methods used for human DC isolation and allow the separation of human cDC into two subsets. However, DC purification with these antibodies probably results in overlapping of the subsets described by the Hart studies. It should also be noted that although the BDCA-1$^+$ and BDCA-3$^+$ cDC in blood and tonsils share some surface markers, the extensive microarray analyses presented by Lindstedt et al. (2005) demonstrate that at the transcriptome level these cells are substantially different in the two different environments (Lindstedt et al., 2005). Recent analyses of DC from human lung also hint at heterogeneous DC subsets defined by BDCA-1 (CD1c) and BDCA-3 (Demedts et al., 2005; Masten et al., 2006).

Studies in the human thymus indicate that the expression of CD11b is able to delineate (at least) two different subsets of cDC (Vandenabeele et al., 2001). Those cDC that do not express CD11b are major producers of bioactive IL-12p70, reminiscent of the CD8$^+$CD11b$^-$ cDC in the mouse. Freshly isolated CD11b$^+$ cDC express high levels of MIP-1α mRNA, as do the CD8$^-$ cDC of mouse. Further evidence linking mouse and human cDC subsets comes from the recent finding that an antibody to Nectin-like protein 2 (Necl2), a molecule specific for BDCA3$^+$ human cDC in blood and T cell areas in spleen, also specifically recognizes the CD8$^+$ cDC in mouse spleen (Galibert et al., 2005). From the published data it is not yet clear whether the BDCA3$^+$ Necl2$^+$ cDC are also CD11b$^-$, and whether these cells are also the major producers of IL-12 in thymus, spleen, and other lymphoid organs. Nor is it clear whether the BDCA3$^+$Necl2$^+$ cells, like the mouse CD8$^+$ cDC, have a potent ability to cross-present antigen.

3 Relationship of Mouse DC Subsets to Rat DC

According to surface phenotype, the rat pDC appear as a hybrid between human and mouse pDC (Hubert et al., 2004). Similar to mouse pDC, rat pDC express the CD45R (B220) surface molecule. Like human pDC and unlike mouse pDC, the rat pDC do not express CD8α and all are positive for CD4.

The cDC in rat spleen can be separated into $CD4^+$ and $CD4^-$ cells, with no rat cDC expressing CD8. It has recently been shown that rat $CD4^-$ cDC are also CD172 $(Sirp-\alpha)^{-/lo}$ and rat $CD4^+$ cDC are $CD172^{hi}$. This correlates well with the mouse cDC, where $CD8^-CD4^+$ and $CD8^-CD4^-$ DC express high levels of CD172, whereas $CD8^+$ cDC express very low levels. The location of $CD4^-Sirp\alpha^{lo}$ rat cDC to the T cell areas of spleen, taken together with the evidence that these cells also produce high levels of IL-12 and induce Th1 responses in $CD4^+$ T cells (Voisine et al., 2002), correlates well with the notion that this subset represents the equivalent of mouse $CD8\alpha^+$ cDC.

4 DC Generated *In Vitro*

The difficulties inherent in dealing with human tissues have biased human DC studies towards DC generated *in vitro*. Monocyte-derived cDC can be generated from PBMC or bone marrow cells in the presence of GM-CSF and IL-4 (Sallusto and Lanzavecchia, 1994). These *in vitro* cultures generate high numbers of cDC and are similar to cDC generated from mouse BM cells with GM-CSF (Inaba et al., 1992; Scheicher et al., 1992). In both species the resultant "monocyte-derived cDC" are similar to one another, they are relatively mature cells with high levels of MHC and co-stimulatory molecules. Certainly the use of these *in vitro* generated cDC have enhanced the knowledge of DC biology, but it remains to be demonstrated that they do not appear to correlate with the relatively immature steady state cDC *in vivo* (Wilson et al., 2003). Another indication for this is that knockout mice lacking either GM-CSF or a receptor component of the GM-CSF receptor had only minor reductions of cDC numbers in spleen and thymus (Vremec et al., 1997). These *in vitro*-generated, monocyte-derived cDC most likely represent DC generated *in vivo* upon an inflammatory stimulus, although the molecular evidence to prove this is still lacking.

Dendritic cells that resemble $CD1a^+$ Langerhans cells and dermal or interstitial cDC, and that are clearly distinct from the monocyte-derived cDC, can be generated from $CD34^+$ hematopoietic progenitors that are often first enhanced in patients *in vivo* with G-CSF. A cocktail of cytokines including GM-CSF, TNF-α, c-kit, and Flt3-L, with the addition of TGF-β for Langerhans cell generation, or IL-4 for interstitial DC generation, is used.

Another DC culture system utilises Flt3-L to drive mouse bone marrow DC precursors into cDC and pDC (Brasel et al., 2000; Brawand et al., 2002; Gilliet et al., 2002; Hochrein et al., 2002). This recently described system generates high numbers of immature cDC and pDC and has been instrumental in defining the mouse pDC in particular. The recent finding that the cDC within these cultures closely resemble the $CD8^+$ and $CD8^-$ subsets of mouse spleen (Naik et al., 2005b) certainly promotes the use of this system to corroborate *in vivo* studies. Given that human pDC and cDC can also be driven from $CD34^+$ hematopoietic precursors with Flt3-L (Blom et al., 2000) it remains to be seen whether a closer comparison of human and mouse cDC can be made by comparing the cDC generated in the Flt3-L driven system. Our recent data indicate that pDC and cDC development can also be driven from bone marrow cells *in vitro* with M-CSF (CSF-1), independently of Flt3-L (unpublished observations).

5 Toll-Like Receptors and Pathogen Recognition

Members of the ancient pathogen receptor family, the Toll-like receptors (TLR), were initially implicated in the recognition of bacterial and fungal patterns (reviewed in Beutler et al., 2003; Pasare and Medzhitov, 2005; Takeda and Akira, 2004). More recently, TLR have also been implicated in autoimmunity (see Chapter 8 in this volume) and their manipulation has been seen to be extremely important in immunotherapies (see Chapter 11). However, a large body of evidence has also accumulated to show recognition of viruses via TLR (summarized in Figure 1).

The experimental evidence for recognition of a certain virus and a defined TLR is rarely direct, but instead has been shown by a lack of responsiveness using cells

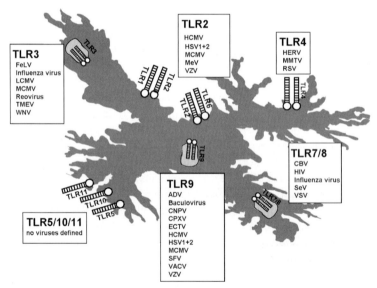

Fig. 1 TLR implicated in viral recognition. ADV: adenovirus; CBV: Coxsackie B virus; CNPV: canarypox virus; CPXV: cowpox virus; ECTV: ectromelia virus; FeLV: feline leukemia virus; HCMV: human cytomegalovirus; HERV: human endogenous retroviruses; HIV: human immunodeficiency virus; HSV: herpes simplex virus; LCMV: lymphocytic choriomeningitis virus; MCMV: murine cytomegalovirus; MMTV: mouse mammary tumor virus; MeV: measles virus; RSV: respiratory syncytial virus; SeV: Sendai virus; SFV: Shope fibroma virus; TMEV: Theiler's murine encephalomyelitis virus; VACV: Vaccinia virus; VSV: vesicular stomatitis virus; VZV: varicella zoster virus; WNV: West Nile virus

from TLR- or adapter molecule-deficient animals. Exceptions to this are the viral protein components recognized by TLR2 and TLR4. In some cases the argument for viral recognition via a certain TLR was shown by higher susceptibility of TLR-deficient animals.

The hemagglutinin protein of the measles virus (MeV) and the envelope glycoproteins B and H of the human cytomegaloviruses (HCMV) are recognized via TLR2 (Bieback et al., 2002; Boehme et al., 2006). TLR2 was also implicated in the recognition of herpes simplex virus (HSV), murine cytomegaloviruses (MCMV) and varicella-zoster virus (VZV) (Aravalli et al., 2005; Compton et al., 2003; Kurt-Jones et al., 2004; Sato et al., 2006; Szomolanyi-Tsuda et al., 2006; Wang et al., 2005).

TLR4 was shown to recognize protein components of the respiratory syncytial virus (RSV), mouse mammary tumour virus (MMTV), and human endogenous retroviruses (HERV) (Burzyn et al., 2004; Haynes et al., 2001; Kurt-Jones et al., 2000; Rassa et al., 2002; Rolland et al., 2006).

TLR3 has been implicated in the recognition of a large panel of different RNA and DNA viruses. Among these are MCMV, influenza virus, lymphocytic choriomeningitis virus (LCMV), feline leukaemia virus (FeLV), reovirus, Theiler's murine encephalomyelitis virus (TMEV), and West Nile virus (WNV) (Abujamra et al., 2006; Alexopoulou et al., 2001; Guillot et al., 2005; So et al., 2006; Tabeta et al., 2004; Town et al., 2006; Wang et al., 2004; Zhou et al., 2005). However, a prominent protective role for TLR3 in the recognition of MCMV, reovirus, LCMV, and VSV has recently been questioned (Edelmann et al., 2004).

TLR7 and 8 have been associated with the recognition of influenza, human immunodeficiency virus (HIV), Coxsackie B virus (CBV), Sendai virus (SeV) and vesicular stomatitis virus (VSV) (Beignon et al., 2005; Diebold et al., 2004; Heil et al., 2004; Lund et al., 2004; Melchjorsen et al., 2005; Triantafilou et al., 2005).

For TLR9 a panel of DNA viruses have been described including; adenovirus (AdV), HSV, HCMV, MCMV, VZV, and baculovirus (Abe et al., 2005b; Basner-Tschakarjan et al., 2006; Delale et al., 2005; Hochrein et al., 2004; Iacobelli-Martinez and Nemerow, 2007; Krug et al., 2004b; Krug et al., 2004a; Lund et al., 2003; Tabeta et al., 2004; Wang et al., 2005). Furthermore, we have experimental evidence for the involvement of TLR9 in the recognition of several members of the poxvirus family including vaccinia viruses (VACV), canarypox virus (CNPV), cowpox virus (CPXV), ectromelia virus (ECTV) and Shope fibroma virus (SFV) (Hochrein et al., unpublished).

5.1 DC and TLR

The separation of DC into multiple subsets based on phenotype also correlates in many instances with a difference in function. How these functional differences amongst the subsets are induced is of major importance in understanding and manipulating the immune response to pathogens, tumors, and the immune response in autoimmune diseases. The responses to pathogens and indeed the immune responses resulting in many autoimmune pathologies involve direct stimulation via the ancient, highly conserved family of TLR. DC link the ancient innate and "modern" adaptive immune systems and a major basis for this is their expression of multiple members of this ancient TLR family.

As it happens, the functionally distinct DC subsets also express distinct members of the TLR family. Table 2 illustrates the data known on TLR expression by the known subsets of mouse, human, and rat *ex vivo* isolated and *in vitro* generated DC.

5.2 cDC Subsets are Geared for Recognition of Extracellular Bacteria and Some Viruses

As shown in Table 2 the cDC subsets all express an array of extracellular and intracellular TLR. In common all cDC of mouse, rat, and humans express at least TLR2, 4, and 6, gearing them with the tools to recognize extracellular bacterial products such as lipopeptides and LPS and also potentially some viral coat proteins (Figure 1).

The TLR3, 7, 8, and 9 are all nucleic acid receptors (dsRNA, ssRNA, ssRNA, and DNA, respectively) and responsible for a large proportion of viral recognition (Figure 1) and also nucleic-acid mediated autoimmune disease (Deane and Bolland, 2006).

All mouse and rat cDC express TLR9. In humans it has been vastly reported that cDC do not respond to TLR9 ligands, although some reports show the expression of mRNA for TLR9 in human cDC and recent reports also demonstrate responsiveness to CpG motifs containing oligonucleotides (CpG-ODN) (Hoene et al., 2006; Kadowaki et al., 2001). A potential problem with these types of analyses could be small numbers of contaminating responder cells like B-cells or pDC in an isolated cDC fraction, or, on the other hand, the unrecognized contamination of a single TLR ligand with another, i.e., endotoxin contaminations within a CpG-ODN. To complicate the issue, TLR-independent recognition mechanisms can potentially incorrectly indicate functional TLR responsiveness; i.e., CpG-ODN can be seen by TLR9 and also by yet unidentified TLR-independent pathways if delivered under conditions of enhanced uptake (Yasuda et al., 2005).

In mice only the CD8$^+$ cDC express high levels of TLR3 mRNA and indeed they appear to be the only mouse cDC subset that responds to TLR3 ligands with cytokine or chemokine production. Similarly the rat CD4$^-$ cDC (putative mouse CD8$^+$ DC equivalents) express about ten-fold more TLR3 than their CD4$^+$ counterparts. On the other hand, they express low levels of TLR7 and no TLR8. The stimulation of CD8$^+$ cDC by TLR3 greatly enhances cross-presentation (Schulz et al., 2005), and it is tempting to speculate that the CD4$^-$ rat cDC are also cross-presenting cells and that both are adapt at responding to dsRNA viruses or to virus induced dsRNA intermediates.

Table 2 Variation of TLR expression amongst different DC subsets of mouse, rat, and human. Data are grouped in species and according to publication with differences between reports likely due to impurities and different methods used to separate the DC subsets and to detect TLR expression

Mouse DC	TLR1	TLR2	TLR3	TLR4	TLR5	TLR6	TLR7	TLR8	TLR9	TLR10 not in mouse
(Edwards et al., 2003b)										
spleen CD4+	++	++	+	+	++	+++	++	++	++	/
spleen CD8+	++	++	+++	+	low	++	neg	++	++	/
spleen CD4− CD8−	++	++	++	+	+	++	++	++	++	/
spleen pDC	++	++	low	+	+	++	+++	++	+++	/
(Okada et al., 2003)										
thymic pDC		low	+	low			++		++	/
thymic cDC		+	++	low			neg		+	/
(Naik et al., 2005b)										
spleen pDC			neg	neg			+++		+++	/
spleen cDC CD24high			++	++			neg		+	/
spleen cDC CD11bhigh			neg	+++			+		++	/
FL-pDC			neg	neg			++		+++	/
FL-cDC CD24high			+++	+			neg		++	/
FL-cDC CD11bhigh			neg	++			+		++	/
(Applequist et al., 2002)										
DC line FSDC	++	++	+++	+++	+	++	++		+++	/
DC line CB-1	low	+	++	++	neg	low	++		+	/
DC line D2SC/1	+++	+++	+++	+++	++	+++	+++		+++	/
Rat DC	TLR1	TLR2	TLR3	TLR4	TLR5	TLR6	TLR7	TLR8	TLR9	TLR10
(Hubert et al., 2006)										
spleen pDC	low	+	low	low	low	neg	++	low	++	neg
spleen CD4+	++	++	++	+	++	+	++	low	+	+
spleen CD4−	++	++	+++	low	+	+	low	neg	+	++
(Muzio et al., 2000)										
Mo-DC	+	+	++	++	+					

(continued)

Table 2 (continued)

Human DC	TLR1	TLR2	TLR3	TLR4	TLR5	TLR6	TLR7	TLR8	TLR9	TLR10
(Jarrossay et al., 2001)										
blood pDC	neg	neg	neg	neg	neg	neg	+	neg	++	
blood cDC	neg	++	low	low	+	low	neg	low	neg	
Mo-DC	low	++	low	++	low	low	neg	+	neg	
(Kadowaki et al., 2001)										
blood CD11c pos	++	++	++	neg	low	low	neg	low	neg	low
blood pDC	low	neg	neg	neg	neg	low	++	neg	+	low
(Krug et al., 2001)										
blood cDC	+	+	+	+	+	+	+	low	neg	
blood pDC	++	low	neg	neg	low	low	+	neg	+	
(Visintin et al., 2001)										
Mo-DC	+	+	low	+	neg	+				
(Hornung et al., 2002)										
blood pDC	low	neg	neg	neg	neg	low	+	neg	++	low
(Ito et al., 2002)										
blood cDC				+			++		neg	
blood pDC				neg			++		+	
(Matsumoto et al., 2003)										
blood pDC		neg	neg	neg						
blood cDC		++	++	++						
Mo-DC		++	++	++						
(Means et al., 2003)										
Mo-DC	++	++	++	+	+	+	+	low	neg	neg
(Kokkinopoulos et al., 2005)										
Mo-DC	neg	low	neg	+	++	neg	neg	+	low	+
(Flacher et al., 2006)										
Langerhans cells	++	+	+	neg	low	++	low	low	neg	++
blood pDC	+	neg	low	neg		++	+++	low	+++	+++
blood cDC	+	++	++	+		++	++	++	low	+++
(Renn et al., 2006)										
LC like in vitro generated	+	+++	++	++	++	low	++	++	+	++
Mo-DC	low	+++	++	++	++	+	++	++	neg	+

Unseparated human blood cDC and also Langerhans cells also express TLR3 and low levels of TLR7, although it is not known whether there is differential expression of these TLR amongst the different subsets of human cDC that have been identified to date.

5.3 pDC are Geared for Recognition of Intracellular Viruses

Table 2 shows clearly that pDC of all species largely lack the plasma membrane-expressed TLR family members, and instead specifically express TLR7–TLR9, which are TLR that recognize ribo- (TLR7, 8) and deoxyribo- (TLR9) nucleic acids and that are located on intracellular membranes. All mouse cDC subsets also express TLR9, and mouse $CD8^-$ cDC also express TLR7. However, in mice, humans, rats, and also pigs (Guzylack-Piriou et al., 2004) it is the pDC that is uniquely able to produce high levels of type I IFNs via these TLR. The recent evidence that several viruses are specifically recognized by TLR7/8 or TLR9 (Figure 1) highlights the importance of pDC in the immune response and, importantly, the innate type I IFN response to these viruses.

The production of type I IFN by pDC in response to TLR7 or 9 activation is also implicated in the etiology of autoimmune diseases such as psoriasis and systemic lupus erythematosus (see Chapter 7 in this volume).

6 Perspectives

It is clear that the expression of TLR by DC can strongly dictate the immune response. It is also clear that DC subsets separated by function, for example the $CD8\alpha^+$ cDC, express a defined subset of TLR, suggesting that the TLR expression either plays a role in dictating the DC function or alternatively has evolved along with the DC subset to complement the functional properties of these cells. The correlation of TLR expression amongst species aligns well with the pDC and indicates a conserved function of viral recognition. Defining the TLR expression amongst the many subpopulations of cDC may aid in understanding the functions of these subsets and, importantly, to cross-correlate functional attributes of DC subsets between species.

References

Abe M, Wang Z, de CA, Thomson AW (2005a) Plasmacytoid dendritic cell precursors induce allogeneic T-cell hyporesponsiveness and prolong heart graft survival. Am J Transplant 5: 1808–1819

Abe T, Hemmi H, Miyamoto H, Moriishi K, Tamura S, Takaku H, Akira S, Matsuura Y (2005b) Involvement of the Toll-like receptor 9 signaling pathway in the induction of innate immunity by baculovirus. J Virol 79: 2847–2858

Abujamra AL, Spanjaard RA, Akinsheye I, Zhao X, Faller DV, Ghosh SK (2006) Leukemia virus long terminal repeat activates NFkappaB pathway by a TLR3-dependent mechanism. Virology 345: 390–403

Alexopoulou L, Holt AC, Medzhitov R, Flavell RA (2001) Recognition of double-stranded RNA and activation of NF-kappaB by Toll-like receptor 3. Nature 413: 732–738

Allan RS, Smith CM, Belz GT, van Lint AL, Wakim LM, Heath WR, Carbone FR (2003) Epidermal viral immunity induced by CD8{alpha}+ dendritic cells but not by Langerhans cells. Science 301: 1925–1928

Applequist SE, Wallin RP, Ljunggren HG (2002) Variable expression of Toll-like receptor in murine innate and adaptive immune cell lines. Int Immunol 14: 1065–1074

Aravalli RN, Hu S, Rowen TN, Palmquist JM, Lokensgard JR (2005) Cutting edge: TLR2-mediated proinflammatory cytokine and chemokine production by microglial cells in response to herpes simplex virus. J Immunol 175: 4189–4193

Asselin-Paturel C, Brizard G, Pin JJ, Briere F, Trinchieri G (2003) Mouse strain differences in plasmacytoid dendritic cell frequency and function revealed by a novel monoclonal antibody. J Immunol 171: 6466–6477

Barchet W, Blasius A, Cella M, Colonna M (2005a) Plasmacytoid dendritic cells: In search of their niche in immune responses. Immunol Res 32: 75–83

Barchet W, Cella M, Colonna M (2005b) Plasmacytoid dendritic cells—Virus experts of innate immunity. Semin Immunol 17: 253–261

Basner-Tschakarjan E, Gaffal E, O'Keeffe M, Tormo D, Limmer A, Wagner H, Hochrein H, Tuting T (2006) Adenovirus efficiently transduces plasmacytoid dendritic cells resulting in TLR9-dependent maturation and IFN-alpha production. J Gene Med 8: 1300–1306

Beignon AS, McKenna K, Skoberne M, Manches O, Dasilva I, Kavanagh DG, Larsson M, Gorelick RJ, Lifson JD, Bhardwaj N (2005) Endocytosis of HIV-1 activates plasmacytoid dendritic cells via Toll-like receptor-viral RNA interactions. J Clin Invest 115: 3265–3275

Belz GT, Shortman K, Bevan MJ, Heath WR (2005) CD8{alpha}+ dendritic cells selectively present MHC class I-restricted noncytolytic viral and intracellular bacterial antigens in vivo. J Immunol 175: 196–200

Belz GT, Smith CM, Eichner D, Shortman K, Karupiah G, Carbone FR, Heath WR (2004a) Cutting edge: conventional CD8 alpha+ dendritic cells are generally involved in priming CTL immunity to viruses. J Immunol 172: 1996–2000

Belz GT, Smith CM, Kleinert L, Reading P, Brooks A, Shortman K, Carbone FR, Heath WR (2004b) Distinct migrating and nonmigrating dendritic cell populations are involved in MHC class I-restricted antigen presentation after lung infection with virus. Proc Natl Acad Sci USA 101: 8670–8675

Belz GT, Vremec D, Febbraio M, Corcoran L, Shortman K, Carbone FR, Heath WR (2002) CD36 is differentially expressed by CD8+ splenic dendritic cells but is not required for cross-presentation in vivo. J Immunol 168: 6066–6070

Beutler B, Hoebe K, Du X, Ulevitch RJ (2003) How we detect microbes and respond to them: The Toll-like receptors and their transducers. J Leukoc Biol 74: 479–485

Bieback K, Lien E, Klagge IM, Avota E, Schneider–Schaulies J, Duprex WP, Wagner H, Kirschning CJ, Ter Meulen V, Schneider-Schaulies S (2002) Hemagglutinin protein of wild-type measles virus activates Toll-like receptor 2 signaling. J Virol 76: 8729–8736

Blom B, Ho S, Antonenko S, Liu YJ (2000) Generation of interferon alpha-producing predendritic cell (Pre-DC)2 from human CD34(+) hematopoietic stem cells. J Exp Med 192: 1785–1796

Boehme KW, Guerrero M, Compton T (2006) Human cytomegalovirus envelope glycoproteins B and H are necessary for TLR2 activation in permissive cells. J Immunol 177: 7094–7102

Brasel K, De Smedt T, Smith JL, Maliszewski CR (2000) Generation of murine dendritic cells from flt3-ligand-supplemented bone marrow cultures. Blood 96: 3029–3039

Brawand P, Fitzpatrick DR, Greenfield BW, Brasel K, Maliszewski CR, De Smedt T (2002) Murine plasmacytoid pre-dendritic cells generated from Flt3 ligand-supplemented bone marrow cultures are immature APCs. J Immunol 169: 6711–6719

Burzyn D, Rassa JC, Kim D, Nepomnaschy I, Ross SR, Piazzon I (2004) Toll-like receptor 4-dependent activation of dendritic cells by a retrovirus. J Virol 78: 576–584

Chung Y, Chang JH, Kweon MN, Rennert PD, Kang CY (2005) CD8alpha-11b+ dendritic cells but not CD8alpha+ dendritic cells mediate cross-tolerance toward intestinal antigens. Blood 106: 201–206

Ciavarra RP, Stephens A, Nagy S, Sekellick M, Steel C (2006) Evaluation of immunological paradigms in a virus model: Are dendritic cells critical for antiviral immunity and viral clearance? J Immunol 177: 492–500

Compton T, Kurt-Jones EA, Boehme KW, Belko J, Latz E, Golenbock DT, Finberg RW (2003) Human cytomegalovirus activates inflammatory cytokine responses via CD14 and Toll-like receptor 2. J Virol 77: 4588–4596

Cresswell P, Ackerman AL, Giodini A, Peaper DR, Wearsch PA (2005) Mechanisms of MHC class I-restricted antigen processing and cross-presentation. Immunol Rev 207: 145–157

de Heer HJ, Hammad H, Soullie T, Hijdra D, Vos N, Willart MA, Hoogsteden HC, Lambrecht BN (2004) Essential role of lung plasmacytoid dendritic cells in preventing asthmatic reactions to harmless inhaled antigen. J Exp Med 200: 89–98

Deane JA, Bolland S (2006) Nucleic acid-sensing TLRs as modifiers of autoimmunity. J Immunol 177: 6573–6578

Delale T, Paquin A, Asselin–Paturel C, Dalod M, Brizard G, Bates EE, Kastner P, Chan S, Akira S, Vicari A, Biron CA, Trinchieri G, Briere F (2005) MyD88-dependent and -independent murine cytomegalovirus sensing for IFN-alpha release and initiation of immune responses in vivo. J Immunol 175: 6723–6732

Demedts IK, Brusselle GG, Vermaelen KY, Pauwels RA (2005) Identification and characterization of human pulmonary dendritic cells. Am J Respir Cell Mol Biol 32: 177–184

den Haan JM, Bevan MJ (2002) Constitutive versus activation-dependent cross-presentation of immune complexes by CD8(+) and CD8(−) dendritic cells in vivo. J Exp Med 196: 817–827

den Haan JM, Lehar SM, Bevan MJ (2000) CD8(+) but not CD8(−) dendritic cells cross-prime cytotoxic T cells in vivo. J Exp Med 192: 1685–1696

Diebold SS, Kaisho T, Hemmi H, Akira S, Reis e Sousa C (2004) Innate antiviral responses by means of TLR7mediated recognition of single-stranded RNA. Science 303: 1529–1531

Edelmann KH, Richardson-Burns S, Alexopoulou L, Tyler KL, Flavell RA, Oldstone MB (2004) Does Toll-like receptor 3 play a biological role in virus infections? Virology 322: 231–238

Edwards AD, Chaussabel D, Tomlinson S, Schulz O, Sher A, Reis e Sousa C (2003a) Relationships among murine CD11c(high) dendritic cell subsets as revealed by baseline gene expression patterns. J Immunol 171: 47–60

Edwards AD, Diebold SS, Slack EM, Tomizawa H, Hemmi H, Kaisho T, Akira S, Reis e Sousa C (2003b) Toll-like receptor expression in murine DC subsets: Lack of TLR7 expression by CD8 alpha+ DC correlates with unresponsiveness to imidazoquinolines. Eur J Immunol 33: 827–833

Flacher V, Bouschbacher M, Verronese E, Massacrier C, Sisirak V, Berthier-Vergnes O, de Saint-Vis B, Caux C, Zutter-Dambuyant C, Lebecque S, Valladeau J (2006) Human Langerhans cells express a specific TLR profile and differentially respond to viruses and Gram-positive bacteria. J Immunol 177: 7959–7967

Flores-Langarica A, Meza-Perez S, Calderon-Amador J, Estrada-Garcia T, Macpherson G, Lebecque S, Saeland S, Steinman RM, Flores-Romo L (2005) Network of dendritic cells within the muscular layer of the mouse intestine. Proc Natl Acad Sci USA 102: 19039–19044

Fuchsberger M, Hochrein H, O'Keeffe M (2005) Activation of plasmacytoid dendritic cells. Immunol Cell Biol 83: 571–577

Fugier-Vivier IJ, Rezzoug F, Huang Y, Graul-Layman AJ, Schanie CL, Xu H, Chilton PM, Ildstad ST (2005) Plasmacytoid precursor dendritic cells facilitate allogeneic hematopoietic stem cell engraftment. J Exp Med 201: 373–383

Galibert L, Diemer GS, Liu Z, Johnson RS, Smith JL, Walzer T, Comeau MR, Rauch CT, Wolfson MF, Sorensen RA, Van der Vuurst de Vries AR, Branstetter DG, Koelling RM, Scholler J,

Fanslow WC, Baum PR, Derry JM, Yan W (2005) Nectin-like protein 2 defines a subset of T-cell zone dendritic cells and is a ligand for class-I-restricted T-cell-associated molecule. J Biol Chem 280: 21955–21964

Geissmann F, Prost C, Monnet JP, Dy M, Brousse N, Hermine O (1998) Transforming growth factor beta1, in the presence of granulocyte/macrophage colony-stimulating factor and interleukin 4, induces differentiation of human peripheral blood monocytes into dendritic Langerhans cells. J Exp Med 187: 961–966

Gilliet M, Boonstra A, Paturel C, Antonenko S, Xu XL, Trinchieri G, O'Garra A, Liu YJ (2002) The development of murine plasmacytoid dendritic cell precursors is differentially regulated by FLT3-ligand and granulocyte/macrophage colony-stimulating factor. J Exp Med 195: 953–958

Groothuis TAM, Neefjes J (2005) The many roads to cross-presentation. J Exp Med 202: 1313–1318

Guillot L, Le Goffic R, Bloch S, Escriou N, Akira S, Chignard M, Si-Tahar M (2005) Involvement of Toll-like receptor 3 in the immune response of lung epithelial cells to double-stranded RNA and influenza A virus. J Biol Chem 280: 5571–5580

Guzylack-Piriou L, Balmelli C, McCullough KC, Summerfield A (2004) Type-A CpG oligonucleotides activate exclusively porcine natural interferon-producing cells to secrete interferon–alpha, tumour necrosis factor-alpha and interleukin-12. Immunology 112: 28–37

Hammad H, de Vries VC, Maldonado-Lopez R, Moser M, Maliszewski C, Hoogsteden HC, Lambrecht BN (2004) Differential capacity of CD8+ alpha or CD8− alpha dendritic cell subsets to prime for eosinophilic airway inflammation in the T-helper type 2-prone milieu of the lung. Clin Exp Allergy 34: 1834–1840

Hartmann G, Weiner GJ, Krieg AM (1999) CpG DNA: a potent signal for growth, activation, and maturation of human dendritic cells. Proc Natl Acad Sci USA 96: 9305–9310

Haynes LM, Moore DD, Kurt-Jones EA, Finberg RW, Anderson LJ, Tripp RA (2001) Involvement of Toll-like receptor 4 in innate immunity to respiratory syncytial virus. J Virol 75: 10730–10737

Heil F, Hemmi H, Hochrein H, Ampenberger F, Kirschning C, Akira S, Lipford G, Wagner H, Bauer S (2004) Species-specific recognition of single-stranded RNA via Toll–like receptor 7 and 8. Science 303: 1526–1529

Henri S, Vremec D, Kamath A, Waithman J, Williams S, Benoist C, Burnham K, Saeland S, Handman E, Shortman K (2001) The dendritic cell populations of mouse lymph nodes. J Immunol 167: 741–748

Hochrein H, O'Keeffe M, Wagner H (2002) Human and mouse plasmacytoid dendritic cells. Hum Immunol 63: 1103–1110

Hochrein H, Schlatter B, O'Keeffe M, Wagner C, Schmitz F, Schiemann M, Bauer S, Suter M, Wagner H (2004) Herpes simplex virus type-1 induces IFN-alpha production via Toll-like receptor 9-dependent and -independent pathways. Proc Natl Acad Sci USA 101: 11416–11421

Hochrein H, Shortman K, Vremec D, Scott B, Hertzog P, O'Keeffe M (2001) Differential production of IL-12, IFN-alpha, and IFN-gamma by mouse dendritic cell subsets. J Immunol 166: 5448–5455

Hoene V, Peiser M, Wanner R (2006) Human monocyte-derived dendritic cells express TLR9 and react directly to the CpG-A oligonucleotide D19. J Leukoc Biol 80: 1328–1336

Hornung V, Rothenfusser S, Britsch S, Krug A, Jahrsdorfer B, Giese T, Endres S, Hartmann G (2002) Quantitative expression of Toll-like receptor 1–10 mRNA in cellular subsets of human peripheral blood mononuclear cells and sensitivity to CpG oligodeoxynucleotides. J Immunol 168: 4531–4537

Hubert FX, Voisine C, Louvet C, Heslan JM, Ouabed A, Heslan M, Josien R (2006) Differential pattern recognition receptor expression but stereotyped responsiveness in rat spleen dendritic cell subsets. J Immunol 177: 1007–1016

Hubert FX, Voisine C, Louvet C, Heslan M, Josien R (2004) Rat plasmacytoid dendritic cells are an abundant subset of MHC class II+ CD4+CD11b−. J Immunol 172: 7485–7494

Hunger RE, Sieling PA, Ochoa MT, Sugaya M, Burdick AE, Rea TH, Brennan PJ, Belisle JT, Blauvelt A, Porcelli SA, Modlin RL (2004) Langerhans cells utilize CD1a and langerin to efficiently present nonpeptide antigens to T cells. J Clin Invest 113: 701–708

Iacobelli-Martinez M, Nemerow GR (2007) Preferential activation of Toll-like receptor nine by CD46-utilizing adenoviruses. J Virol 81: 1305–1312

Ichikawa E, Hida S, Omatsu Y, Shimoyama S, Takahara K, Miyagawa S, Inaba K, Taki S (2004) Defective development of splenic and epidermal CD4+ dendritic cells in mice deficient for IFN regulatory factor-2. PNAS 101: 3909–3914

Iezzi G, Frohlich A, Ernst B, Ampenberger F, Saeland S, Glaichenhaus N, Kopf M (2006) Lymph Node Resident Rather Than Skin-Derived Dendritic Cells Initiate Specific T Cell Responses after *Leishmania major* Infection. J Immunol 177: 1250–1256

Inaba K, Inaba M, Romani N, Aya H, Deguchi M, Ikehara S, Muramatsu S, Steinman RM (1992) Generation of large numbers of dendritic cells from mouse bone marrow cultures supplemented with granulocyte/macrophage colony-stimulating factor. J Exp Med 176: 1693–1702

Ito T, Amakawa R, Kaisho T, Hemmi H, Tajima K, Uehira K, Ozaki Y, Tomizawa H, Akira S, Fukuhara S (2002) Interferon-alpha and interleukin-12 are induced differentially by Toll-like receptor 7 ligands in human blood dendritic cell subsets. J Exp Med 195: 1507–1512

Jang MH, Sougawa N, Tanaka T, Hirata T, Hiroi T, Tohya K, Guo Z, Umemoto E, Ebisuno Y, Yang BG, Seoh JY, Lipp M, Kiyono H, Miyasaka M (2006) CCR7 is critically important for migration of dendritic cells in intestinal lamina propria to mesenteric lymph nodes. J Immunol 176: 803–810

Jarrossay D, Napolitani G, Colonna M, Sallusto F, Lanzavecchia A (2001) Specialization and complementarity in microbial molecule recognition by human myeloid and plasmacytoid dendritic cells. Eur J Immunol 31: 3388–3393

Jung S, Unutmaz D, Wong P, Sano G, De los Santos K, Sparwasser T, Wu S, Vuthoori S, Ko K, Zavala F, Pamer EG, Littman DR, Lang RA (2002) In vivo depletion of CD11c(+) dendritic cells abrogates priming of CD8(+) T cells by exogenous cell–associated antigens. Immunity 17: 211–220

Kadowaki N, Ho S, Antonenko S, Malefyt RW, Kastelein RA, Bazan F, Liu YJ (2001) Subsets of human dendritic cell precursors express different Toll–like receptors and respond to different microbial antigens. J Exp Med 194: 863–869

Kamath AT, Henri S, Battye F, Tough DF, Shortman K (2002) Developmental kinetics and lifespan of dendritic cells in mouse lymphoid organs. Blood 100: 1734–1741

Kamath AT, Pooley J, O'Keeffe MA, Vremec D, Zhan Y, Lew AM, D'Amico A, Wu L, Tough DF, Shortman K (2000) The development, maturation, and turnover rate of mouse spleen dendritic cell populations. J Immunol 165: 6762–6770

Kamogawa-Schifter Y, Ohkawa J, Namiki S, Arai N, Arai K, Liu Y (2005) Ly49Q defines 2 pDC subsets in mice. Blood 105: 2787–2792

Kissenpfennig A, Henri S, Dubois B, Laplace–Builhe C, Perrin P, Romani N, Tripp CII, Douillard P, Leserman L, Kaiserlian D, Saeland S, Davoust J, Malissen B (2005) Dynamics and function of Langerhans cells *in vivo*: dermal dendritic cells colonize lymph node areas distinct from slower migrating Langerhans cells. Immunity 22: 643–654

Kissenpfennig A, Malissen B (2006) Langerhans cells—Revisiting the paradigm using genetically engineered mice. Trends Immunol 27: 132–139

Kokkinopoulos I, Jordan WJ, Ritter MA (2005) Toll-like receptor mRNA expression patterns in human dendritic cells and monocytes. Mol Immunol 42: 957–968

Krug A, French AR, Barchet W, Fischer JA, Dzionek A, Pingel JT, Orihuela MM, Akira S, Yokoyama WM, Colonna M (2004a) TLR9-dependent recognition of MCMV by IPC and DC generates coordinated cytokine responses that activate antiviral NK cell function. Immunity 21: 107–119

Krug A, Luker GD, Barchet W, Leib DA, Akira S, Colonna M (2004b) Herpes simplex virus type 1 activates murine natural interferon-producing cells through Toll-like receptor 9. Blood 103: 1433–1437

Krug A, Towarowski A, Britsch S, Rothenfusser S, Hornung V, Bals R, Giese T, Engelmann H, Endres S, Krieg AM, Hartmann G (2001) Toll-like receptor expression reveals CpG DNA as a unique microbial stimulus for plasmacytoid dendritic cells which synergizes with CD40 ligand to induce high amounts of IL-12. Eur J Immunol 31: 3026–3037

Kurt-Jones EA, Popova L, Kwinn L, Haynes LM, Jones LP, Tripp RA, Walsh EE, Freeman MW, Golenbock DT, Anderson LJ, Finberg RW (2000) Pattern recognition receptors TLR4 and CD14 mediate response to respiratory syncytial virus. Nat Immunol 1: 398–401

Kurt-Jones EA, Sandor F, Ortiz Y, Bowen GN, Counter SL, Wang TC, Finberg RW (2004) Use of murine embryonic fibroblasts to define Toll–like receptor activation and specificity. J Endotoxin Res 10: 419–424

Lahoud MH, Proietto AI, Gartlan KH, Kitsoulis S, Curtis J, Wettenhall J, Sofi M, Daunt C, O'Keeffe M, Caminschi I, Satterley K, Rizzitelli A, Schnorrer P, Hinohara A, Yamaguchi Y, Wu L, Smyth G, Handman E, Shortman K, Wright MD (2006) Signal regulatory protein molecules are differentially expressed by CD8- dendritic cells. J Immunol 177: 372–382

Le Borgne M, Etchart N, Goubier A, Lira SA, Sirard JC, van Rooijen N, Caux C, Ait-Yahia S, Vicari A, Kaiserlian D, Dubois B (2006) Dendritic cells rapidly recruited into epithelial tissues via CCR6/CCL20 are responsible for CD8+ T cell crosspriming *in vivo*. Immunity 24: 191–201

Lian ZX, Okada T, He XS, Kita H, Liu YJ, Ansari AA, Kikuchi K, Ikehara S, Gershwin ME (2003) Heterogeneity of dendritic cells in the mouse liver: identification and characterization of four distinct populations. J Immunol 170: 2323–2330

Lindstedt M, Lundberg K, Borrebaeck CA (2005) Gene family clustering identifies functionally associated subsets of human in vivo blood and tonsillar dendritic cells. J Immunol 175: 4839–4846

Liu CH, Fan YT, Dias A, Esper L, Corn RA, Bafica A, Machado FS, Aliberti J (2006a) Cutting edge: Dendritic cells are essential for in vivo IL-12 production and development of resistance against *Toxoplasma gondii* infection in mice. J Immunol 177: 31–35

Liu L, Fuhlbrigge RC, Karibian K, Tian T, Kupper TS (2006b) Dynamic programming of CD8+ T cell trafficking after live viral immunization. Immunity 25: 511–520

Liu YJ (2005) IPC: Professional type 1 interferon-producing cells and plasmacytoid dendritic cell precursors. Annu Rev Immunol 23: 275–306

Lund J, Sato A, Akira S, Medzhitov R, Iwasaki A (2003) Toll-like receptor 9-mediated recognition of Herpes simplex virus-2 by plasmacytoid dendritic cells. J Exp Med 198: 513–520

Lund JM, Alexopoulou L, Sato A, Karow M, Adams NC, Gale NW, Iwasaki A, Flavell RA (2004) Recognition of single-stranded RNA viruses by Toll-like receptor 7. Proc Natl Acad Sci USA 101: 5598–5603

MacDonald KP, Munster DJ, Clark GJ, Dzionek A, Schmitz J, Hart DN (2002) Characterization of human blood dendritic cell subsets. Blood 100: 4512–4520

Maldonado-Lopez R, De Smedt T, Michel P, Godfroid J, Pajak B, Heirman C, Thielemans K, Leo O, Urbain J, Moser M (1999) CD8alpha+ and CD8alpha- subclasses of dendritic cells direct the development of distinct T helper cells *in vivo*. J Exp Med 189: 587–592

Masten BJ, Olson GK, Tarleton CA, Rund C, Schuyler M, Mehran R, Archibeque T, Lipscomb MF (2006) Characterization of myeloid and plasmacytoid dendritic cells in human lung. J Immunol 177: 7784–7793

Matsumoto M, Funami K, Tanabe M, Oshiumi H, Shingai M, Seto Y, Yamamoto A, Seya T (2003) Subcellular localization of Toll-like receptor 3 in human dendritic cells. J Immunol 171: 3154–3162

Maurer T, Heit A, Hochrein H, Ampenberger F, O'Keeffe M, Bauer S, Lipford GB, Vabulas RM, Wagner H (2002) CpG-DNA aided cross-presentation of soluble antigens by dendritic cells. Eur J Immunol 32: 2356–2364

Means TK, Hayashi F, Smith KD, Aderem A, Luster AD (2003) The Toll-like receptor 5 stimulus bacterial flagellin induces maturation and chemokine production in human dendritic cells. J Immunol 170: 5165–5175

Melchjorsen J, Jensen SB, Malmgaard L, Rasmussen SB, Weber F, Bowie AG, Matikainen S, Paludan SR (2005) Activation of innate defense against a paramyxovirus is mediated by RIG-I and TLR7 and TLR8 in a cell-type-specific manner. J Virol 79: 12944–12951

Muzio M, Bosisio D, Polentarutti N, D'amico G, Stoppacciaro A, Mancinelli R, van't Veer C, Penton-Rol G, Ruco LP, Allavena P, Mantovani A (2000) Differential expression and regulation of Toll-like receptors (TLR) in human leukocytes: selective expression of TLR3 in dendritic cells. J Immunol 164: 5998–6004

Naik SH, Corcoran LM, Wu L (2005a) Development of murine plasmacytoid dendritic cell subsets. Immunol Cell Biol 83: 563–570

Naik SH, Proietto AI, Wilson NS, Dakic A, Schnorrer P, Fuchsberger M, Lahoud MH, O'Keeffe M, Shao QX, Chen WF, Villadangos JA, Shortman K, Wu L (2005b) Cutting edge: generation of splenic CD8+ and CD8− dendritic cell equivalents in Fms-like tyrosine kinase 3 ligand bone marrow cultures. J Immunol 174: 6592–6597

O'Keeffe M, Grumont RJ, Hochrein H, Fuchsberger M, Gugasyan R, Vremec D, Shortman K, Gerondakis S (2005) Distinct roles for the NF-kappaB1 and c-Rel transcription factors in the differentiation and survival of plasmacytoid and conventional dendritic cells activated by TLR-9 signals. Blood 106: 3457–3464

O'Keeffe M, Hochrein H, Vremec D, Caminschi I, Miller JL, Anders EM, Wu L, Lahoud MH, Henri S, Scott B, Hertzog P, Tatarczuch L, Shortman K (2002a) Mouse plasmacytoid cells: Long-lived cells, heterogeneous in surface phenotype and function, that differentiate into CD8(+) dendritic cells only after microbial stimulus. J Exp Med 196: 1307–1319

O'Keeffe M, Hochrein H, Vremec D, Pooley J, Evans R, Woulfe S, Shortman K (2002b) Effects of administration of progenipoietin 1, Flt-3 ligand, granulocyte colony-stimulating factor, and pegylated granulocyte-macrophage colony-stimulating factor on dendritic cell subsets in mice. Blood 99: 2122–2130

O'Keeffe M, Hochrein H, Vremec D, Scott B, Hertzog P, Tatarczuch L, Shortman K (2003) Dendritic cell precursor populations of mouse blood: Identification of the murine homologues of human blood plasmacytoid pre–DC2 and CD11c+ DC1 precursors. Blood 101: 1453–1459

Ochando JC, Homma C, Yang Y, Hidalgo A, Garin A, Tacke F, Angeli V, Li Y, Boros P, Ding Y, Jessberger R, Trinchieri G, Lira SA, Randolph GJ, Bromberg JS (2006) Alloantigen-presenting plasmacytoid dendritic cells mediate tolerance to vascularized grafts. Nat Immunol 7: 652–662

Okada T, Lian ZX, Naiki M, Ansari AA, Ikehara S, Gershwin ME (2003) Murine thymic plasmacytoid dendritic cells. Eur J Immunol 33: 1012–1019

Omatsu Y, Iyoda T, Kimura Y, Maki A, Ishimori M, Toyama–Sorimachi N, Inaba K (2005) Development of murine plasmacytoid dendritic cells defined by increased expression of an inhibitory NK receptor, Ly49Q. J Immunol 174: 6657–6662

Ortner U, Inaba K, Koch F, Heine M, Miwa M, Schuler G, Romani N (1996) An improved isolation method for murine migratory cutaneous dendritic cells. J Immunol Methods 193: 71–79

Pasare C, Medzhitov R (2005) Toll-like receptors: Linking innate and adaptive immunity. Adv Exp Med Biol 560: 11–18

Pooley JL, Heath WR, Shortman K (2001) Cutting edge: intravenous soluble antigen is presented to CD4 T cells by CD8- dendritic cells, but cross-presented to CD8 T cells by CD8+ dendritic cells. J Immunol 166: 5327–5330

Proietto AI, O'Keeffe M, Gartlan K, Wright MD, Shortman K, Wu L, Lahoud MH (2004) Differential production of inflammatory chemokines by murine dendritic cell subsets. Immunobiology 209: 163–172

Rassa JC, Meyers JL, Zhang Y, Kudaravalli R, Ross SR (2002) Murine retroviruses activate B cells via interaction with Toll-like receptor 4. Proc Natl Acad Sci USA 99(2): 2281–2286

Renn CN, Sanchez DJ, Ochoa MT, Legaspi AJ, Oh CK, Liu PT, Krutzik SR, Sieling PA, Cheng G, Modlin RL (2006) TLR activation of Langerhans cell-like dendritic cells triggers an antiviral immune response. J Immunol 177(2): 298–305

Rolland A, Jouvin-Marche E, Viret C, Faure M, Perron H, Marche PN (2006) The envelope protein of a human endogenous retrovirus-W family activates innate immunity through CD14/TLR4 and promotes Th1-like responses. J Immunol 176: 7636–7644

Saeki H, Moore AM, Brown MJ, Hwang ST (1999) Cutting edge: secondary lymphoid–tissue chemokine (SLC) and CC chemokine receptor 7 (CCR7) participate in the emigration pathway of mature dendritic cells from the skin to regional lymph nodes. J Immunol 162: 2472–2475

Salazar-Gonzalez RM, Niess JH, Zammit DJ, Ravindran R, Srinivasan A, Maxwell JR, Stoklasek T, Yadav R, Williams IR, Gu X, McCormick BA, Pazos MA, Vella AT, Lefrancois L, Reinecker HC, McSorley SJ (2006) CCR6-mediated dendritic cell activation of pathogen-specific T cells in Peyer's patches. Immunity 24: 623–632

Sallusto F, Lanzavecchia A (1994) Efficient presentation of soluble antigen by cultured human dendritic cells is maintained by granulocyte/macrophage colony-stimulating factor plus interleukin 4 and downregulated by tumor necrosis factor alpha. J Exp Med 179: 1109–1118

Sato A, Linehan MM, Iwasaki A (2006) Dual recognition of herpes simplex viruses by TLR2 and TLR9 in dendritic cells. Proc Natl Acad Sci USA 103: 17343–17348

Scheicher C, Mehlig M, Zecher R, Reske K (1992) Dendritic cells from mouse bone marrow: in vitro differentiation using low doses of recombinant granulocyte-macrophage colony-stimulating factor. J Immunol Methods 154: 253–264

Scheinecker C, McHugh R, Shevach EM, Germain RN (2002) Constitutive presentation of a natural tissue autoantigen exclusively by dendritic cells in the draining lymph node. J Exp Med 196: 1079–1090

Schnorrer P, Behrens GMN, Wilson NS, Pooley JL, Smith CM, El-Sukkari D, Davey G, Kupresanin F, Li M, Maraskovsky E, Belz GT, Carbone FR, Shortman K, Heath WR, Villadangos JA (2006) The dominant role of CD8+ dendritic cells in cross-presentation is not dictated by antigen capture. PNAS 103: 10729–10734

Schuler G, Steinman RM (1985) Murine epidermal Langerhans cells mature into potent immunostimulatory dendritic cells *in vitro*. J Exp Med 161: 526–546

Schulz O, Diebold SS, Chen M, Naslund TI, Nolte MA, Alexopoulou L, Azuma YT, Flavell RA, Liljestrom P, Reis e Sousa C (2005) Toll-like receptor 3 promotes cross-priming to virus-infected cells. Nature 433: 887–892

Shen L, Rock KL (2006) Priming of T cells by exogenous antigen cross-presented on MHC class I molecules. Curr Opin Immunol 18: 85–91

Shortman K, Liu YJ (2002) Mouse and human dendritic cell subtypes. Nat Rev Immunol 2: 151–161

Smith CM, Belz GT, Wilson NS, Villadangos JA, Shortman K, Carbone FR, Heath WR (2003) Cutting edge: Conventional CD8 alpha+ dendritic cells are preferentially involved in CTL priming after footpad infection with herpes simplex virus-1. J Immunol 170: 4437–4440

So EY, Kang MH, Kim BS (2006) Induction of chemokine and cytokine genes in astrocytes following infection with Theiler's murine encephalomyelitis virus is mediated by the Toll-like receptor 3. Glia 53: 858–867

Soos TJ, Sims TN, Barisoni L, Lin K, Littman DR, Dustin ML, Nelson PJ (2006) CX3CR1+ interstitial dendritic cells form a contiguous network throughout the entire kidney. Kidney Int 70: 591–596

Soumelis V, Liu YJ (2006) From plasmacytoid to dendritic cell: morphological and functional switches during plasmacytoid pre-dendritic cell differentiation. Eur J Immunol 36: 2286–2292

Steinman RM (1991) The dendritic cell system and its role in immunogenicity. Annu Rev Immunol 9: 271–296

Strobl H, Bello-Fernandez C, Riedl E, Pickl WF, Majdic O, Lyman SD, Knapp W (1997) flt3 ligand in cooperation with transforming growth factor-beta1 potentiates in vitro development of Langerhans-type dendritic cells and allows single-cell dendritic cell cluster formation under serum-free conditions. Blood 90: 1425–1434

Summers KL, Hock BD, McKenzie JL, Hart DN (2001) Phenotypic characterization of five dendritic cell subsets in human tonsils. Am J Pathol 159: 285–295

Sung SS, Fu SM, Rose CE Jr, Gaskin F, Ju ST, Beaty SR (2006) A Major Lung CD103 ({alpha}E)-beta7 Integrin-Positive Epithelial Dendritic Cell Population Expressing Langerin and Tight Junction Proteins. J Immunol 176: 2161–2172

Szomolanyi-Tsuda E, Liang X, Welsh RM, Kurt-Jones EA, Finberg RW (2006) Role for TLR2 in NK cell-mediated control of murine cytomegalovirus *in vivo*. J Virol 80: 4286–4291

Tabeta K, Georgel P, Janssen E, Du X, Hoebe K, Crozat K, Mudd S, Shamel L, Sovath S, Goode J, Alexopoulou L, Flavell RA, Beutler B (2004) Toll-like receptors 9 and 3 as essential components of innate immune defense against mouse cytomegalovirus infection. Proc Natl Acad Sci USA 101: 3516–3521

Takeda K, Akira S (2004) Microbial recognition by Toll-like receptors. J Dermatol Sci 34: 73–82

Tamura T, Tailor P, Yamaoka K, Kong HJ, Tsujimura H, O'Shea JJ, Singh H, Ozato K (2005) IFN regulatory factor-4 and -8 govern dendritic cell subset development and their functional diversity. J Immunol 174: 2573–2581

Town T, Jeng D, Alexopoulou L, Tan J, Flavell RA (2006) Microglia recognize double-stranded RNA via TLR3. J Immunol 176: 3804–3812

Triantafilou K, Orthopoulos G, Vakakis E, Ahmed MA, Golenbock DT, Lepper PM, Triantafilou M (2005) Human cardiac inflammatory responses triggered by Coxsackie B viruses are mainly Toll-like receptor (TLR) 8-dependent. Cell Microbiol 7: 1117–1126

Vandenabeele S, Hochrein H, Mavaddat N, Winkel K, Shortman K (2001) Human thymus contains 2 distinct dendritic cell populations. Blood 97: 1733–1741

Visintin A, Mazzoni A, Spitzer JH, Wyllie DH, Dower SK, Segal DM (2001) Regulation of Toll-like receptors in human monocytes and dendritic cells. J Immunol 166: 249–255

Voisine C, Hubert FX, Trinite B, Heslan M, Josien R (2002) Two phenotypically distinct subsets of spleen dendritic cells in rats exhibit different cytokine production and T cell stimulatory activity. J Immunol 169: 2284–2291

Vremec D, Lieschke GJ, Dunn AR, Robb L, Metcalf D, Shortman K (1997) The influence of granulocyte/macrophage colony-stimulating factor on dendritic cell levels in mouse lymphoid organs. Eur J Immunol 27: 40–44

Vremec D, O'Keeffe M, Hochrein H, Fuchsberger M, Caminschi I, Lahoud M, Shortman K (2007) Production of interferons by dendritic cells, plasmacytoid cells, natural killer cells, and interferon-producing killer dendritic cells. Blood 109: 1165–1173

Vremec D, Pooley J, Hochrein H, Wu L, Shortman K (2000) CD4 and CD8 expression by dendritic cell subtypes in mouse thymus and spleen. J Immunol 164: 2978–2986

Wang JP, Kurt-Jones EA, Shin OS, Manchak MD, Levin MJ, Finberg RW (2005) Varicella-zoster virus activates inflammatory cytokines in human monocytes and macrophages via Toll-like receptor 2. J Virol 79: 12658–12666

Wang T, Town T, Alexopoulou L, Anderson JF, Fikrig E, Flavell RA (2004) Toll-like receptor 3 mediates West Nile virus entry into the brain causing lethal encephalitis. Nat Med 10: 1366–1373

Watanabe N, Wang YH, Lee HK, Ito T, Wang YH, Cao W, Liu YJ (2005) Hassall's corpuscles instruct dendritic cells to induce CD4+CD25+ regulatory T cells in human thymus. Nature 436: 1181–1185

Wilson NS, El Sukkari D, Belz GT, Smith CM, Steptoe RJ, Heath WR, Shortman K, Villadangos JA (2003) Most lymphoid organ dendritic cell types are phenotypically and functionally immature. Blood 102: 2187–2194

Worbs T, Bode U, Yan S, Hoffmann MW, Hintzen G, Bernhardt G, Forster R, Pabst O (2006) Oral tolerance originates in the intestinal immune system and relies on antigen carriage by dendritic cells. J Exp Med 203: 519–527

Wu L, Shortman K (2005) Heterogeneity of thymic dendritic cells. Semin Immunol 17: 304–312

Yasuda K, Yu P, Kirschning CJ, Schlatter B, Schmitz F, Heit A, Bauer S, Hochrein H, Wagner H (2005) Endosomal translocation of vertebrate DNA activates dendritic cells via TLR9-dependent and -independent pathways. J Immunol 174: 6129–6136

Zhou S, Kurt-Jones EA, Mandell L, Cerny A, Chan M, Golenbock DT, Finberg RW (2005) MyD88 is critical for the development of innate and adaptive immunity during acute lymphocytic choriomeningitis virus infection. Eur J Immunol 35: 822–830

Structure of Toll-Like Receptors

Nicholas J. Gay(✉) and Monique Gangloff

Abstract The ten human Toll-like receptors are able to respond to an extremely diverse range of microbial products ranging from di- and tri-acylated lipids to nucleic acids. An understanding of the molecular structure adopted by the receptor extracellular, transmembrane, and cytoplasmic domains and the way in which these structures interact with ligands and downstream signaling adapters can explain how recognition and signal transduction are achieved at a molecular level. In this article we discuss how the leucine-rich repeats of the receptor ectodomain have evolved to bind a wide variety of biological molecules. We also discuss how ligand binding induces dimerization of two receptor chains and initiates a series of protein conformational changes that lead to a signaling event in the cytoplasm of the immune system cell. Thus, the signaling process of the TLRs can be viewed as a unidirectional molecular switch.

Nicholas J. Gay

University of Cambridge, 80, Tennis Court Rd., Cambridge, CB2 1GA, UK

njg11@mole.bio.cam.ac.uk

S. Bauer, G. Hartmann (eds.), *Toll-Like Receptors (TLRs) and Innate Immunity.*
Handbook of Experimental Pharmacology 183.
© Springer-Verlag Berlin Heidelberg 2008

1 Introduction

The human Toll-like receptors (hTLR) were originally isolated by hybridization
or from expressed sequence tag libraries prepared from a variety of tissues (Rock
et al., 1998). The DNA sequence of these clones revealed that the proteins they
encoded had a modular structure similar to that of the *Drosophila* Toll, a type I
transmembrane receptor that functions in dorsoventral patterning and innate immunity in the insect (Belvin and Anderson, 1996; Imler and Hoffmann, 2001). This
initial study identified five hTLRs, but completion of the human genome project
revealed a total of ten. In common with *Drosophila* Toll, hTLRs have a signal
sequence for secretion to the endoplasmic reticulum followed by an extracellular
domain (ectodomain) made up of "typical" leucine-rich repeats (LRRs). Leucine-
rich repeats are about 24 amino acids long and are found in a large, functionally
diverse superfamily of proteins found in all cellular and extracellular compartments
(Buchanan and Gay, 1996). There are 250 LRR proteins currently identified in the
human genome sequence[1]. In the hTLRs, the blocks of LRRs are usually flanked at
the N and C termini by capping structures stabilized by disulfide bonds. The number
of LRR repeats in the hTLRs varies from 20 in TLR1, 2, 6, and 10 to 27 in TLR7,
8, and 9. Another important feature of the TLR ectodomains is that they are glycosylated. Again the level of glycosylation is variable with four sites identified in
TLR2 (Weber et al., 2004) and 11 in TLR3 (Bell et al., 2005). The ectodomains are
connected to the cytoplasm by a hydrophobic transmembrane sequence of about 22
amino acids, which probably form into an α-helix. The cytoplasmic domain of the
receptor consists of a linker, which connects the membrane to a globular fold called
the Toll/interleukin 1 receptor (TIR) domain. The TIR domain consists of about
200 amino acids and folds into an $\alpha - \beta$ structure similar to that of the bacterial
chemotaxis protein CheY (see Section 3.2).

The *Drosophila* genome also encodes multiple homologues of the Toll receptor, and a phylogenetic analysis of the receptors from humans and *Drosophila*
reveals a number of interesting features. First, except for dToll9, the *Drosophila*
Tolls are more related to each other than to the human receptors (Figure 1). This
suggests that, although related evolutionarily, this receptor family has become
specialized for different functions in vertebrates and invertebrates. Thus, whereas
all of the hTLRs function in innate immune recognition, only one fulfils this role
in *Drosophila* (Tauszig et al., 2000). Similarly, the *Drosophila* but not the human
receptors function in ontogenesis and cell adhesion. These functional differences
are reflected in the way that the receptors recognize activating stimuli. *Drosophila*
Tolls respond to an endogenous protein ligand generated outside of the cell by a
proteolytic cascade. By contrast, the human receptors sense microbial stimuli in a
more direct fashion, either by direct binding or by the use of co-receptor proteins
(Gangloff et al., 2005). Another interesting feature revealed by this phylogenetic
analysis is the clustering of the human TLRs into two broad groups. The TLRs that
respond to bacterial stimuli (1, 2, 4, 5, 6) fall into one group and those that recognize

---

[1] see http://www.ensembl.org/Homo_sapiens/domainview?domainentry=IPR003591

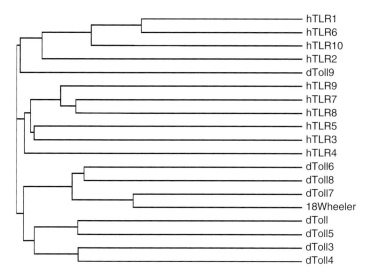

Fig. 1 Phylogenetic tree of *Drosophila* and human Tolls. The tree was generated using the program CLUSTAL W (Thompson et al., 1994)

nucleic acid like molecules (3, 7, 8, and 9) another. This indicates that there may be common mechanisms for the recognition of bacterial structures (principally lipids and lipopeptides) and nucleic acids, respectively. In this regard a recent study has revealed that TLR7, 8, and 9 have a higher order repeat at their N-termini. Remarkably, the first 9 LRRs in these receptors are a triplication of an ancestral 3 LRR unit (Matsushima et al., 2007).

2 Extracellular Domains

2.1 Secondary Structure Elements

The TLR ectodomains consist of three discrete secondary structure elements, the LRR, N-capping, and C- capping structures (Figure 2). TLRs have, on the whole, "typical" LRR repeats of about 24 amino acids (as opposed to "long" repeats as found in ribonuclease inhibitor (Kobe and Deisenhofer, 1993) or the "short" repeats characteristic of prokaryotic LRRs such as the *Listeria* protein internalin (Schubert et al., 2002)). Each repeat has conserved leucines, or often other hydrophobic residues such as isoleucine and valine, at positions 1, 4, 7, 9, 14, 17 and 22 (Figure 2a).

A single asparagine residue at position 12 is nearly invariant although occasionally other amino acids can be accommodated at this position. The structures of about 20 leucine-rich repeat proteins have now been solved, including that for the ectodomain of TLR3 (Bell et al., 2005; Choe et al., 2005). This structure reveals that the LRRs fold into an extended rather than a globular structure. Each LRR has

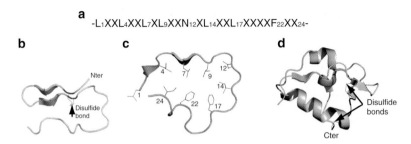

a

-L₁XXL₄XXL₇XL₉XXN₁₂XL₁₄XXL₁₇XXXXF₂₂XX₂₄-

Fig. 2 Secondary structure elements of the TLR ectodomains. **a** Primary consensus sequence of a typical LRR. **b** N-cap of TLR3 ectodomain (PDB code 2A0Z) stabilized by one disulfide bridge. **c** LRR from TLR3 (LRR7 from residue 196 to 220). The side chains of conserved residues are shown. **d** C-cap of TLR3 stabilized by two disulfide bonds

a short region of β-sheet, a turn, and then a more variable secondary structure. The conserved leucine residues pack together to form a hydrophobic core and the asparagine is required for the turn that connects the two secondary structure elements. The individual LRR units fold together to form a solenoidal structure with a characteristic curvature (Figure 3). The fold is stabilized by the formation of a parallel β sheet, with one strand being contributed by each LRR; this forms the internal or convex surface of the solenoid. The variable region of the repeat forms the concave surface of the structure and can be α-helix, 3_{10} helix, β sheet, or other extended types of conformation. The nature of the variable region determines the curvature of the solenoid. For example, ribonuclease inhibitor (Kobe and Deisenhofer, 1993) has a regular α-helix and this causes a sharp curvature, whereas other structures, for example the platelet glycoprotein 1b (Gp1b) (Huizinga et al., 2002), are much flatter.

In the TLRs and other extracellular LRR proteins, the repeat blocks are often flanked by cysteine-rich capping structures. The purpose of these may be to shield the hydrophobic residues of the terminal repeats but there is also evidence that they participate in protein-protein interactions. In Gp1b the C-capping structure makes a large contribution to binding of the adhesion molecule von Willebrand factor (vWF) "A" domain. A loop of the C-cap structure is induced to form an antiparallel β strand on binding by vWF (Huizinga et al., 2002). The functional importance of these structures is shown by the properties of type 1 dominant mutations of the *Drosophila* Toll receptor (Schneider et al., 1991). These proteins have mutations in the cysteine residues of the C-cap which cause the receptor to become constitutively active (see Section 5). The N-caps also have both structural and functional roles. In TLR4 this element is required for association of the co-receptor protein MD-2 (Nishitani et al., 2006) and preliminary evidence suggests that it is also important for association of the Spätzle protein ligand with *Drosophila* Toll.

The LRR C-cap, exemplified by that of TLR3, has a sequence with four cysteine residues and these are conserved in most extracellular LRR proteins. The connectivity of the disulfide bonds (CI-CIII and CII-CIV) is invariant but the spacing of the cysteine residues is quite variable (between 22 and 52 residues). The C-cap has an α/ß structure, with an α-helix, several short 3_{10}-helices and β-strands capping the hydrophobic core and forming hydrogen bonds with the last repeat (Figure 2d, (Bell et al., 2005)). In fact the first two cysteines of the LRR C-cap motif occur in the middle of the last repeat at positions 15 and 17, respectively. In contrast to the C-caps, the structure of the N-cap is simpler, with one disulfide bond that stabilizes the amino-terminus end and a compact β-hairpin structure. The single disulfide between cysteines CI and CIII forms "a small knot" and holds the amino-terminal loopy end in a closed conformation on top of the tandem segments of LRRs (Figure 2b).

2.2 Three-Dimensional Structure of TLR Extracellular Domains

Despite a considerable effort by a number of laboratories only the structure of TLR3 has been solved to date (Figure 3) (Bell et al., 2005; Choe et al., 2005). As expected, the 23 leucine-rich repeats fold into a solenoidal structure, but unlike other LRR structures it lacks a twist across the solenoid axis. This causes the structure to adopt a flat conformation and may facilitate the interactions with ligand that are required for dimerization or oligomerization during the signaling process. The lack of twist may be caused by the presence of several irregular repeats and two loops that protrude from the solenoid structure at LRR12 and 20. Another striking feature of the TLR 3 ectodomain is the presence of 11 N-linked glycosylations representing about 35% of the total mass (Sun et al., 2006). These modifications are concentrated on one side of the solenoid leaving the other lateral surface available for interaction

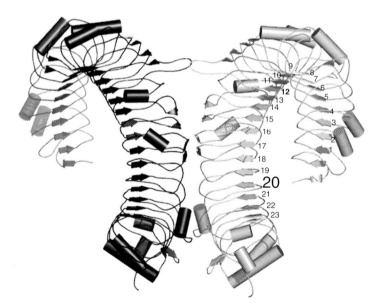

Fig. 3 TLR3 ectodomain. The domain contains 23 repeats, as indicated. In the crystal structures TLR3 forms a dimer with protein-protein contacts between LRR12 and LRR20. Residues from LRR20 have been shown to be involved in double-stranded RNA ligand binding

with the putative ligand, double-stranded RNA (dsRNA). The presence of loops and extensive N-linked glycan is characteristic of TLR family members and both of these features are critical for receptor biogenesis or function (see below).

A low-resolution structure of *Drosophila* Toll generated by 3-dimensional image reconstruction of negatively stained electron micrographs shows a very similar arrangement to that observed for TLR3. Unlike TLR3, *Drosophila* Toll has two discrete blocks of LRRs and capping structures. This causes a discontinuity in the solenoid structure that is visible in the EM reconstruction (Gay and Gangloff, unpublished).

3 Transmembrane and Cytoplasmic Domains

3.1 Transmembrane Domains

An alignment of the transmembrane (TM) and juxta-membrane sequences from the human TLRs is presented in Figure 4.

Like other type I receptors TLRs have a short region of about 22 uncharged amino acids predicted to form a membrane spanning α-helix. Apart from being apolar the sequences are not conserved, and five of them have glycines, an amino acid not usually accommodated in α-helices. The linker between the C-terminal

```
               10        20        30        40        50        60
        ....|....|....|....|....|....|....|....|....|....|....|....|
hTLR1   CTCELGEFVKNIDQVSSEVLEGWPDSYKCDYPESYRGTLLKDFHMSELSCNIT-------
hTLR6   CTCELREFVKNIDQVSSEVLEGWPDSYKCDYPESYRGSPLKDFHMSELSCNIT-------
hTLR10  CTCELKNFIQ-LETYSEVMMVGWSDSYTCEYPLNLRGIRLKDVHLHELSCNTA-------
hTLR2   CSCEFLSFTQEQQ-ALAKVLIDWPANYLCDSPSHVRGQQVQDVRLSVSECHRT-------
hTLR9   CACGAAFMDFLLE--VQAAVPGLPSRVKCGSPGQLQGLSIFAQDLRL--CLDEALSWDC-
hTLR8   CTCDIGDFRRWMDEHLNVKIPRLV-DVICASPGDQRGKSIVSLELTT--CVSDVT-----
hTLR7   CTCDAVWFVWWVN-HTEVTIPYLATDVTCVGPGAHKGQSVISLDLYT--CELDLTN----
hTLR5   CECELSTFINWLN-HTNVTIAGPPADIYCVYPDSFSGVSLFSLSTEG--CDEEEVLKSLK
hTLR4   CTCEHQSFLQWIK--DQRQLLVEVERMECATPSDKQGMPVLSLNIT---CQMNK------
hTLR3   CTCESIAWFVNWINETHTNIPELSSHYLCNTPPHYIIGFPVRLFDTSS--CKDSAPFEL--

                   LRR C-terminal cap                    Linker

               70        80        90        100       110
        ....|....|....|....|....|....|....|....|....|....|....|....|
hTLR1   LLIVTIVATMLVLAVTVTSLCIYLDLPWYLRMVCQWTQTRRR-ARNIPLEELQRN    634
hTLR6   LLIVTIGATMLVLAVTVTSLCIYLDLPWYLRMVCQWTQTRRR-ARNIPLEELQRN    639
hTLR10  LLIVTIVVIMLVLGLAVAFCCLHFDLPWYLRMLGQCTQTWHR-VRKTTQEQLKRN    631
hTLR2   ALVSGMCCALFLLILLTGVLCHRFHGLWYMKMMWAWLQAKRK-PRKAPSRN----    638
hTLR9   FALSLLAVALGLGVPMLHHLC----G-WDLWYCFHLCLAWLP-WRGRQSGRDEDA    867
hTLR8   AVILFFFTFFITTMVMLAALAHHLFY-WDVWFIYNVCLAKVKGYRSLSTSQ----    877
hTLR7   LILFLSLSISVSLFLMVMMT-ASHLYF-WDVWYIYHFCKAKIKGYQRLISPD----    888
hTLR5   FSLFIVCTVTLTLFLMTILTVTKFRG---FCFICYKTAQRLV-FKDHPQGTEPDM    690
hTLR4   TIIGVSVLSVLVVSVVAVLVY---------KFYFHLMLLAGCIK-YGRGE-----    671
hTLR3   FFMINTSILLIFIFIVLLIHF---EG-WRISFYWNVSVHRVLGFKEIDRQTEQ--    753

            Transmembrane region           Intracellular linker
```

Fig. 4 Sequence alignment of human TLRs trans- and juxta-membrane regions. The sequence starts at the conserved cysteine residues from the C-caps and includes the intracellular linkers to the TIR domains. The latter is not shown

capping structure of the ectodomain and the membrane is very short. The cysteine residue that forms the second disulfide bond of the capping structure is between the 2 and 5 amino acids from the first residue that is predicted to be embedded in the membrane. In TLR3 the capping structure is packed tightly against the last LRR and the short linker may serve to position the ectodomain correctly and ensure a rigid connection with the membrane. On the cytoplasmic side of the membrane there is a much longer linker connecting the TM sequence to the first secondary structure element of the TIR domain, varying from 20 amino acids in TLR4 to 30 in TLR5. There is some sequence conservation in this juxta-membrane sequence; for example, a tryptophan residue close to the membrane surface and a cluster of basic amino acids. It is unclear whether this linker adopts a fixed conformation or has a fixed orientation with respect to the ectodomain and transmembrane helix.

3.2 The TIR Domains

The TIR domain is found in 25 human proteins, which can be subdivided into two groups. The first group consist of type I transmembrane receptors, the ten TLRs and the interleukin 1 receptor (IL-1R) family. The eight IL-1R family members have different ectodomains made up immunoglobulin type modules rather than LRRs (Sims 2002). They function in the second phase of the innate immune response and although evolutionarily related to TLRs are not found in insects. The second group constitute the signaling adapters for the TLRs of which there are five (Mal/TIRAP, MyD88, SARM, TRAM, and TRIF) (O'Neill et al., 2003). MyD88 also functions as the exclusive adapter for signaling by IL-1R family members. TIR domains are also found in bacteria, viruses, and plants, being particularly abundant in *Arabidopsis*, where they fulfil roles in both development and disease resistance (Jebanathirajah et al., 2002). Thus it is conceivable that TIR domains evolved as general protein-protein interaction domains that later acquired some specialized functions in development and in immune processes.

The primary sequences of TIR domains are characterised by three conserved sequence boxes, designated Box 1, 2, and 3, spread across the length of the module. Outside these boxes TIR domains are very divergent with sequence similarities of 20—30% among superfamily members. Box 1, the most conserved of the three, has the signature sequence **F/YDAF–Y**. Mutational studies over this region suggest disruption but not total abrogation of signal transduction. Box 2 has the consensus sequence **G–LC–RD–PG**. Mutational studies have mostly mapped residues crucial for receptor signaling to this region (Slack et al., 2000). Mutation of the conserved proline in box 2 to histidine in murine TLR4 renders mice insensitive to LPS (Poltorak et al., 1998). A similar mutation in TLR2 abrogates signal transduction in response to yeast and Gram-positive bacterial stimulation. Changing the conserved arginine to alanine in human IL-1 receptor abolishes Toll/IL-1 signaling (Heguy et al., 1992). Box 3 is characterised by the conserved **FW** motif.

As originally predicted by Bazan (Rock et al., 1998), the TIR domain adopts an $\alpha - \beta$ fold very similar to that of the bacterial chemotaxis protein CheY (Stock

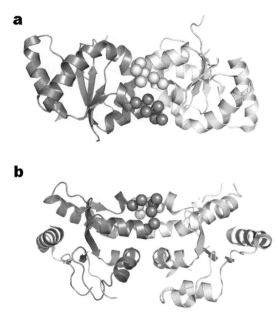

Fig. 5 TIR domain structure. (a) Top and (b) side views of TLR10 dimer (PDB code 2J67) in ribbon representation. Carbon alpha atoms from the BB loop are shown in sphere representation

et al., 1989). CheY proteins consist of a single regulatory domain that is activated by conformational change induced by a phospho-transfer reaction from a histidine kinase to a conserved aspartyl residue. Although structural superposition of CheY and TIR domains shows remarkable topological and tertiary structure conservation, especially over the central beta sheet region, TLRs do not have a phosphotransferase activity. To date there are x-ray structures for isolated TIR domains from TLR1, 2, and 10 and also from the interleukin-1 receptor accessory protein (Xu et al., 2000; Khan et al., 2004) (Figure 5). The fold consists of 4 or 5 parallel β sheets surrounded by five α-helical segments. As with the LRRs, sequence conservation reflects the structural requirements of the fold. By contrast a comparison of the surface electrostatic properties of the crystal structures and models of other TIR domains from TLRs and cognate adapter proteins reveal substantial differences in the surface charge distribution, which may confer specificity for adapter binding and downstream signaling (Dunne et al., 2003).

4 Molecular Mechanisms of Ligand Recognition

There is now considerable evidence that the basic mechanism of signal transmission by TLRs and many other type I receptors is ligand-induced dimerization (Gay et al., 2006). This extracellular crosslinking is transmitted across the membrane and causes rearrangement of the cytoplasmic domain, which in turn generates a downstream signal, for example cross-phosphorylation in the case of receptor tyrosine kinases. Unlike other type I receptors, activated TLRs do not have an enzymatic activity. Instead the rearranged TIRs act as a scaffold for the recruitment of downstream signal transducers such as adapters and non-receptor protein kinases.

4.1 Diverse Nature of the Stimuli

An important characteristic of the TLRs is the chemically diverse nature of the stimuli that activate them. These fall into four general categories and are illustrated in Figure 6. (1) Endogenous and exogenous protein ligands. These include the dimeric cytokine ligand Spätzle that activates the *Drosophila* Toll pathway in the insect immune response (Weber et al., 2003), microbial products such as flagellin (TLR5) (Smith et al., 2003) and the "F" protein of the respiratory syncytial virus (TLR4) (Haynes et al., 2001). (2) Lipids and lipopeptides. Examples include

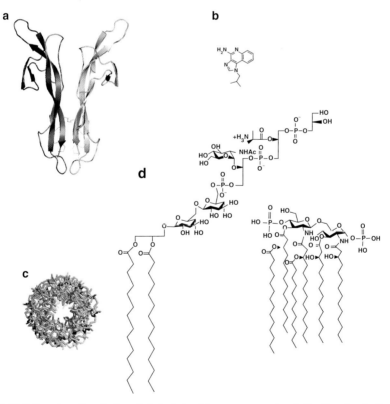

Fig. 6 TLR ligands. **a** Protein ligand: Spätzle in ribbon representation. **b** Small molecule ligand: Imiquimod. **c** Nucleic acid ligand: double-stranded RNA shown in its cross section (PDB code 1QC0). **d** Lipidic ligands: LTA on the left and lipid A on the right

lipopolysaccharide (LPS) (TLR4), a component of the outer membrane from Gram-negative bacteria and lipoteichoic acid (Poltorak et al., 1998; Qureshi et al., 1999), a diacylated lipid from the cytoplasmic membrane of Gram-positive bacteria (TLR2) (Morath et al., 2002). (3) Non-self nucleic acids derived form bacteria and viruses. TLR9 responds to DNA containing unmethylated CpG dinucleotides (Bauer et al., 2001). TLR7 and 8 are activated by GU-rich single-stranded RNA (Diebold et al., 2004; Lund et al., 2004) and TLR3 by double-stranded RNA (Alexopoulou et al., 2001). These molecules are produced in the course of viral infections. (4) A group of synthetic small drug molecules can also stimulate TLR7 and TLR8 signaling (Hemmi et al., 2002; Gorden et al., 2005). For example, the imidazoquinolines are used for treatment of basal cell carcinoma and human papilloma virus infection (Geisse et al., 2004). Other molecules chemically similar to guanosine nucleotides, such as loxoribene, are also effective agonists of TLR7 and 8 (Lee et al., 2003).

4.2 Direct Versus Indirect Activation of TLR Signaling

The activation of type I receptors by protein ligands involves high affinity binding with dissociation constants (K_d) in the order of 1nM (Schlessinger, 2002; Weber et al., 2003). At a structural level, interactions between receptor and ligand involve extensive interfaces between the proteins that are stabilized by the hydrophobic effect, hydrogen bonds, and salt bridges. For TLRs that bind to endogenous or exogenous protein ligands, such as *Drosophila* Toll and Spätzle ($K_d = 0.4$nM) and TLR5 and flagellin, this also seems to be the case. On the other hand, if high affinity binding is a prerequisite for the formation of receptor dimers, how can small molecules such as imidazoquinolines crosslink two receptor chains into a functional signaling complex? One possibility is that the receptors do not bind directly to the ligand but require and accessory or co-receptor protein.

As described in detail in 4.4, TLR4 requires a co-receptor MD-2 to sense LPS (Nagai et al., 2002). In addition to MD-2, signaling in response to LPS requires other accessory proteins that are not stably associated with the receptor. LBP (LPS-binding protein) (Jack et al., 1997) is a circulating glycoprotein that extracts and opsonizes LPS from infecting Gram-negative bacteria and transfers it to CD14, an extrinsic outer membrane protein found on the surface of immune system cells such as macrophages (Tobias et al., 1995). CD14 is also an LRR protein and is able to bind a fairly broad spectrum of lipids (Kim et al., 2007). Thus CD14 can also enhance signaling by tri-acylated lipopeptides through TLR2 and TLR1 (Manukyan et al., 2005). Two other accessory proteins enhance responses through TLR2. Oblivious/CD36 is a scavenger receptor required for inflammatory responses to tri-acylated lipopeptides (Hoebe et al., 2005). Secondly, Dectin-1, a lectin family receptor for β-glucans derived from fungi, collaborates with TLRs in recognizing microbes and enhances TLR2 signaling in macrophages and dendritic cells (Gantner et al., 2005; Taylor et al., 2007).

4.3 Binding and Activation of Drosophila Toll by Spätzle

The protein ligand for *Drosophila* Toll is a dimer of the C-terminal 106 amino acids, cleaved proteolytically from an inactive pro-protein. The dimer has a single, intramolecular disulfide bond and the subunits have a "cysteine knot" fold (Mizuguchi et al., 1998) (Figure 6). In this fold there is a long antiparallel β sheet that is held together by three intersecting disufide bonds. Spätzle C106 is able to bind and crosslink two Toll receptor molecules, and this dimerization event is sufficient to establish signal transduction. Purified Toll ectodomains can also bind Spätzle in solution and forms either a 2:1 complex, a 2:2 or a 1:1 complex, depending on the conditions used (Weber et al., 2005; Gangloff and Gay, unpublished results). This result suggests that the binding events that lead to the signalling complex are nonequivalent and that the binding reaction probably involves negative cooperativity.

A low resolution structure of the 1:1 complex of Toll and Spätzle generated by 3D image reconstruction of EM images shows that the ligand binds close to the N-terminus of the solenoid (Gangloff and Gay, unpublished results). This binding probably involves the N-capping structure and initial LRRs. Further insight into the nature of the interaction between Toll and Spätzle comes from a structure of the nerve growth factor (NGF), a cysteine knot growth factor related to Spätzle, with the p75 neurotrophin receptor. In this structure (He and Garcia, 2004) 24 residues of the NGF monomer contribute to binding and these are localized in two discrete regions of the molecules including the N-terminus. Interestingly, a number of residues in both sites are conserved or are charge reversals (Weber et al., 2007). This suggests that binding of Spätzle C-106 to the Toll ectodomain is analogous to that of NGF to p75, involving the burial of hydrophobic surfaces together with electrostatic complementarity provided by surrounding salt bridges and hydrogen bonds. It is also of note that the structure solved was of a 1:1 receptor:NGF complex rather than the 2:1 complex formed during signaling (Aurikko et al., 2005), suggesting that like Toll/Spätzle NGF/p75 shows negative cooperativity. In fact, in this structure NGF has two discontinuous sites of interaction with p75 and the unbound, symmetry-related pseudo-sites show a certain amount of structural distortion as a consequence of the first binding event. This suggests that compared to the first binding event the second will be energetically unfavorable. In conclusion, the ectodomain of *Drosophila* Toll binds to an endogenous protein ligand in a manner analogous to the vertebrate neurotrophin receptor binding to NGF.

4.4 The TLR4/MD2 Co-Receptor Complex

Genetic studies in mice have established the essential role played by TLR4 and MD-2 in LPS signaling (Nagai et al., 2002). Since these initial findings, biochemical studies have shown that TLR4 and MD-2 are expressed as a noncovalent complex on the cell surface (Re and Strominger, 2002; Akashi et al., 2003; Gioannini et al., 2004). Lipid A, the active moiety of LPS, is usually hexa acylated (Figure 6) but there is considerable variation both in chain number and length depending on the species of Gram-negative bacteria from which the LPS is derived (Heinrichs et al., 1998). Lipid A binds to TLR4/MD-2 on the cell surface and causes oligomerization of the receptor/co-receptor complexes (Saitoh et al., 2004; Kobayashi et al., 2006). Thus, MD-2 is analogous to Spätzle as it binds specifically to the TLR4 ectodomain although it functions as an endogenous co-receptor rather than a protein ligand. The structure of TLR4 has not been determined but it is likely to fold into a solenoid similar to that of TLR3 (see Figure 3 and (Rallabhandi et al., 2006)). A recent study suggests that like Spätzle MD-2 binds to the N-terminus of the ectodomain. In particular, the integrity of the N-terminal capping structure (24–47) is essential both for MD-2 binding and function (Nishitani et al., 2006). Mutations in the two cysteine residues that form a stabilizing disulfide bond in the N-cap abolish MD-2 binding.

Despite some superficial similarities between Spätzle and MD-2, their three-dimensional structures are very different. MD-2 consists of about 144 amino acids and belongs to a family of lipid-binding proteins that include the mite dust allergen Derp2 and the GM-2 activator protein (termed the ML family) (Inohara and Nunez, 2002). These proteins have a β-sandwich or immunoglobulin-type fold consisting of six antiparallel β-strands. Lipids bind to ML members by intercalating acyl chains into the hydrophobic core of the fold. On the basis of the known structure of the mite dust allergen and other ML family members it is possible to construct a homology model of MD-2 (Figure 7) (Gangloff and Gay, 2004; Gruber et al., 2004).[2]

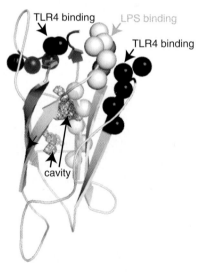

Fig. 7 Model of MD-2. The structure shows the internal cavity in a wire-frame representation. Spheres indicate the localization of residues involved in LPS binding (in white) and TLR4 binding (in black)

---

[2] Since submission high resolution structures of MD-2 and MD-2 in complex with TLR4 have been publishes (Ohto et al., 2007; Kim et al., 2007)

This model predicts that lipid will bind to MD-2 by inserting one or more acyl chains into an internal cavity in the structure and that this binding event is likely to cause a large conformational change in MD-2. At the mouth of this cavity is a loop structure containing two basic amino acids, residues that are essential for LPS signaling (Visintin et al., 2003). It is likely that these side-chains make electrostatic contacts with the glucosamine phosphate head group of the lipid A and thereby stabilize LPS binding. In fact, MD-2 has been the subject of extensive mutagenesis studies that have also identified regions required for binding of MD-2 to TLR4 (57–79; 108–135) (Viriyakosol et al., 2006). This approach has also identified residues that account for species-specific differences observed in responsiveness to lipid A variants. For example, lipid IVa (a tetracylated form) acts as an agonist in mice but an antagonist in humans. Specific residues in MD-2 have been identified that confer these variations and, interestingly, these lie in the regions required for association with TLR4 (Muroi and Tanamoto, 2006).

4.5 The Nucleic Acid-Binding TLRs

The TLR3, 7, 8, and 9 group all respond to nucleic acid derivatives or small molecules with structural similarities to purine nucleotides. In addition, unlike other TLRs, this group localizes not to the cell surface but to intracellular compartments (Latz et al., 2004; Gibbard et al., 2006). Although mainly localized to the endoplasmic reticulum, they function in acidified compartments, the late endosome and lysosome. Thus, there must be constitutive or regulated trafficking of these receptors from the ER to acid compartments. Intracellular localization may also be important to prevent activation of immune responses by self-nucleic acids. The elucidation of the TLR3 ectodomain structure has led to significant advances in our understanding of nucleic acid recognition by these receptors and the evidence suggests that binding is likely to be direct and does not require a co-receptor like MD-2.

Two recent papers describe mutagenesis studies of the TLR 3 ectodomain and have identified a number of residues that are required both for binding of double-stranded RNA and signaling. Bell et al., (Bell et al., 2006) identified only two residues—H539 and N541 in the 20th LRR—that abolished signaling and also showed that mutant ectodomains were no longer able to bind dsRNA *in vivo*. These residues lie on a lateral surface of the solenoid (Figure 3) that is free from glycoyslation and the authors suggest that the asaparagine residue might accept a hydrogen bond from the 2′ ribose of the dsRNA. This interaction may provide specificity for ribonucleic acid and explain why deoxyribonucleotides, which lack a hydroxyl group at the 2′ position, do not activate the pathway or bind to the ectodomain. This result also suggests that dsRNA could induce symmetrical oligomers of TLR3 ectodomains. A more recent paper extended this analysis and found a number of additional amide residues in LRRs 18–20 that have a profound effect on TLR3 signaling function (Ranjith-Kumar et al., 2007). These are located on the same glycan-free lateral surface and suggest a more extensive binding interface for dsRNA involving side-chain amides. These authors also show that the TLR3 ectodomain exists as a dimer in solution and that many of the mutants can exert dominant negative effects when co-expressed with wild-type receptor. This indicates that the signaling process involves not only protein: RNA binding but also protein-protein interactions occur between two receptor chains.

In the case of TLR9, which responds to unmethylated CpG DNA, there is also evidence for direct binding between the nucleic acid and receptor. Rutz et al. (2004) showed that the TLR9 ectodomain bound to CpG DNA with high affinity (ca 60nM) and that this binding is pH-dependent. They also showed that ectodomains with mutations in LRR 17 lost the ability to bind DNA. Thus, as with TLR3, TLR9 has a surface located towards the C-terminal of the ectodomain that can bind nucleic acid. The equivalent region of the TLR8 ectodomain is also important for signaling in response to both single-stranded RNA and the imidazoquinoline resiquimod (Gibbard et al., 2006). The involvement of negatively charged residues has led to the suggestion there are pH-dependent changes in the ligands that enable binding. For example, the imidazo group of resiquimod has a pK_a of about 6.7 and so will be largely uncharged at pH 7 but will become protonated at pH 5. Thus, binding of the positively charged ligand by a negatively charged region of the ectodomain may promote association of two receptor chains by hydrophobic stacking interactions between the ring structures of the imidazoquinoline.

5 Mechanism of Signal Transduction

As discussed above, the basic mechanism of signaling by the TLRs is ligand-induced dimerization or oligomerization. The evidence for this comes from experiments with *Drosophila* Spätzle that demonstrate both *in vivo* and *in vitro* that this cytokine binds and triggers the crosslinks of two Toll receptor ectodomains. Domain swap experiments in which the TLR4 ectodomain is replaced by that of *Drosophila* Toll signal in response to Spätzle with similar biochemical characteristics (Weber et al., 2003), suggesting that the basic mechanism is highly conserved. However, recent studies have shown that the process of activation is likely to be more complex than simple crosslinking and to involve concerted protein conformational changes (Weber et al., 2005). Like TLR3, the full-length *Drosophila* Toll ectodomain is able to form unstable dimers in solution, but truncations at the N-terminus allows the formation of a stable dimeric complex, suggesting that sequences at the C-terminus of the ectodomain are able to mediate receptor-receptor interactions. The importance of these juxtamembrane regions is emphasised by findings that point mutations in the cysteine residues of the C-terminal cap structure (Figure 2) cause constitutive activation of the receptor (Schneider et al., 1991). Thus the N-terminal region of the ectodomain acts as an auto-inhibitor and may provide structural hindrance that prevents unregulated dimerization (Hu et al., 2004). Furthermore, in the Toll-TLR4 domain swap experiments; chimeric receptors with the *Drosophila* Toll transmembrane helix are tightly regulated in response to Spätzle but chimeras with the TLR4 transmembrane helix are constitutively active (Weber et al., 2005). As the interaction site for Spätzle is located at the extreme N-terminus of the ectodomain, initial ligand-induced dimerization and receptor-receptor interaction are not directly coupled.

Taken together the results outlined above suggest that receptor activation is a concerted, sequential and irreversible process. Ligand binding induces a conformational change in the C- terminal region of the ectodomain that enables stable receptor-receptor interactions and this in turn arranges the transmembrane helices of the receptor dimer in a manner that allows downstream signaling to occur (Figure 8). The structure of the isolated TLR3 ectodomain provides support for the activation scheme outlined above (see Section 4) (Bell et al., 2005; Choe et al., 2005). In the crystal structure two molecules are arranged as dimers (Figure 3). The dimer interface is on the convex surface at the C-terminus and this arrangement may reflect the conformation adopted by the ectodomain dimer prior to binding of dsRNA.

As noted above, the immediate juxtamembrane and transmembrane regions are critical for transmission of the signal to the cytoplasm. The cytoplasmic TIR domain is required for coupling extracellular dimerization to downstream signal transduction. The evidence suggests that active TLRs recruit specific sets of adapter proteins into multitypic complexes (O'Neill et al., 2003). These adapters also contain TIR domains and receptor dimerization must in some way create a new scaffold that provides the binding specificity required for recruitment of the appropriate adapter combinations by the TLR. The surface properties of the receptor and adapter TIRs are distinct, and it has been proposed that surface complementarity is the basis of TLR-specific adapter recruitment (Dunne et al., 2003). The most complex adapter

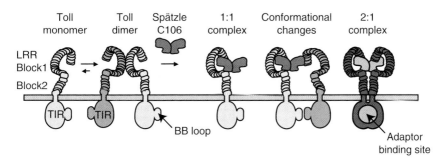

Fig. 8 Mechanism for binding of ligand and signaling by *Drosophila* Toll. In the absence of ligand, Toll ectodomains are found in equilibrium between monomers and dimers with a dissociation constant of about 2μM (Weber et al., 2005). This interaction may be mediated by the first block of leucine-rich repeats (LRRs) and resemble the dimeric crystal structure observed for Toll-like receptor 3 (TLR3). The second block of LRRs forms strong dimer contacts that are prevented by the first block. Spätzle dissociates Toll dimers to form a 1:1 complex. Recruitment of a second receptor molecule in the 2:1 complex displays negative cooperativity, which implies conformational rearrangement in the receptor-ligand and receptor-receptor interactions. The BB loop of the signaling TIR (define) domain is likely to be involved in receptor-receptor contacts. The signaling complex is proposed to generate a new interface for adapter recruitment

usage is shown by TLR4, which recruits four adapters in response to LPS stimulation and couples to two different downstream pathways leading to activation of NF-κB (requires Mal and MyD88) and the interferon regulatory factor 3 (IRF-3) (TRAM and TRIF), respectively (Fitzgerald et al., 2003).

With regard to the signaling mechanism, two characteristics of the receptor assemblies are likely to be crucial: first, the connections that link the ectodomain to the TIR are rigid, and second, because of the homodimeric nature of the signaling complex, the assemblies induced by the ligand binding must be symmetrical. This means that symmetry-related surfaces of the receptor TIR will be forced into association and are likely to undergo a structural rearrangement as a consequence. In TLR4 signaling, residues centred on a surface structural feature called the "BB" loop may be involved in symmetric homodimerization of the receptor TIRs. A mutation of a residue in this flexible loop is the basis of LPS hyporesponsiveness in C3H/Hej mice (Poltorak et al., 1998), and this allele is also a dominant negative, suggesting that it may interfere with receptor dimerization. It is interesting to note that the crystal structure of the TLR10 TIR domain, recently solved as part a structural genomics project, is a symmetrical homodimer (Figure 5). The dimer interface is extensive and involves the proline residue of the BB loop (or Box 2) that is implicated in receptor-receptor interactions. Thus this structure may represent a physiologically relevant conformation. Site-directed mutagenesis also shows that other residues in this surface region are absolutely required for signaling (Ronni et al., 2003). Recent work in this lab also indicates that distinct surface areas of the TLR4 TIR domain are required to couple signaling through the Mal adaptor to NFκB and the TRAM adapter to interferon β respectively. In conclusion, homodimerization of the receptor TIRs may provide a new surface that is able to recruit the specific adapters that are required for downstream signal transduction.

References

Akashi S, Saitoh S, Wakabayashi Y, Kikuchi T, Takamura N, Nagai Y, Kusumoto Y, Fukase K, Kusumoto S, Adachi Y, Kosugi A, Miyake K (2003) Lipopolysaccharide interaction with cell surface Toll-like receptor 4-MD-2: Higher affinity than that with MD-2 or CD14. J Exp Med 198: 1035–1042

Alexopoulou L, Holt AC, Medzhitov R, Flavell RA (2001) Recognition of double-stranded RNA and activation of NF-kappa B by Toll-like receptor 3. Nature 413: 732–738

Aurikko JP, Ruotolo BT, Grossmann JG, Moncrieffe MC, Stephens E, Leppanen VM, Robinson CV, Saarma M, Bradshaw RA, Blundell TL (2005) Characterization of symmetric complexes of nerve growth factor and the ectodomain of the pan-neurotrophin receptor, p75NTR. J Biol Chem 280: 33453–33460

Bauer S, Kirschning CJ, Hacker H, Redecke V, Hausmann S, Akira S, Wagner H, Lipford GB (2001) Human TLR9 confers responsiveness to bacterial DNA via species-specific CpG motif recognition. Proc Natl Acad Sci USA 98: 9237–9242

Bell JK, Askins J, Hall PR, Davies DR, Segal DM (2006) The dsRNA binding site of human Toll-like receptor 3. Proc Natl Acad Sci USA 103: 8792–8797

Bell JK, Botos I, Hall PR, Askins J, Shiloach J, Segal DM, Davies DR (2005) The molecular structure of the Toll-like receptor 3 ligand-binding domain. Proc Natl Acad Sci USA 102: 10976–10980

Belvin MP, Anderson KV (1996) A conserved signaling pathway: The *Drosophila* Toll-Dorsal pathway. Ann Rev Cell Dev Biol 12: 393–416

Buchanan SGS, Gay NJ (1996) Structural and functional diversity in the leucine rich repeat family of proteins. Prog Biophys Mol Biol 65: 1–44

Choe J, Kelker MS, Wilson IA (2005) Crystal structure of human toll-like receptor 3 (TLR3) ectodomain. Science 309: 581–585

Diebold SS, Kaisho T, Hemmi H, Akira S, Reis e Sousa C (2004) Innate antiviral responses by means of TLR7-mediated recognition of single-stranded RNA. Science 303: 1529–1531.

Dunne A, Ejdeback M, Ludidi P, O'Neill LAJ, Gay NJ (2003) Structural complementarity of Toll/interleukin 1 receptor identity regions in Toll-like receptors and the adaptors Mal and MyD88. J Biol Chem 278: 41443–41451

Fitzgerald KA, Rowe DC, Barnes BJ, Caffrey DR, Visintin A, Latz E, Monks B, Pitha PM, Golenbock DT (2003) LPS-TLR4 signaling to IRF-3/7 and NF-kappaB involves the toll adapters TRAM and TRIF. J Exp Med 198: 1043–1055

Gangloff M, Gay NJ (2004) MD-2: The Toll 'gatekeeper' in endotoxin signalling. Trends Biochem Sci 29: 294–300

Gangloff M, Weber AN, Gay NJ (2005) Conserved mechanisms of signal transduction by Toll and Toll-like receptors. J Endotoxin Res 11: 294–298

Gantner BN, Simmons RM, Underhill DM (2005) Dectin-1 mediates macrophage recognition of *Candida albicans* yeast but not filaments. EMBO J 24: 1277–1286

Gay N, Gangloff M, Weber A (2006) Toll-like receptors as molecular switches. Nature Rev Immunol. 6: 693–698

Geisse J, Caro I, Lindholm J, Golitz L, Stampone P, Owens M (2004) Imiquimod 5% cream for the treatment of superficial basal cell carcinoma: Results from two phase III, randomized, vehicle-controlled studies. J Am Acad Dermatol 50: 722–733

Gibbard RJ, Morley PJ, Gay NJ (2006) Conserved features in the extracellular domain of human Toll-like receptor 8 are essential for pH-dependent signaling. J Biol Chem 281: 27503–27511

Gioannini TL, Teghanemt A, Zhang D, Coussens NP, Dockstader W, Ramaswamy S, Weiss JP (2004) Isolation of an endotoxin-MD-2 complex that produces Toll-like receptor 4-dependent cell activation at picomolar concentrations. Proc Natl Acad Sci USA 101: 4186–4191

Gorden KB, Gorski KS, Gibson SJ, Kedl RM, Kieper WC, Qiu X, Tomai MA, Alkan SS, Vasilakos JP (2005) Synthetic TLR agonists reveal functional differences between human TLR7 and TLR8. J Immunol 174: 1259–1268

Gruber A, Mancek M, Wagner H, Kirschning CJ, Jerala R (2004) Structural model of MD-2 and functional role of its basic amino acid clusters involved in cellular lipopolysaccharide recognition. J Biol Chem 279: 28475–28482

Haynes LM, Moore DD, Kurt-Jones EA, Finberg RW, Anderson LJ, Tripp RA (2001) Involvement of Toll-like receptor 4 in innate immunity to respiratory syncytial virus. J Virol 75: 10730–10737

He XL, Garcia KC (2004) Structure of nerve growth factor complexed with the shared neurotrophin receptor p75. Science 304: 870–875

Heguy A, Baldari CT, Macchia G, Telford JL, Melli M (1992) Amino-acids conserved in interleukin-1 receptors (Il-1rs) and the *Drosophila* Toll protein are essential for Il-1r signal transduction. J Biol Chem 267: 2605–2609

Heinrichs DE, Yethon JA, Whitfield C (1998) Molecular basis for structural diversity in the core regions of the lipopolysaccharides of *Escherichia coli* and *Salmonella enterica*. Mol Microbiol 30: 221–232

Hemmi H, Kaisho T, Takeuchi O, Sato S, Sanjo H, Hoshino K, Horiuchi T, Tomizawa H, Takeda K, Akira S (2002) Small anti-viral compounds activate immune cells via the TLR7 MyD88-dependent signaling pathway. Nature Immunol 3: 196–200

Hoebe K, Georgel P, Rutschmann S, Du X, Mudd S, Crozat K, Sovath S, Shamel L, Hartung T, Zahringer U, Beutler B (2005) CD36 is a sensor of diacylglycerides. Nature 433: 523–527

Hu X, Yagi Y, Tanji T, Zhou S, Ip YT (2004) Multimerization and interaction of Toll and Spätzle in *Drosophila*. Proc Natl Acad Sci USA 101: 9369–9374

Huizinga EG, Tsuji S, Romijn RAP, Schiphorst ME, de Groot PG, Sixma JJ, Gros P (2002) Structures of glycoprotein Ib alpha and its complex with von Willebrand factor A1 domain. Science 297: 1176–1179

Imler JL, Hoffmann JA (2001) Toll receptors in innate immunity. Trends Cell Biol 11: 304–311

Inohara N, Nunez G (2002) ML – A conserved domain involved in innate immunity and lipid metabolism. Trends Biochem Sci 27: 219–221

Jack RS, Fan XL, Bernheiden M, Rune G, Ehlers M, Weber A, Kirsch G, Mentel R, Furll B, Freudenberg M, Schmitz G, Stelter F, Schutt C (1997) Lipopolysaccharide-binding protein is required to combat a murine Gram-negative bacterial infection. Nature 389: 742–745

Jebanathirajah JA, Peri S, Pandey A (2002) Toll and interleukin-1 receptor (TIR) domain-containing proteins in plants: a genomic perspective. Trends Plant Sci 7: 388–391

Khan JA, Brint EK, O'Neill LA, Tong L (2004) Crystal structure of the Toll/interleukin-1 receptor domain of human IL-1RAPL. J Biol Chem 279: 31664–31670

Kim JI, Lee CJ, Jin MS, Lee CH, Paik SG, Lee H, Lee JO (2005) Crystal structure of CD14 and its implications for lipopolysaccharide signaling. J Biol Chem 280: 11347–11351

Kim HM, Park BS, Kim JI, Kim SE, Lee J, et al. (2007) Crystal Structure of the TLR4-MD-2 Complex with Bound Endotoxin Antagonist Eritoran. Cell 130: 906–917

Kobayashi M, Saitoh S, Tanimura N, Takahashi K, Kawasaki K, Nishijima M, Fujimoto Y, Fukase K, Akashi-Takamura S, Miyake K (2006) Regulatory roles for MD-2 and TLR4 in ligand-induced receptor clustering. J Immunol 176: 6211–6218

Kobe B, Deisenhofer J (1993) Crystal structure of porcine ribonuclease inhibitor, a protein with leucine-rich repeats. Nature 366: 751–756

Latz E, Schoenemeyer A, Visintin A, Fitzgerald KA, Monks BG, Knetter CF, Lien E, Nilsen NJ, Espevik T, Golenbock DT (2004) TLR9 signals after translocating from the ER to CpG DNA in the lysosome. Nat Immunol 5: 190–198

Lee J, Chuang TH, Redecke V, She LP, Pitha PM, Carson DA, Raz E, Cottam HB (2003) Molecular basis for the immunostimulatory activity of guanine nucleoside analogs: Activation of Toll-like receptor 7. Proc Natl Acad Sci USA 100: 6646–6651

Lund JM, Alexopoulou L, Sato A, Karow M, Adams NC, Gale NW, Iwasaki A, Flavell RA (2004) Recognition of single-stranded RNA viruses by Toll-like receptor 7. Proc Natl Acad Sci USA 101: 5598–5603

Manukyan M, Triantafilou K, Triantafilou M, Mackie A, Nilsen N, Espevik T, Wiesmuller KH, Ulmer AJ, Heine H (2005) Binding of lipopeptide to CD14 induces physical proximity of CD14, TLR2 and TLR1. Eur J Immunol 35: 911–921

Matsushima N, Tanaka T, Enkhbayar P, Mikami T, Taga M, et al. (2007) Comparative sequence analysis of leucine-rich repeats (LRRs) within vertebrate toll-like receptors. BMC Genomics 8: 124

Mizuguchi K, Parker JS, Blundell TL, Gay NJ (1998) Getting knotted: A model for the structure and activation of Spätzle. Trends Biochem Sci 23: 239–242

Morath S, Stadelmaier A, Geyer A, Schmidt RR, Hartung T (2002) Synthetic lipoteichoic acid from *Staphylococcus aureus* is a potent stimulus of cytokine release. J Exp Med 195: 1635–1640

Muroi M, Tanamoto K (2006) Structural regions of MD-2 that determine the agonist-antagonist activity of lipid IVa. J Biol Chem 281: 5484–5491

Nagai Y, Akashi S, Nagafuku M, Ogata M, Iwakura Y, Akira S, Kitamura T, Kosugi A, Kimoto M, Miyake K (2002) Essential role of MD-2 in LPS responsiveness and TLR4 distribution. Nat Immunol 3: 667–672

Nishitani C, Mitsuzawa H, Sano H, Shimizu T, Matsushima N, Kuroki Y (2006) Toll-like receptor 4 region Glu24-Lys47 is a site for MD-2 binding: Importance of CYS29 and CYS40. J Biol Chem 281: 38322–38329

Ohto U, Fukase K, Miyake K, Satow Y (2007) Crystal structures of human MD-2 and its complex with antiendotoxic lipid IVa. Science 316: 1632–1634

O'Neill LAJ, Fitzgerald KA, Bowie AG (2003) The Toll-IL-1 receptor adaptor family grows to five members. Trends in Immunol 24: 287–290

Poltorak A, He XL, Smirnova I, Liu MY, Van Huffel C, Du X, Birdwell D, Alejos E, Silva M, Galanos C, Freudenberg M, Ricciardi-Castagnoli P, Layton B, Beutler B (1998) Defective LPS signaling in C3H/HeJ and C57BL/10ScCr mice: Mutations in Tlr4 gene. Science 282: 2085–2088

Qureshi ST, Lariviere L, Leveque G, Clermont S, Moore KJ, Gros P, Malo D (1999) Endotoxin-tolerant mice have mutations in toll-like receptor 4 (Tlr4). J Exp Med 189: 615–625

Rallabhandi P, Bell J, Boukhvalova MS, Medvedev A, Lorenz E, Arditi M, Hemming VG, Blanco JC, Segal DM, Vogel SN (2006) Analysis of TLR4 polymorphic variants: New insights into TLR4/MD-2/CD14 stoichiometry, structure, and signaling. J Immunol 177: 322–332

Ranjith-Kumar CT, Miller W, Xiong J, Russell WK, Lamb R, Santos J, Duffy KE, Cleveland L, Park M, Bhardwaj K, Wu Z, Russell DH, Sarisky RT, Mbow ML, Kao CC (2007) Biochemical and functional analyses of the human Toll-like receptor 3 ectodomain. J Biol Chem

Re F, Strominger JL (2002) Monomeric recombinant MD-2 binds Toll-like receptor 4 tightly and confers lipopolysaccharide responsiveness. J Biol Chem 277: 23427–23432

Rock FL, Hardiman G, Timans JC, Kastelein RA, Bazan JF (1998) A family of human receptors structurally related to Drosophila Toll. Proc Natl Acad Sci USA 95: 588–593

Ronni T, Agarwal V, Haykinson M, Haberland ME, Cheng G, Smale ST (2003) Common interaction surfaces of the Toll-like receptor 4 cytoplasmic domain stimulate multiple nuclear targets. Mol Cell Biol 23: 2543–2555

Rutz M, Metzger J, Gellert T, Luppa P, Lipford GB, Wagner H, Bauer S (2004) Toll-like receptor 9 binds single-stranded CpG-DNA in a sequence- and pH-dependent manner. Eur J Immunol 34: 2541–2550

Saitoh S, Akashi S, Yamada T, Tanimura N, Kobayashi M, Konno K, Matsumoto F, Fukase K, Kusumoto S, Nagai Y, Kusumoto Y, Kosugi A, Miyake K (2004) Lipid A antagonist, lipid IVa, is distinct from lipid A in interaction with Toll-like receptor 4 (TLR4)-MD-2 and ligand-induced TLR4 oligomerization. Int Immunol 16: 961–969

Schlessinger J (2002) Ligand-induced, receptor-mediated dimerization and activation of EGF receptor. Cell 110: 669–672

Schneider DS, Hudson KL, Lin TY, Anderson KV (1991) Dominant and recessive mutations define functional domains of Toll, a transmembrane protein required for Dorsal Ventral polarity in the Drosophila embryo. Genes Dev 5: 797–807

Schubert WD, Urbanke C, Ziehm T, Beier V, Machner MP, Domann E, Wehland J, Chakraborty T, Heinz DW (2002) Structure of internalin, a major invasion protein of Listeria monocytogenes, in complex with its human receptor E-cadherin. Cell 111: 825–836

Sims JE (2002) IL-1 and IL-18 receptors, and their extended family. Curr Opin Immunol 14: 117–122

Slack JL, Schooley K, Bonnert TP, Mitcham JL, Qwarnstrom EE, Sims JE, Dower SK (2000) Identification of two major sites in the type I interleukin-1 receptor cytoplasmic region responsible for coupling to pro-inflammatory signaling pathways. J Biol Chem 275: 4670–4678

Smith KD, Andersen-Nissen E, Hayashi F, Strobe K, Bergman MA, Barrett SL, Cookson BT, Aderem A (2003) Toll-like receptor 5 recognizes a conserved site on flagellin required for protofilament formation and bacterial motility. Nat Immunol 4: 1247–1253

Stock AM, Mottonen JM, Stock JB, Schutt CE (1989) Three-dimensional structure of CheY, the response regulator of bacterial chemotaxis. Nature 337: 745–749

Sun J, Duffy KE, Ranjith-Kumar CT, Xiong J, Lamb RJ, Santos J, Masarapu H, Cunningham M, Holzenburg A, Sarisky RT, Mbow ML, Kao C (2006) Structural and functional analyses of the human Toll-like receptor 3. Role of glycosylation. J Biol Chem 281: 11144–11151

Tauszig S, Jouanguy E, Hoffmann JA, Imler JL (2000) Toll-related receptors and the control of antimicrobial peptide expression in Drosophila. Proc Natl Acad Sci USA 97: 10520-10525

Taylor PR, Tsoni SV, Willment JA, Dennehy KM, Rosas M, Findon H, Haynes K, Steele C, Botto M, Gordon S, Brown GD (2007) Dectin-1 is required for beta-glucan recognition and control of fungal infection. Nat Immunol 8: 31–38

Thompson JD, Higgins DG, Gibson TJ (1994) Clustal-W – Improving the sensitivity of progressive multiple sequence alignment through sequence weighting, position-specific gap penalties and weight matrix choice. Nucleic Acids Res 22: 4673–4680

Tobias PS, Soldau K, Gegner JA, Mintz D, Ulevitch RJ (1995) Lipopolysaccharide-binding protein-mediated complexation of lipopolysaccharide with soluble Cd14. J Biol Chem 270: 10482–10488

Viriyakosol S, Tobias PS, Kirkland TN (2006) Mutational analysis of membrane and soluble forms of human MD-2. J Biol Chem 281: 11955–11964

Visintin A, Latz E, Monks BG, Espevik T, Golenbock DT (2003) Lysines 128 and 132 enable lipopolysaccharide binding to MD-2, leading to Toll-like receptor-4 aggregation and signal transduction. J Biol Chem 278: 48313–48320

Weber A, Tauszig-Delamasure S, Hoffmann J, Lelièvre E, Gascan H, Ray K, Morse M, Imler J, Gay N (2003) Binding of the *Drosophila* cytokine Spätzle to Toll is direct and establishes signaling. Nature Immunol 4: 794–800

Weber AN, Moncrieffe MC, Gangloff M, Imler JL, Gay NJ (2005) Ligand-receptor and receptor-receptor interactions act in concert to activate signaling in the *Drosophila* toll pathway. J Biol Chem 280: 22793–22799

Weber AN, Morse MA, Gay NJ (2004) Four N-linked glycosylation sites in human Toll-like receptor 2 cooperate to direct efficient biosynthesis and secretion. J Biol Chem 279: 34589–34594

Weber ANR, Gangloff M, Moncrieffe MC, Hyvert Y, Imler JL, Gay NJ (2007) Role of Spätzle pro-domain in the generation of an active Toll receptor ligand. J Biol Chem 282 (in press)

Xu YW, Tao X, Shen BH, Horng T, Medzhitov R, Manley JL, Tong L (2000) Structural basis for signal transduction by the Toll/interleukin-1 receptor domains. Nature 408: 111–115

Toll-Like Receptor-Agonists in the Treatment of Skin Cancer: History, Current Developments and Future Prospects

Joerg Wenzel, Damia Tormo, and Thomas Tüting(✉)

Abstract This review will briefly cover some important aspects of skin structure and function before touching upon fundamental principles of neoplastic cell growth in the skin and some of the important molecular pathways involved. After presenting evidence for a role of the immune system in shaping the development of skin cancer, concepts for tumor immunotherapy with TLR-agonists are introduced from a historical point of view. Subsequently, the use of synthetic DNA, synthetic RNA and synthetic small immunostimulatory molecules for immunotherapy of early forms of epithelial carcinoma (actinic keratoses) and melanoma (lentigo maligna), as well as for advanced metastatic melanoma, is comprehensively presented. Finally, current developments and future prospects for immunotherapy of occult or unresectable melanoma metastastases, the most important clinical problem today, are discussed.

Thomas Tüting

Department of Dermatology, University of Bonn, Sigmund-Freud-Strasse 25, 53105 Bonn, Germany

`thomas.tueting@ukb.uni-bonn.de`

S. Bauer, G. Hartmann (eds.), *Toll-Like Receptors (TLRs) and Innate Immunity.*
Handbook of Experimental Pharmacology 183.
© Springer-Verlag Berlin Heidelberg 2008

1 A Primer of Skin Biology

The skin is the largest organ of the body with many important functions (see Figure 1). At the barrier to the environment it prevents loss of body fluids, protects the organism against noxious chemical substances, physical trauma, and UV-irradiation and provides the first line of immunological defense against pathogens such as bacteria, viruses, and fungi. Furthermore, it regulates body temperature and helps in metabolic homeostasis. Last but not least, it acts as a sensory organ and is of great importance for social communication. To fulfill these various tasks the skin contains a large variety of different cell types with a complex organization. The outermost layer of the skin, the epidermis, consists primarily of keratinocytes, which continuously proliferate and form a stratified epithelium with a water-impermeable cornified lipid structure at the surface. At its base, melanocytes produce pigments, which they pass on to keratinocytes for UV-protection. Scattered throughout the epidermis are specialized cells of the immune system such as antigen-presenting

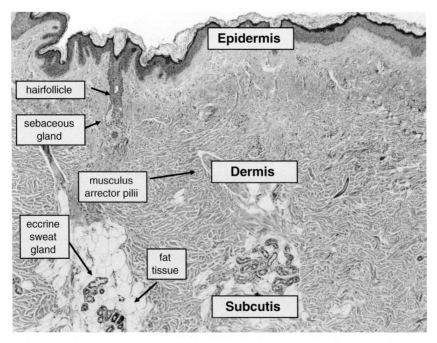

Fig. 1 Structural components of the skin. The human skin is a complex organ system acting as the barrier of the organism to the external environment. It is composed of three layers. The epidermis is a squamous epithelium, which produces and carries the stratum corneum, an impermeable horny lipid-rich protective layer of the skin surface. Additionally, the epidermis contains melanocytes, intraepithelial lymphocytes, and Langerhans cells. The dermis consists of a connective tissue framework and contains blood vessels, nerves, as well as several types of skin appendages (various hair follicles, sebaceous, and sweat glands). The subcutis is a fat cushion that separates the dermis from deeper tissues such as muscle fasciae, joint cartilage, or bone

Langerhans cells and intraepidermal T lymphocytes, which provide the first line of immunological defense. The epidermis is anchored to a flexible connective tissue framework, the dermis, which is primarily generated by fibroblasts producing extracellular matrix components. These include ground substance, collagen, and elastic fibers. Dermal dendritic cells, macrophages, mast cells, and lymphocytes represent the second line of immunological defense against pathogens. The dermis is highly vascularized with large numbers of capillary vessels made by endothelial cells in the upper (papillary) dermis, which are connected to arteries and veins of different caliber below. An intricate network of different nerve structures provides afferent sensory information and enables efferent control of blood flow as well as immune functions. The dermis rests on a fat cushion, the subcutis, which separates the skin from deeper muscles, tendons, cartilage, and bone. Depending on the body site, various epithelial organs such as hair follicles with sebaceous glands and pilar muscle fibers, as well as eccrine and apocrine sweat glands (adnexial structures of the skin), protrude from the epidermis into the dermis and subcutis.

2 Fundamental Principles of Physiologic, Benign, and Malignant Cell Growth in the Skin

Development, regeneration, and maintenance of the complex architecture of the skin requires not only precise control of growth, differentiation, and death of various cell types but also coordinated cell migration, positioning, and polarization. If developmental processes are not properly regulated, hamartomas and congenital nevi may appear in the skin. Common examples are congenital moles or haemangiomas observed in newborns, which result from abnormal proliferations of melanocytes or endothelial cells, respectively. Similar harmless neoplastic lesions can also derive from keratinocytes in the epidermis, from fibroblast, muscle, and nerve cells in the dermis, or from adnexial structures. Regeneration of skin structures is required during wound healing where keratinocytes, endothelial cells, fibroblasts, and cells of the immune system need to rapidly proliferate in a coordinated fashion. The appearance of benign tumors such as eruptive angioma or hypertrophic keloid scars, which consist of proliferating endothelial cells or fibroblasts, respectively, shows that this process is not always properly orchestrated. Skin tumors can also appear as a result of abnormal cell growth or cell death during physiologic tissue maintenance. This is exemplified by common viral warts, which are mostly seen in children and young adults. Viral proteins stimulate keratinocyte growth and simultaneously prevent normal differentiation and cell death leading to benign epithelial tumors. Acquired pigmented moles may result from abnormal proliferation of melanocytes following UV-stimulation. Benign tumors can also develop *de novo* from every other cell type in the skin leading to a large number of histologically diverse skin lesions. Errors in the regulation of cell growth, differentiation, and death and in the orchestration of cell migration, positioning, and polarization are considered the common denominator for aberrant cell growth. Fortunately, a number of different mechanisms can eventually arrest erroneous cell growth in benign skin tumors. Occasionally, tumor growth in the skin is not stopped and neoplastic cells continue to grow, fail to differentiate, loose their polarization, invade adjacent structures, enter lymphatic and blood vessels, migrate to other tissues, and form metastatic lesions. Malignant skin tumors most commonly originate from epithelial cells (basal cell carcinoma and squamous cell carcinoma) and melanocytes (malignant melanoma), but they can derive from any other cell type in the skin.

3 Important Molecular Pathways Involved in the Development of Skin Cancer

A large body of experimental evidence collectively demonstrates that both benign and malignant cell growth generally result from acquired or inherited genetic changes in key molecules of growth signaling pathways (oncogenes) and control mechanisms for cell cycle progression, apoptosis, or senescence (tumor suppressor genes). Furthermore, structural chromosomal changes due to genetic instability are an important feature of malignant cells. When several different and cooperating genetic changes accumulate, neoplastic cells show an increasingly malignant behavior. The concept of multistep carcinogenesis has been investigated for skin tumors both in experimental animal models as well as in man (see Figure 2).

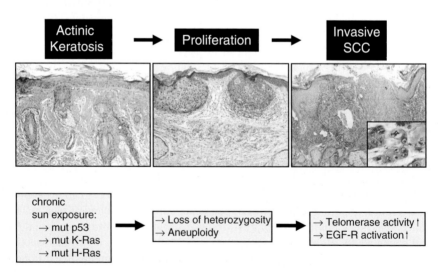

Fig. 2 Multistep pathogenesis of invasive squamous cell carcinoma. Squamous cell carcinoma (SCC) develops in sun damaged areas of the skin from early actinic lesions, proliferating actinic keratosis (carcinoma *in situ*) into invasively growing tumors. Shown are characteristic histological and genetic changes thought to be associated with the individual stages of evolution. Early lesions present with genetic mutations characteristic for UV-dependent DNA-damage. Advanced lesions are associated with genomic instability and loss of heterozygosity (17p, 17q, 9p, 9q). Model adapted from (Dlugosz JID, 2002)

Neoplastic transformation of keratinocytes progresses from actinic keratoses, which represent early forms of an intraepithelial carcinoma *in situ* towards later forms of invasive squamous cell carcinoma with dedifferentiation and metastatic spread. This form of skin cancer is associated with chronic UV irradiation of the skin and consequently appears predominantly in sun-exposed skin areas (forehead, nose, ear, lower lip) in men and women aged 70 years and above. The incidence of actinic keratoses and squamous cell carcinomas is increasing worldwide, particularly in fair-skinned people (Memon et al., 2000). Squamous cell carcinomas metastasize via lymphatic or blood vessels and may eventually lead to death. Fortunately, this is a comparatively rare event. UV-induced mutations in the tumor suppressor protein p53 appear to be important for the initial development of intraepithelial carcinoma *in situ* (actinic keratoses). p53 functions as the "gate keeper" for epithelial cancer development. Subsequently, mutations in oncogenic signaling cascades, such as the Ras family, and alterations in telomerase activity promote cellular transformation and genetic instability leading to invasive cell growth. Undifferentiated and metastatic squamous cell carcinoma eventually show chromosomal translocations, deletions, and amplifications as the latest step in epithelial carcinogenesis (Boukamp, 2005).

Neoplastic transformation of melanocytes in the skin begins in the basal epidermal layer with abnormal proliferations of atypical cells, which form nests and spread horizontally throughout the epidermis (melanoma *in situ*). Intermittent highdose UV irradiation during childhood is considered to be the most important etiologic factor for melanoma development. Malignant melanoma progresses when cells acquire the ability to invade the dermal compartment and subsequently to migrate towards regional lymph nodes and distal organs such as lungs, liver, bone, or brain, where metastases are formed. Melanoma accounts for only about 4% of all skin cancers. However, it causes the greatest number of skin cancer-related deaths because disseminated melanoma metastases can only rarely be cured. Studies in families with hereditary melanoma susceptibility have shown that genetic alterations in the inhibitor of cyclin-dependent kinases INK4a/p16 and one of its target molecules, the cyclin-dependent kinase 4, predispose for aberrant growth of melanocytes. These observations were complemented by reports describing acquired chromosomal deletions or epigenetic silencing of the INK4a/p16 locus as well as amplifications of the cyclin-dependent kinase 4 locus. Furthermore, large-scale sequencing of melanoma genes unraveled somatic mutations in the signaling molecules N-Ras and B-Raf in melanomas (Chin et al., 2006).

4 Role of the Immune System in the Development of Skin Cancer

The primary—and from an evolutionary point of view probably most important—role for the immune system is thought to be protection against harmful pathogens. This can be illustrated by considering an infection with herpes simplex virus (HSV), a common and well known blistering skin disease. Upon first contact, HSV usually

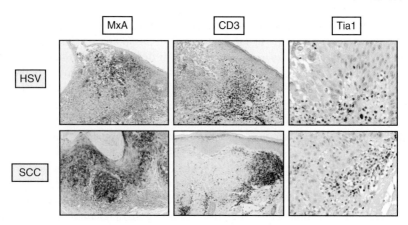

Fig. 3 Similarities of type I interferon associated cytotoxic inflammation in herpes simplex infection and invasive squamous cell carcinoma. The type I Interferon system plays an important role in antiviral immune defense. Viral DNA stimulates the innate immune system via TLR-dependent and -independent mechanisms and induce type I IFN production. This leads to the lesional production of IFN-inducible antiviral proteins, such as the myxovirus protein A (MxA), but also supports the development of an antigen-specific cellular response of the adaptive immune system. Infiltrating CD3+ lymphocytes carrying Tia1+ cytotoxic granules recognize and kill virus-affected keratinocytes by induction of apoptosis. Interestingly, invasive squamous cell carcinoma also frequently shows endogenous activation of the type I IFN system accompanied by infiltration with Tia1+ cytotoxic CD3+ T lymphocytes

replicates and destroys epithelial keratinocytes in the oropharynx or the genital mucosa (Figure 3). Activation of the type I IFN system along with recruitment of plasmacytoid DC and NK cells provide the first line of innate immune defense. Antigen-specific CD8+ cytotoxic T cells subsequently arrive, destroy virally infected cells, and clear the acute infection. However, HSV manages to persist in the body in a latent form, particularly in cells of the nervous system, and can cause recurrent localized blistering upon reactivation in some individuals, in particular following immunosuppression.

The immune system is also involved in controlling viral warts, which are benign skin tumors most commonly caused by human papilloma viruses (HPV). Similar to HSV infection, both innate and adaptive immunity with type I IFNs and cytotoxic CD8+ T cells are thought to be required to successfully combat HPV infections. Children with a history of hay fever and atopic dermatitis are particularly susceptible to developing viral warts caused by HPV. Interestingly, patients with hay fever and atopic dermatitis also frequently show recurrent blistering skin disease due to reactivation of HSV. This clinical observation suggests a common genetic basis in the regulation of innate and adaptive antiviral immunity against persistent viral pathogens in the skin and supports the notion that a similar cytotoxic inflammatory response is important for disease control.

In the last 15 years it has become clear that antigen-specific CD8+ cytotoxic T cells are also able to detect and potentially destroy transformed cells in the skin. Primary melanomas of the skin as well as actinic keratoses and invasive squamous cell carcinomas are frequently infiltrated by lymphocytes. Spontaneous regressions of clinically apparent melanomas have been well documented over decades. Lymphocytic infiltrations surrounding and penetrating skin tumors are composed of CD8+ cytotoxic T cells, NK cells, and plasmacytoid DCs. The cellular immune response is accompanied by endogenous activation of the type I IFN system. This pattern of cytotoxic inflammation bears marked similarity to that observed in viral infection (Wenzel et al., 2005b). It has been amply demonstrated that infiltrating CD8+ cytotoxic T cells in melanoma specifically recognize cells of the melanocytic lineage. Tumor-specific T lymphocytes from melanoma patients have been shown to detect oncogenic mutations involved in molecular pathogenesis (Wenzel et al., 2005b). Similarly, CD8+ cytotoxic T cells infiltrating squamous cell carcinomas have been shown to specifically recognize mutated epitopes of p53 involved in keratinocyte transformation (Black and Ogg, 2003). Melanoma patients with tumor-infiltrating lymphocytes in the primary skin tumor survived statistically longer than patients without tumor-infiltrating lymphocytes, providing some evidence for the prognostic significance of cellular antitumor immune responses (Clark, Jr. et al., 1989; Clemente et al., 1996).

MacFarlane Burnet hypothesized many years ago that the immune system is able to detect and eliminate transformed cells (Burnet, 1970). This "immunosurveillance hypothesis" has been controversially debated for many years (Dunn et al., 2004). Recently, two lines of evidence support an important role for the immune system in controlling cancer development in the skin. Firstly, genetically engineered mice that lacked genes encoding for interferon receptors or for interferon receptor signaling molecules such as STAT1 not only succumb to experimental viral infections but are also much more prone to develop carcinogen-induced epithelial or mesenchymal tumors (Shankaran et al., 2001; Dunn et al., 2005). Mice without T and B cells due to deletion of the recombination-activating gene 1 (RAG-1) or RAG-2, which are responsible for rearrangement of lymphocyte antigen receptors, also developed carcinogen-induced sarcomas in the skin more rapidly and with greater frequency than genetically matched wild-type controls (Shankaran et al., 2001). Furthermore, mice without $\gamma\delta$ T cells due to deletion of the TCR δ-chain also showed a greater susceptibility to carcinogen-induced epithelial tumors with a higher incidence of papilloma-to-carcinoma progression than wild-type mice (Girardi et al., 2001).

Clinical observations in organ transplant recipients requiring long-term systemic immunosuppressive therapy to prevent allograft rejection provide a second line of evidence for a role of the immune system in skin cancer development. Immunosuppressed patients show a significantly increased incidence of viral warts, actinic keratoses, squamous cell carcinoma, basal cell carcinomas, and melanomas. In particular, squamous cell carcinomas occur 65 to 250 times more frequently and appear to grow more aggressively in transplant recipients than in the general population. Furthermore, their incidence increases with the duration of immunosuppressive therapy (Euvrard et al., 2003). Interestingly, neoplastic skin lesions may regress when therapeutic immunosuppression is relieved. Taken together, the results of animal experiments and clinical investigations in organ transplant recipients suggest that the immune system is actively involved in controlling neoplastic cell growth in the skin. Importantly, these observations have spurred attempts to therapeutically stimulate the ability of the immune system to detect and eliminate transformed cells.

5 Early Attempts at Tumor Immunotherapy

Almost a century ago, physicians observed that patients with sarcoma who accidentally contracted erysipelas sometimes exhibited regression of the neoplasm. The surgeon William Coley pioneered the use of killed bacterial extracts from *Streptococcus pyogenes* and *Serratia marcescens* as a treatment for inoperable cases of advanced sarcomas in the early 20th century (Coley, 1991). "Coley's toxin," which was usually applied in conjunction with radiotherapy, can be considered one of the earliest forms of tumor immunotherapy. It showed well-documented tumor regressions in some patients. Spontaneous tumor regressions were on very rare occasions also observed following acute viral infections. In the 1950s patients with inoperable cervical carcinomas were treated with wild-type adenoviruses (Huebner et al., 1956). More than half the patients treated with live virus exhibited tumor regression, whereas the control patients treated with inactivated virus showed no response. The initial tumor regression, though, was soon followed by tumor progression in all patients. The idea of using either live or killed bacteria or viruses for cancer therapy has precipitated countless experimental and clinical studies over the past 50 years.

In the 1960s and 1970s extracts from bacteria such as Bacillus Calmette–Guerin (BCG) (a weakened form of mycobacteria tuberculosis) and from *Corynebacterium parvum* were investigated for the prevention and treatment of metastatic disease in melanoma patients. Previously, studies in mice showed that BCG, *Listeria monocytogenes, Corynebacterium parvum*, or *Bordetella pertussis* inhibited the growth of transplanted B16 melanoma cells *in vivo* (Chee and Bodurtha, 1974; Youdim, 1976; Purnell et al., 1975). The principal effect of bacterial extracts was thought to be due to the induction of immunostimulatory cytokines such as IFNs. In the 1980s genes coding for IFN-alpha were cloned and expressed as recombinant proteins in bacteria. Purified, recombinant IFN-alpha showed efficacy in the treatment of various skin tumors such as viral warts, squamous cell carcinoma, and melanoma. In the 1990s, recombinant IFN-alpha showed clinical efficacy in the adjuvant treatment of melanoma patients with a high risk for recurrence and was subsequently approved by the FDA for this indication.

6 Synthetic DNA Oligonucleotides for Tumor Immunotherapy: The CpG Story

Many researchers were interested in understanding the mechanisms underlying the immunotherapeutic effects of bacterial lysates. In 1984 Japanese researchers fractionated extracts from BCG and showed that the bacterial DNA was responsible for its antitumor action (Tokunaga et al., 1984). It was subsequently demonstrated that bacterial but not mammalian DNA could induce interferons and activate cells of the immune system (Yamamoto et al., 1992). This immunostimulatory activity could be mimicked with synthetic oligonucleotides containing palindromic sequence motifs (Yamamoto et al., 1994). In 1995, Arthur Krieg reported that the immunostimulatory property of bacterial DNA was caused by the presence of motifs consisting of an unmethylated cytidine-guanosine dinucleotide (CpG) flanked by two 5' purines and two 3' pyrimidines (Krieg et al., 1995). His group was interested in manipulating gene expression in B cell lymphomas with synthetic antisense oligonucleotides and accidentally observed that certain control sequences induced B cell proliferation and immunoglobulin synthesis. This activity was similar to that of bacterial DNA. Further investigations showed that B cell activation was restricted to CpG motifs that are unmethylated in synthetic DNA oligonucleotides as well as in most of bacterial DNA. In contrast, vertebrate DNA mostly contains methylated CpG motifs.

It quickly became apparent that defined synthetic oligodeoxynucleotides containing appropriate CpG sequences (CpG-ODN) could substitute for undefined bacterial lysates in therapeutic approaches to stimulate interferons and cellular as well as humoral immunity. Sequence optimization and chemical modifications such as phosphorothioate modifications in the backbone of synthetic DNA were able to significantly enhance their stability and improve the therapeutic effect of CpG-ODN *in vivo*. In a mouse model for B cell lymphoma, injections of CpG-ODN were able to enhance anti-idiotypic immune responses against the malignant tumor cells (Weiner et al., 1997). Repeated intra- and peritumoral injections of optimized CpG-ODN were also able to strengthen the efficacy of cellular antitumor immune responses in transplantable mouse models for other tumor types including the C26 colon carcinoma and the B16 melanoma (Heckelsmiller et al., 2002; Kunikata et al., 2004; Kawarada et al., 2001). The classical approach of William Coley, who combined his bacterial toxin with irradiation for tumor treatment, could likewise be effectively repeated in experimental mouse models (Milas et al., 2004; Garbi et al., 2004). Further investigations demonstrated that injections of CpG-ODN supported the infiltration of tumors with lymphocytes. Activation of both innate and adaptive cellular immunity appeared to be required for the therapeutic efficacy of intra- and peritumoral injections of CpG-ODN since antibody-mediated elimination of CD8+ T cells and NK cells significantly abrogated the antitumor response. In recent years, therapeutic application of CpG-ODN has been advanced for clinical applications by delineation and optimization of sequence motifs for the human immune system (Hartmann et al., 2000). A recent phase II trial of a CpG oligonucleotide in patients with metastatic melanoma has shown promising results with limited adverse events, and with 5 of 20 patients with a partial response (Pashenkov et al., 2006).

Bacterial CpG motifs also turned out to be of central importance for the efficacy of plasmid DNA-based genetic vaccines. Researchers in the field of gene therapy noticed in the early 1990s that injection of eukaryotic expression plasmids into skin or muscle stimulated a significant immune response against the encoded transgene gene (Tang et al., 1992; Ulmer et al., 1996). It subsequently was shown that the presence of CpG-ODN in the bacterial plasmids was required for the immunogenicity of plasmid (Sato et al., 1996). Several research groups soon recognized, that CpG-ODN were able to activate antigen-presenting dendritic cells (DC) (Sparwasser et al., 1998; Jakob et al., 1998; Hartmann et al., 1999). It became evident that CpG-ODN also was a powerful adjuvant for antigen-specific vaccines with recombinant proteins or synthetic peptides (Lipford et al., 1997; Vabulas et al., 2000). CpG-ODN strongly supported the induction of Th1-biased cellular immunity with IFN-g-producing CD4+ helper T cells and CD8+ cytotoxic T cells (Roman et al., 1997; Chu et al., 1997). Not surprisingly, it could be shown that CpG-ODN were able to significantly enhance the induction of cellular antitumor immunity against B16 melanoma and other transplantable tumors using peptide vaccines in animal tumor models (Davila and Celis, 2000; Miconnet et al., 2002; Davila et al., 2003). Adjuvant administration of CpG-ODN also showed considerable efficacy in boosting the induction of CD8+ T cells with synthetic melanoma peptides (Speiser et al., 2005; Appay et al., 2006).

7 Synthetic RNA for Tumor Immunotherapy: The Poly I:C Story

It had been noted many years ago that synthetic double-strandedRNA such as polyriboinosinic-polyribocytidylic acid (poly I:C) was able to mimic the effect of viral infection on the production of interferons and promote an antiviral state of cells in culture (Field et al., 1967; De et al., 1970). Poly I:C was also demonstrated to induce interferon in mammalian cells (Baron et al., 1969). Subsequently, poly I:C was used successfully to inhibit the growth of various transplantable rodent skin tumors, including those known to be induced by virus and those that are apparently spontaneous in origin (Kreider and Benjamin, 1972; Gelboin and Levy, 1970; Zeleznick and Bhuyan, 1969; Bart et al., 1971). An examination of poly I:C in a phase 1 and 2 trial against various solid tumors, including metastatic melanoma, revealed that while the complex had been a good IFN inducer as well as an antitumor agent in rodents, it proved to be a poor interferon inducer in humans, had no detectable antitumor effect, and was not clinically useful at any dosage (Robinson et al., 1976). It was recognized that primate serum contains high levels of hydrolytic activity (nuclease) against poly I:C. Therefore, rapid hydrolysis appeared to be responsible for the absence of clinical activity (Nordlund et al., 1970). A stabilized poly I:C complex consisting of high molecular weight poly I:C and low molecular weight poly L-lysine and carboxymethylcellulose poly I:C-LC was ten times more resistance to hydrolysis by pancreatic RNAses. Poly I:C-LC was the first consistent inducer of high serum interferon levels in humans (Levine et al., 1979). However, no antitumor responses occurred in 16 patients with metastatic malignant melanoma after treatment with poly I:C-LC, although IFN was consistently detected in the serum 8 hours after a single injection (Hawkins et al., 1985).

8 Synthetic Nucleic Acid Derivatives for Tumor Immunotherapy: The Imiquimod Story

The imidazoquinoline compounds imiquimod and R-848 were discovered as antiviral agents in a screen of small molecules with activity as antimetabolites in a guinea pig model for herpes simplex virus infection. Subsequent investigations showed that the therapeutic antiviral effect was due to the stimulation of interferons and other cytokines *in vivo* (Miller et al., 1999). Because of its antiviral activity, imiquimod was first clinically investigated for the treatment of viral warts in the genital and anal mucosa (*Condylomata acuminata*) caused by HPV. Based on results of extensive preclinical testing, topical imiquimod 5% cream was approved by the US FDA for the treatment of this comparatively frequent sexually transmitted condition (Beutner et al., 1998; Tyring, 2001). Its activity is thought to be due to the local induction of cytokines, which ultimately lead to a reduction of viral load and immune mediated viral wart regression (Jacobs et al., 2004; Sauder, 2000; Hober et al., 2005).

Imiquimod was subsequently also clinically tested for the treatment of actinic keratoses in UV-damaged skin. Several randomized double-blind trials confirmed a reduction or complete clearance of the majority of actinic keratoses following topical application of 5% imiquimod cream (Hadley et al., 2006). Immunohistochemical studies and gene expression analyses showed that imiquimod induces intralesional expression of type I interferons and type I interferon-induced genes, which are associated with the recruitment of DC and cytotoxic T cells and a Th1-associated cytotoxic inflammatory response (Lysa et al., 2004; Urosevic et al., 2005; Wenzel et al., 2005a; Wolf et al., 2005; Todd et al., 2004; Stary et al., 2007). As a consequence, topical imiquimod was recently approved by the US FDA and later also by the corresponding European regulatory authorities for the treatment of actinic keratoses.

Topical imiquimod has also been used for the treatment of lentigo maligna, a comparatively rare subset of melanoma *in situ* arising in sun-damaged skin primarily in the face and which can be considered a precursor for invasive lentigo maligna melanoma. In 2000 the first case report described a clinical and histological cure in one patient with lentigo maligna following long-term application of imiquimod 5% cream (Ahmed and Berth-Jones, 2000). A meta analysis published in 2006 identified a total of 11 case reports and 4 open-label studies, including a total of 67 lentigo maligna patients treated with topical imiquimod. Most patients experienced complete clinical remissions (Rajpar and Marsden, 2006). Immunohistological investigations revealed an increased infiltration of skin lesion with CD8+ cytotoxic T cells, suggesting that imiquimod was able to locally stimulate cellular immunity against premalignant melanocytes (Michalopoulos et al., 2004; Wolf et al., 2005). Topical imiquimod was also used in a clinical study in patients with cutaneous melanoma metastases in conjunction with a peptide vaccine with little success (Shackleton et al., 2004).

Topical application of imiquimod for the treatment of melanoma has also been investigated in mouse models for melanoma in order to better understand the mechanisms involved in its antitumor activity. In mice, imiquimod has been shown to enhance cellular immune responses against established transplanted melanoma cells in the skin by increasing lesional infiltration of the tumor with plasmacytoid DC and cytotoxic T lymphocytes (Palamara et al., 2004). Imiquimod has also proven to be effective against metastatic growth of B16 melanoma when applied in combination with an antigen-specific vaccine consisting of recombinant Listeria expressing a defined melanoma antigen (Craft et al., 2005). Several compounds that are structurally related to imiquimod are currently under investigation for the systemic treatment of metastatic melanoma both in experimental animal models as well as in early clinical trials.

9 The Role of TLRs for the Treatment of Skin Cancer with Immunostimulatory Nucleic Acids

Almost a decade ago the discovery of the family of Toll-like receptors as germline-encoded receptors for the molecular recognition of pathogens has initiated a new era for research in the mechanisms of innate immunity. At the beginning it was shown by the group of Charley Janeway that TLR2 and 4 were responsible for the detection of bacterial cell wall components such as endotoxin in mice (Medzhitov et al., 1997; Medzhitov and Janeway, Jr., 2002; Janeway, Jr., and Medzhitov, 2002). In 2000, TLR-9 was identified as the receptor for bacterial DNA as well as synthetic CpG-ODN using gene knock-out strategies (Hemmi et al., 2002; Takeshita et al., 2001). In a similar manner, TLR3 was shown to recognize double-stranded viral or synthetic RNA such as poly I:C in 2001 (Alexopoulou et al., 2001). Furthermore, TLR7 and 8 could be demonstrated to detect single-stranded RNA as well as small antiviral compunds such as imiquimod (Hemmi et al., 2002). Subsequent studies unraveled the subcellular localization of the TLRs as well as the signaling cascades and transcription factors mediating the immunostimulatory effects following TLR activation. These are discussed in great detail in other chapters of this book. Knowledge of the molecular mechanisms underlying the interaction of synthetic nucleic acids with the immune system greatly increased the interest in applying them for tumor immunotherapy. The skin is a well-suited target because not only resident skin DCs but also epidermal keratinocytes of both mouse and man express several functional TLR 3 and 9 (Lebre et al., 2006; Flacher et al., 2006). The regulation of TLRs during infection and tumor development in the skin are currently under investigation.

10 Current Developments and Future Prospects for the Treatment of Skin Tumors with Immunostimulatory Nucleic Acids

The treatment of occult or unresectable metastatic melanoma represents the most important challenge in skin cancer therapy today. In experimental animal models, immunostimulatory CpG-ODN are currently being successfully combined with other forms of immunotherapy such as recombinant cytokines. For example, CpG-ODN show synergistic effects with recombinant IL-2 or IL-18 for the treatment of B16 melanoma (Kochenderfer et al., 2006; Chaudhry et al., 2006). Furthermore, CpG-ODN have been combined with chemotherapeutic strategies with considerable success (Bourquin et al., 2006). Of particular interest has been the idea of combining different TLR-agonists for additive effects on DC activation and stimulation of T cells. The combinatorial code of TLR-ligand interactions with DC was first functionally evaluated *in vitro* by the group of Lanzavecchia (Napolitani et al., 2005). The simultaneous application of CpG-ODN with poly I:C showed superior therapeutic efficacy in the B16 melanoma lung metastases model *in vivo* (Whitmore et al., 2004). Intra- and peritumoral injections of both CpG-ODN and poly I:C were also able to enhance the therapeutic efficacy of a recombinant viral vaccine against growth of B16 melanoma in the skin (Tormo et al., 2006a). As an alternative approach, CpG-ODN have been combined with DC-based melanoma vaccines (Pilon-Thomas et al., 2006). Based on the observation that TLR8-agonists were able to override the influence of regulatory T cells for the control of T cell responses, it was suggested that tumor-specific tolerance mechanisms could potentially be circumvented by choosing appropriate combinations of TLR-agonists (Pasare and Medzhitov, 2003; Wang, 2006).

The seminal discovery of RNA interference has stimulated great interest in the use of synthetic short interfering RNA (siRNA) to therapeutically abrogate the expression of genes involved in neoplastic transformation (Schlee et al., 2006). The recent identification of sequence-specific recognition of single-stranded RNA by TLR7 further expands the possibilites for combinatorial design of therapeutic strategies using synthetic oligonucleotides (Hornung et al., 2005). In principle, siRNA can now be designed and synthesized in such a way that they directly attack molecular pathways involved in transformation and are able to simultaneously stimulate the immune system. Advances in pharmacology and biotechnology may enable appropriate chemical modifications ensuring stability of siRNA *in vivo* and pave the road for the development of innovative delivery methods using engineered recombinant viruses or synthetic virus-like particles. Novel genetic models for mouse melanoma which recapitulate the molecular pathogenesis of melanoma are currently being established and will be of great importance to guide the preclinical and clinical development of such treatment strategies (Tormo et al., 2006b; Chin et al., 2006).

One of the most exciting recent developments is the identification of cytosolic pattern recognition receptors which are able to detect viral or bacterial as well as synthetic nucleic acids inside the cells. It could be shown that RNA viruses or synthetic RNA are not only recognized by TLR3, 7, or 8 in endosomal compartments but also by the helicases RIG-I and MDA-5 in the cytosol (Kato et al., 2006). RIG-I recognizes viral RNA with a triphosphate group at the $5'$ end (so-called 3p-RNA) (Hornung et al., 2006). Most importantly, TLR-independent immunostimulatory effects mediated by cytosolic pathogen recognition receptors such as RIG-I or MDA-5 can be observed in many cell types including tumor cells because helicases are ubiquitously expressed. In contrast, the expression of the endosomal TLRs 3, 7, 8, and 9, which are able to detect nucleic acids, is restricted to subsets of immune cells

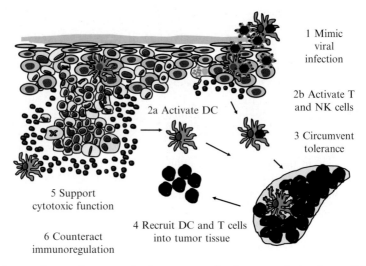

Fig. 4 Immunotherapeutic concept for the treatment of melanoma and other forms of skin cancer by stimulation of the innate and the adaptive arm of the immune system. TLR agonists mimic a local viral infection, activate DC and, subsequently, NK and T cells, circumvent mechanisms maintaining peripheral immune tolerance, recruit lymphocytes into tumor tissue, support cytotoxic activity, and counteract immunoregulation. This contributes to immunological clearance of malignant cells

with few exceptions. TLR-independent effects most likely mediate some of the direct effects of immunostimulatory nucleic acids on tumor cells, which may involve activation of the type I interferon system and induction of an antiviral state leading to cell cycle arrest, down regulation of protein synthesis and apoptosis (Schon et al., 2004). In the near future we will undoubtedly learn more about how different cells detect viruses and how they respond. This may teach us new ways to therapeutically exploit this knowledge for tumor therapy. We believe that stimulation of antiviral pathways—both systemically in draining lymph nodes as well as locally in the tumor tissue by mimicking a viral infection—will be a prerequisite for effective treatment of metastatic melanoma (Figure 4).

11 Conclusion and Outlook

TLR-agonists have been extensively investigated for different types of skin cancer from preclinical models to routine clinical use in everyday patient care. Topical application of the TLR7-agonist imiquimod, which has initially been clinically developed to eradicate viral warts, is now approved for immunological treatment of actinic keratoses, which represent a frequently observed carcinoma *in situ* in sun-damaged skin with a tendency to progress towards an invasive squamous cell carcinoma. Furthermore, various TLR-agonists are being considered to enhance adjuvant melanoma vaccines that aim at eliminating occult micrometastases in patients with resected primary melanoma and a high risk of recurrence. Finally, TLR-agonists are investigated as part of combinatorial treatment regimens to combat inoperable metastatic melanoma, which can only rarely be cured. Advances in understanding the molecular pathogenesis of melanoma and the regulation of cellular antitumor immune responses are providing the scientific basis for new immunotherapeutic strategies. These will ideally have to synergize with other treatment approaches such as chemotherapy or therapies targeting molecular pathways involved in cellular transformation using small molecules or monoclonal antibodies. Effective novel therapies could help to overcome the current limited treatment options for patients with metastatic melanoma and similar deadly tumor entities.

References

Ahmed I, Berth-Jones J (2000) Imiquimod: A novel treatment for lentigo maligna. Br J Dermatol 143: 843–845

Alexopoulou L, Holt AC, Medzhitov R, Flavell RA (2001) Recognition of double-stranded RNA and activation of NF-kappaB by Toll-like receptor 3. Nature 413: 732–738

Appay V, Jandus C, Voelter V, Reynard S, Coupland SE, Rimoldi D, Lienard D, Guillaume P, Krieg AM, Cerottini JC, Romero P, Leyvraz S, Rufer N, Speiser DE (2006) New generation vaccine induces effective melanoma-specific CD8+ T cells in the circulation but not in the tumor site. J Immunol 177: 1670–1678

Baron S, Bogomolova NN, Billiau A, Levy HB, Buckler CE, Stern R, Naylor R (1969) Induction of interferon by preparations of synthetic single-stranded RNA. Proc Natl Acad Sci USA 64: 67–74

Bart RS, Kopf AW, Silagi S (1971) Inhibition of the growth of murine malignant melanoma by polyinosinic-polycytidylic acid. J Invest Dermatol 56: 33–38

Beutner KR, Tyring SK, Trofatter KF, Jr, Douglas JM, Jr, Spruance S, Owens ML, Fox TL, Hougham AJ, Schmitt KA (1998) Imiquimod, a patient-applied immune-response modifier for treatment of external genital warts. Antimicrob Agents Chemother 42: 789–794

Black AP, Ogg GS (2003) The role of p53 in the immunobiology of cutaneous squamous cell carcinoma. Clin Exp Immunol 132: 379–384

Boukamp P (2005) Non-melanoma skin cancer: what drives tumor development and progression? Carcinogenesis 26: 1657–1667

Bourquin C, Schreiber S, Beck S, Hartmann G, Endres S (2006) Immunotherapy with dendritic cells and CpG oligonucleotides can be combined with chemotherapy without loss of efficacy in a mouse model of colon cancer. Int J Cancer 118: 2790–2795

Burnet FM (1970) The concept of immunological surveillance. Prog Exp Tumor Res 13: 1–27

Chaudhry UI, Kingham TP, Plitas G, Katz SC, Raab JR, DeMatteo RP (2006) Combined stimulation with interleukin-18 and CpG induces murine natural killer dendritic cells to produce IFN-gamma and inhibit tumor growth. Cancer Res 66: 10497–10504

Chee DO, Bodurtha AJ (1974) Facilitation and inhibition of b16 melanoma by BCG *in vivo* and by lymphoid cells from bcg-treated mice *in vitro*. Int J Cancer 14: 137–143

Chin L, Garraway LA, Fisher DE (2006) Malignant melanoma: genetics and therapeutics in the genomic era. Genes Dev 20: 2149–2182

Chu RS, Targoni OS, Krieg AM, Lehmann PV, Harding CV (1997) CpG oligodeoxynucleotides act as adjuvants that switch on T helper 1 (Th1) immunity. J Exp Med 186: 1623–1631

Clark WH, Jr, Elder DE, Guerry D, Braitman LE, Trock BJ, Schultz D, Synnestvedt M, Halpern AC (1989) Model predicting survival in stage I melanoma based on tumor progression. J Natl Cancer Inst 20(81): 1893–1904

Clemente CG, Mihm MC, Jr, Bufalino R, Zurrida S, Collini P, Cascinelli N (1996) Prognostic value of tumor infiltrating lymphocytes in the vertical growth phase of primary cutaneous melanoma. Cancer 77: 1303–1310

Coley WB (1991) The treatment of malignant tumors by repeated inoculations of erysipelas. With a report of ten original cases. 1893. Clin Orthop Relat Res 3–11

Craft N, Bruhn KW, Nguyen BD, Prins R, Lin JW, Liau LM, Miller JF (2005) The TLR7 agonist imiquimod enhances the anti–melanoma effects of a recombinant Listeria monocytogenes vaccine. J Immunol 175: 1983–1990

Davila E, Celis E (2000) Repeated administration of cytosine-phosphorothiolated guanine-containing oligonucleotides together with peptide/protein immunization results in enhanced CTL responses with anti-tumor activity. J Immunol 165: 539–547

Davila E, Kennedy R, Celis E (2003) Generation of antitumor immunity by cytotoxic T lymphocyte epitope peptide vaccination, CpG-oligodeoxynucleotide adjuvant, and CTLA-4 blockade. Cancer Res 63: 3281–3288

De CE, Nuwer MR, Merigan TC (1970) The role of interferon in the protective effect of a synthetic double-strandedpolyribonucleotide against intranasal vesicular stomatitis virus challenge in mice. J Clin Invest 49: 1565–1577

Dunn GP, Bruce AT, Sheehan KC, Shankaran V, Uppaluri R, Bui JD, Diamond MS, Koebel CM, Arthur C, White JM, Schreiber RD (2005) A critical function for type I interferons in cancer immunoediting. Nat Immunol 6: 722–729

Dunn GP, Old LJ, Schreiber RD (2004) The immunobiology of cancer immunosurveillance and immunoediting. Immunity 21: 137–148

Euvrard S, Kanitakis J, Claudy A (2003) Skin cancers after organ transplantation. N Engl J Med 348: 1681–1691

Field AK, Tytell AA, Lampson GP, Hilleman MR (1967) Inducers of interferon and host resistance. II. Multistranded synthetic polynucleotide complexes. Proc Natl Acad Sci USA 58: 1004–1010

Flacher V, Bouschbacher M, Verronese E, Massacrier C, Sisirak V, Berthier-Vergnes O, de Saint-Vis B, Caux C, Dezutter-Dambuyant C, Lebecque S, Valladeau J (2006) Human Langerhans cells express a specific TLR profile and differentially respond to viruses and Gram–positive bacteria. J Immunol 177: 7959–7967

Garbi N, Arnold B, Gordon S, Hammerling GJ, Ganss R (2004) CpG motifs as proinflammatory factors render autochthonous tumors permissive for infiltration and destruction. J Immunol 172: 5861–5869

Gelboin HV, Levy HB (1970) Polyinosinic-polycytidylic acid inhibits chemically induced tumorigenesis in mouse skin. Science 167: 205–207

Girardi M, Oppenheim DE, Steele CR, Lewis JM, Glusac E, Filler R, Hobby P, Sutton B, Tigelaar RE, Hayday AC (2001) Regulation of cutaneous malignancy by gammadelta T cells. Science 19(294): 605–609

Hadley G, Derry S, Moore RA (2006) Imiquimod for actinic keratosis: Systematic review and meta-analysis. J Invest Dermatol 126: 1251–1255

Hartmann G, Weeratna RD, Ballas ZK, Payette P, Blackwell S, Suparto I, Rasmussen WL, Waldschmidt M, Sajuthi D, Purcell RH, Davis HL, Krieg AM (2000) Delineation of a CpG phosphorothioate oligodeoxynucleotide for activating primate immune responses in vitro and in vivo. J Immunol 164: 1617–1624

Hartmann G, Weiner GJ, Krieg AM (1999) CpG DNA: A potent signal for growth, activation, and maturation of human dendritic cells. Proc Natl Acad Sci USA 96: 9305–9310

Hawkins MJ, Levin M, Borden EC (1985) An Eastern Cooperative Oncology Group phase I-II pilot study of polyriboinosinic-polyribocytidylic acid poly-L-lysine complex in patients with metastatic malignant melanoma. J Biol Response Mod 4: 664–668

Heckelsmiller K, Rall K, Beck S, Schlamp A, Seiderer J, Jahrsdorfer B, Krug A, Rothenfusser S, Endres S, Hartmann G (2002) Peritumoral CpG DNA elicits a coordinated response of CD8 T cells and innate effectors to cure established tumors in a murine colon carcinoma model. J Immunol 169: 3892–3899

Hemmi H, Kaisho T, Takeuchi O, Sato S, Sanjo H, Hoshino K, Horiuchi T, Tomizawa H, Takeda K, Akira S (2002) Small anti-viral compounds activate immune cells via the TLR7 MyD88-dependent signaling pathway. Nat Immunol 3: 196–200

Hober D, Ajram L, Chehadeh W, Lazrek M, Goffard A, Dewilde A, Wattre P (2005) Mechanisms of imiquimod indirect antiviral activity. Ann Biol Clin (Paris) 63: 155–163

Hornung V, Ellegast J, Kim S, Brzozka K, Jung A, Kato H, Poeck H, Akira S, Conzelmann KK, Schlee M, Endres S, Hartmann G (2006) 5′-Triphosphate RNA is the ligand for RIG-I. Science 314: 994–997

Hornung V, Guenther-Biller M, Bourquin C, Ablasser A, Schlee M, Uematsu S, Noronha A, Manoharan M, Akira S, de FA, Endres S, Hartmann G (2005) Sequence-specific potent induction of IFN-alpha by short interfering RNA in plasmacytoid dendritic cells through TLR7. Nat Med 11: 263–270

Huebner RJ, Rowe WP, Schatten WE, Smith RR, Thomas LB (1956) Studies on the use of viruses in the treatment of carcinoma of the cervix. Cancer 9: 1211–1218

Jacobs S, Grussendorf-Conen EI, Rosener I, Rubben A (2004) Molecular analysis of the effect of topical imiquimod treatment of HPV 2/27/57-induced common warts. Skin Pharmacol Physiol 17: 258–266

Jakob T, Walker PS, Krieg AM, Udey MC, Vogel JC (1998) Activation of cutaneous dendritic cells by CpG-containing oligodeoxynucleotides: A role for dendritic cells in the augmentation of Th1 responses by immunostimulatory DNA. J Immunol 161: 3042–3049

Janeway CA, Jr, Medzhitov R (2002) Innate immune recognition. Annu Rev Immunol 20:197–216. Epub 2001 Oct 4: 197–216

Kato H, Takeuchi O, Sato S, Yoneyama M, Yamamoto M, Matsui K, Uematsu S, Jung A, Kawai T, Ishii KJ, Yamaguchi O, Otsu K, Tsujimura T, Koh CS, Reis e Sousa, Matsuura Y, Fujita T, Akira S (2006) Differential roles of MDA5 and RIG-I helicases in the recognition of RNA viruses. Nature 441: 101–105

Kawarada Y, Ganss R, Garbi N, Sacher T, Arnold B, Hammerling GJ (2001) NK- and CD8(+) T cell-mediated eradication of established tumors by peritumoral injection of CpG-containing oligodeoxynucleotides. J Immunol 167: 5247–5253

Kochenderfer JN, Chien CD, Simpson JL, Gress RE (2006) Synergism between CpG-containing oligodeoxynucleotides and IL–2 causes dramatic enhancement of vaccine-elicited CD8+ T cell responses. J Immunol 177: 8860–8873

Kreider JW, Benjamin SA (1972) Tumor immunity and the mechanism of polyinosinic-polycytidylic acid inhibition of tumor growth. J Natl Cancer Inst 49: 1303–1310

Krieg AM, Yi AK, Matson S, Waldschmidt TJ, Bishop GA, Teasdale R, Koretzky GA, Klinman DM (1995) CpG motifs in bacterial DNA trigger direct B-cell activation. Nature 374: 546–549

Kunikata N, Sano K, Honda M, Ishii K, Matsunaga J, Okuyama R, Takahashi K, Watanabe H, Tamura G, Tagami H, Terui T (2004) Peritumoral CpG oligodeoxynucleotide treatment inhibits tumor growth and metastasis of B16F10 melanoma cells. J Invest Dermatol 123: 395–402

Lebre MC, van der Aar AM, van Baarsen L, van Capel TM, Schuitemaker JH, Kapsenberg ML, de Jong EC (2006) Human keratinocytes express functional Toll-like receptor 3, 4, 5, and 9. J Invest Dermatol 127: 331–341

Levine AS, Sivulich M, Wiernik PH, Levy HB (1979) Initial clinical trials in cancer patients of polyriboinosinic-polyribocytidylic acid stabilized with poly-L-lysine, in carboxymethylcellulose [poly(ICLC)], a highly effective interferon inducer. Cancer Res 39: 1645–1650

Lipford GB, Bauer M, Blank C, Reiter R, Wagner H, Heeg K (1997) CpG-containing synthetic oligonucleotides promote B and cytotoxic T cell responses to protein antigen: A new class of vaccine adjuvants. Eur J Immunol 27: 2340–2344

Lysa B, Tartler U, Wolf R, Arenberger P, Benninghoff B, Ruzicka T, Hengge UR, Walz M (2004) Gene expression in actinic keratoses: Pharmacological modulation by imiquimod. Br J Dermatol 151: 1150–1159

Medzhitov R, Janeway CA, Jr (2002) Decoding the patterns of self and nonself by the innate immune system. Science 296: 298–300

Medzhitov R, Preston-Hurlburt P, Janeway CA, Jr (1997) A human homologue of the *Drosophila* Toll protein signals activation of adaptive immunity. Nature 388: 394–397

Memon AA, Tomenson JA, Bothwell J, Friedmann PS (2000) Prevalence of solar damage and actinic keratosis in a Merseyside population. Br J Dermatol 142: 1154–1159

Michalopoulos P, Yawalkar N, Bronnimann M, Kappeler A, Braathen LR (2004) Characterization of the cellular infiltrate during successful topical treatment of lentigo maligna with imiquimod. Br J Dermatol 151: 903–906

Miconnet I, Koenig S, Speiser D, Krieg A, Guillaume P, Cerottini JC, Romero P (2002) CpG are efficient adjuvants for specific CTL induction against tumor antigen-derived peptide. J Immunol 168: 1212–1218

Milas L, Mason KA, Ariga H, Hunter N, Neal R, Valdecanas D, Krieg AM, Whisnant JK (2004) CpG oligodeoxynucleotide enhances tumor response to radiation. Cancer Res 64: 5074–5077

Miller RL, Gerster JF, Owens ML, Slade HB, Tomai MA (1999) Imiquimod applied topically: A novel immune response modifier and new class of drug. Int J Immunopharmacol 21: 1–14

Napolitani G, Rinaldi A, Bertoni F, Sallusto F, Lanzavecchia A (2005) Selected Toll-like receptor agonist combinations synergistically trigger a T helper type 1-polarizing program in dendritic cells. Nat Immunol 6: 769–776

Nordlund JJ, Wolff SM, Levy HB (1970) Inhibition of biologic activity of poly I:poly C by human plasma. Proc Soc Exp Biol Med 133: 439–444

Palamara F, Meindl S, Holcmann M, Luhrs P, Stingl G, Sibilia M (2004) Identification and characterization of pDC-like cells in normal mouse skin and melanomas treated with imiquimod. J Immunol 173: 3051–3061

Pasare C, Medzhitov R (2003) Toll pathway-dependent blockade of CD4+ CD25+ T cell-mediated suppression by dendritic cells. Science 299: 1033–1036

Pashenkov M, Goess G, Wagner C, Hormann M, Jandl T, Moser A, Britten CM, Smolle J, Koller S, Mauch C, Tantcheva-Poor I, Grabbe S, Loquai C, Esser S, Franckson T, Schneeberger A, Haarmann C, Krieg AM, Stingl G, Wagner SN (2006) Phase II trial of a Toll-like receptor 9-activating oligonucleotide in patients with metastatic melanoma. J Clin Oncol 20(24): 5716–5724

Pilon-Thomas S, Li W, Briggs JJ, Djeu J, Mule JJ, Riker AI (2006) Immunostimulatory effects of CpG-ODN upon dendritic cell-based immunotherapy in a murine melanoma model. J Immunother 29: 381–387

Purnell DM, Kreider JW, Bartlett GL (1975) Evaluation of antitumor activity of *Bordetella pertussis* in two murine tumor models. J Natl Cancer Inst 55: 123–128

Rajpar SF, Marsden JR (2006) Imiquimod in the treatment of lentigo maligna. Br J Dermatol 155: 653–656

Robbins PF, el-Gamil M, Li YF, Kawakami Y, Loftus D, Appella E, Rosenberg SA (1996) A mutated beta-catenin gene encodes a melanoma-specific antigen recognized by tumor infiltrating lymphocytes. J Exp Med 183: 1185–1192

Robinson RA, DeVita VT, Levy HB, Baron S, Hubbard SP, Levine AS (1976) A phase I-II trial of multiple-dose polyriboinosic-polyribocytidylic acid in patients with leukemia or solid tumors. J Natl Cancer Inst 57: 599–602

Roman M, Martin-Orozco E, Goodman JS, Nguyen MD, Sato Y, Ronaghy A, Kornbluth RS, Richman DD, Carson DA, Raz E (1997) Immunostimulatory DNA sequences function as T helper-1-promoting adjuvants. Nat Med 3: 849–854

Sato Y, Roman M, Tighe H, Lee D, Corr M, Nguyen MD, Silverman GJ, Lotz M, Carson DA, Raz E (1996) Immunostimulatory DNA sequences necessary for effective intradermal gene immunization. Science 19(273): 352–354

Sauder DN (2000) Immunomodulatory and pharmacologic properties of imiquimod. J Am Acad Dermatol 43: S6-11

Schlee M, Hornung V, Hartmann G (2006) siRNA and isRNA: Two edges of one sword. Mol Ther 14: 463–470

Schon MP, Wienrich BG, Drewniok C, Bong AB, Eberle J, Geilen CC, Gollnick H, Schon M (2004) Death receptor-independent apoptosis in malignant melanoma induced by the small-molecule immune response modifier imiquimod. J Invest Dermatol 122: 1266–1276

Shackleton M, Davis ID, Hopkins W, Jackson H, Dimopoulos N, Tai T, Chen Q, Parente P, Jefford M, Masterman KA, Caron D, Chen W, Maraskovsky E, Cebon J (2004) The impact of imiquimod, a Toll-like receptor-7 ligand (TLR7L), on the immunogenicity of melanoma peptide vaccination with adjuvant Flt3 ligand. Cancer Immun 4:9.: 9

Shankaran V, Ikeda H, Bruce AT, White JM, Swanson PE, Old LJ, Schreiber RD (2001) IFNgamma and lymphocytes prevent primary tumour development and shape tumour immunogenicity. Nature 410: 1107–1111

Sparwasser T, Koch ES, Vabulas RM, Heeg K, Lipford GB, Ellwart JW, Wagner H (1998) Bacterial DNA and immunostimulatory CpG oligonucleotides trigger maturation and activation of murine dendritic cells. Eur J Immunol 28: 2045–2054

Speiser DE, Lienard D, Rufer N, Rubio-Godoy V, Rimoldi D, Lejeune F, Krieg AM, Cerottini JC, Romero P (2005) Rapid and strong human CD8+ T cell responses to vaccination with peptide, IFA, and CpG oligodeoxynucleotide 7909. J Clin Invest 115: 739–746

Stary G, Bangert C, Tauber M, Strohal R, Kopp T, Stingl G (2007) Tumoricidal activity of TLR7/8-activated inflammatory dendritic cells. J Exp Med 204: 1441–1451

Takeshita F, Leifer CA, Gursel I, Ishii KJ, Takeshita S, Gursel M, Klinman DM (2001) Cutting edge: Role of Toll-like receptor 9 in CpG DNA-induced activation of human cells. J Immunol 167: 3555–3558

Tang DC, DeVit M, Johnston SA (1992) Genetic immunization is a simple method for eliciting an immune response. Nature 356: 152–154

Todd RW, Steele JC, Etherington I, Luesley DM (2004) Detection of CD8+ T cell responses to human papillomavirus type 16 antigens in women using imiquimod as a treatment for high-grade vulval intraepithelial neoplasia. Gynecol Oncol 92: 167–174

Tokunaga T, Yamamoto H, Shimada S, Abe H, Fukuda T, Fujisawa Y, Furutani Y, Yano O, Kataoka T, Sudo T (1984) Antitumor activity of deoxyribonucleic acid fraction from *Mycobacterium bovis* BCG. I. Isolation, physicochemical characterization, and antitumor activity. J Natl Cancer Inst 72: 955–962

Tormo D, Ferrer A, Bosch P, Gaffal E, Basner-Tschakarjan E, Wenzel J, Tüting T (2006a) Therapeutic efficacy of antigen-specific vaccination and Toll-like receptor stimulation against established transplanted and autochthonous melanoma in mice. Cancer Res 66: 5427–5435

Tormo D, Ferrer A, Gaffal E, Wenzel J, Basner-Tschakarjan E, Steitz J, Heukamp LC, Gutgemann I, Buettner R, Malumbres M, Barbacid M, Merlino G, Tüting T (2006b) Rapid growth of invasive metastatic melanoma in carcinogen-treated hepatocyte growth factor/scatter factor-transgenic mice carrying an oncogenic CDK4 mutation. Am J Pathol 169: 665–672

Tyring S (2001) Imiquimod applied topically: A novel immune response modifier. Skin Therapy Lett 6[6]. Ulmer JB, Sadoff JC, Liu MA (1996) DNA vaccines. Curr Opin Immunol 8: 531–536

Urosevic M, Dummer R, Conrad C, Beyeler M, Laine E, Burg G, Gilliet M (2005) Disease-independent skin recruitment and activation of plasmacytoid predendritic cells following imiquimod treatment. J Natl Cancer Inst 97[15]: 1903

Vabulas RM, Pircher H, Lipford GB, Hacker H, Wagner H (2000) CpG-DNA activates *in vivo* T cell epitope presenting dendritic cells to trigger protective antiviral cytotoxic T cell responses. J Immunol 164: 2372–2378

Wang RF (2006) Regulatory T cells and Toll-like receptors in cancer therapy. Cancer Res 66: 4987–4990

Weiner GJ, Liu HM, Wooldridge JE, Dahle CE, Krieg AM (1997) Immunostimulatory oligodeoxynucleotides containing the CpG motif are effective as immune adjuvants in tumor antigen immunization. Proc Natl Acad Sci USA 94: 10833–10837

Wenzel J, Uerlich M, Haller O, Bieber T, Tüting T (2005a) Enhanced type I interferon signaling and recruitment of chemokine receptor CXCR3-expressing lymphocytes into the skin following treatment with the TLR7-agonist imiquimod. J Cutan Pathol 32: 257–262

Wenzel J, Uerlich M, Worrenkamper E, Freutel S, Bieber T, Tüting T (2005b) Scarring skin lesions of discoid lupus erythematosus are characterized by high numbers of skin-homing cytotoxic lymphocytes associated with strong expression of the type I interferon-induced protein MxA. Br J Dermatol 153: 1011–1015

Whitmore MM, DeVeer MJ, Edling A, Oates RK, Simons B, Lindner D, Williams BR (2004) Synergistic activation of innate immunity by double-stranded RNA and CpG DNA promotes enhanced antitumor activity. Cancer Res 64: 5850–5860

Wolf IH, Cerroni L, Kodama K, Kerl H (2005) Treatment of lentigo maligna (melanoma *in situ*) with the immune response modifier imiquimod. Arch Dermatol 141: 510–514

Wolfel T, Hauer M, Schneider J, Serrano M, Wolfel C, Klehmann-Hieb E, De PE, Hankeln T, Meyer zum Buschenfelde KH, Beach D (1995) A p16INK4a-insensitive CDK4 mutant targeted by cytolytic T lymphocytes in a human melanoma. Science 269: 1281–1284

Yamamoto S, Yamamoto T, Shimada S, Kuramoto E, Yano O, Kataoka T, Tokunaga T (1992) DNA from bacteria, but not from vertebrates, induces interferons, activates natural killer cells and inhibits tumor growth. Microbiol Immunol 36: 983–997

Yamamoto T, Yamamoto S, Kataoka T, Komuro K, Kohase M, Tokunaga T (1994) Synthetic oligonucleotides with certain palindromes stimulate interferon production of human peripheral blood lymphocytes *in vitro*. Jpn J Cancer Res 85: 775–779

Youdim S (1976) Resistance to tumor growth mediated by *Listeria monocytogenes*. Destruction of experimental malignant melanoma by LM-activated peritoneal and lymphoid cells. J Immunol 116: 579–584

Zeleznick LD, Bhuyan BK (1969) Treatment of leukemic (L-1210) mice with double-stranded polyribonucleotides. Proc Soc Exp Biol Med 130: 126–128

Vaccination with Messenger RNA (mRNA)

Steve Pascolo

Abstract Both DNA and mRNA can be used as vehicles for gene therapy. Because the immune system is naturally activated by foreign nucleic acids thanks to the presence of Toll-like Receptors (TLR) in endosomes (TLR3, 7, and 8 detect exogenous RNA, while TLR9 can detect exogenous DNA), the delivery of foreign nucleic acids usually induces an immune response directed against the encoded protein. Many preclinical and clinical studies were performed using DNA-based experimental vaccines. However, no such products are yet approved for the human population. Meanwhile, the naturally transient and cytosolically active mRNA molecules are seen as a possibly safer and more potent alternative to DNA for gene vaccination. Optimized mRNA (improved for codon usage, stability, antigen-processing characteristics of the encoded protein, etc.) were demonstrated to be potent gene vaccination vehicles when delivered naked, in liposomes, coated on particles or transfected in dendritic cells *in vitro*. Human clinical trials indicate that the delivery of mRNA

Steve Pascolo

Institut for Cell Biology, Department of Immunology, University of Tuebingen, Auf der Morgenstelle 15, 72076 Tuebingen, Germany
steve.pascolo@uni-tuebingen.de

S. Bauer, G. Hartmann (eds.), *Toll-Like Receptors (TLRs) and Innate Immunity.*
Handbook of Experimental Pharmacology 183.
© Springer-Verlag Berlin Heidelberg 2008

naked or transfected in dendritic cells induces the expected antigen-specific immune response. Follow-up efficacy studies are on the way. Meanwhile, mRNA can be produced in large amounts and GMP quality, allowing the further development of mRNA-based therapies. This chapter describes the structure of mRNA, its possible optimizations for immunization purposes, the different methods of delivery used in preclinical studies, and finally the results of clinical trial where mRNA is the active pharmaceutical ingredient of new innovative vaccines.

1 Introduction

The seminal article of Wolf et al. shows that naked minimal nucleic acid vectors in the form of plasmid DNA (pDNA) or messenger RNA (mRNA) that code for a protein in an eukaryotic cell are spontaneously taken up and expressed in mouse muscles (Wolff et al., 1990). Thus, *in vivo* injected foreign nucleic acids can somehow penetrate in the cytosole (mRNA) and the nucleus (pDNA) of somatic cells before being degraded by ubiquitous extracellular nucleases. This phenomenon is more surprising for mRNA than for pDNA since the former is degraded within seconds in contact to the abundant extracellular RNases (Probst et al., 2006). The uptake mechanism is saturable and can be competed away for both pDNA—review by (Wolff and Budker, 2005)—and mRNA (Probst et al., Gene Ther. 2007 Aug 14(15): 1175–80). It involves the movement of vesicles and probably specific receptors. Other sites than the skeletal muscle can be used for *in vivo* gene delivery using naked nucleic acids: skin, liver, and heart muscle, for example; review by Nishikawa (Nishikawa and Hashida, 2002). Following Wolff and associate's results, the utilization of minimal nucleic acid vectors for local expression of an antigen to be recognized by the immune system was undertaken as shown with pDNA first (Ulmer et al., 1993) and mRNA thereafter (Conry et al., 1995). The capacity of the immune system to recognize specifically the protein expressed from the foreign nucleic acid is probably linked to the capacity of immune cells such as dendritic cells to sense these exogenous genetic molecules through TLR9 for bacterial DNA or TLR3 and TLR7 or TLR8 for double stranded RNA (dsRNA) and single stranded RNA (ssRNA), respectively.

The utilization of mRNA has several superlative advantages compared to pDNA:

(i) At the peak of expression, the amount of protein produced through injection of naked mRNA is higher than the amount of protein produced by the injection of the same amount of naked pDNA (Probst, Gene Ther. 2007 Aug 14(15): 1175–80)

(ii) Due to its transient nature, mRNA is expressed during a controlled period of few days while pDNA-expression is uncontrolled: Its expression in mice can be transient or last for months depending on the random fate of these stable molecules (the integration of pDNA in the genome could result in the long-term expression of the transgene). This guarantees that long-term expression

and its possible consecutive tolerization of the immune response will not occur
with mRNA-based vaccines.

(iii) Because mRNA cannot modify the genetic information of the host, it is not considered a gene therapy approach by the authorities. Thus, for example, tedious
genotoxicity evaluation in animals can be avoided.

For these reasons, several methods based on mRNA for vaccination were tested
in mice and further evaluated in humans. This chapter summarizes the features of
the mRNA that are needed for vaccine formulation, the different methods that were
developed and validated in mice, and finally the result of phase I/II clinical trials.

2 Messenger RNA: Structure, Production, and Specific Optimizations for Vaccination Purposes

2.1 Messenger RNA for Research

A mature eukaryotic mRNA has three characteristic structural elements: the $5'$ Cap,
the coding sequence starting with usually an ATG codon in a "Kozak" surrounding
and ending at a stop codon, and finally a poly-A tail of several hundred residues.
For vaccination purposes, mRNA can be purified from cells such as tumor cells
and formulated in an immunogenic solution in order to trigger an immune response
against a broad range of antigens. However, for mRNA-based vaccination, *in vitro*
transcribed mRNA is usually used. It is produced through molecular biology methods. First, the gene of interest is cloned in a plasmid vector that contains (i) an
upstream promoter exclusively recognized by processive RNA polymerases available as recombinant proteins such as the T7, S6, or T3 RNA polymerases from
bacteriophages; (ii) a downstream poly A sequence of a minimum of 30 bases; and
(iii) a unique restriction site downstream the poly A-tail. A bacterial clone containing this plasmid is cultured at $37°C$ in an adequate bouillon (usually LB medium
that contains the antibiotic for which the plasmid carries specific resistance). Bacteria are then collected by centrifugation and lysed (usually using sodium hydrox-
ide and SDS). Proteins and bacteria genomic DNA are precipitated by potassium
acetate. The cleared lysate contains the plasmids that can be isolated using, for example, anion exchange columns (see, for example, www.qiagen.com). The eluted
pDNA is highly pure. It can be precipitated by salts (ammonium acetate or sodium
chloride, for example) plus isopropanol or ethanol. The nucleic acid pellet is resuspended in water or tris-EDTA buffer, quantified by spectrophotometry (absorbance
at 260 nm) and stored in the cold ($4°C$ for short term and $-20°C$ or $-80°C$ for long
term). Messenger RNA is produced from pDNA in an *in vitro* transcription reaction. To this end the pDNA is linearized thanks to the unique restriction site that is
downstream of the poly-A tail. After digestion, the proteins are extracted by phenol-
chloroform, the pDNA is recovered by ethanol precipitation, and, after a wash
in ethanol 75%, resuspended in water. The run-off transcription of this linearized

plasmid is performed by the addition of an adequate buffer, the RNA polymerase specific for the upstream promoter (T7, SP6, or T3 RNA polymerase), the four nucleotides in their triphosphate form (ATP, UTP, GTP, and CTP) and a four-fold excess of Cap analogue (the dinucleotide methyl-7-Guanin(5′) PPP(5′) Guanin, in short m7G(5′) ppp(5′)G) compared to GTP. This will guarantee that approximately 80% of the RNA molecules will start with a Cap instead of a G-residue (the first base of the RNA is dictated by the sequence of the promoter and set as a G in T7, SP6, and T3 promoters). After two hours incubation at 37°C, a DNase is added that will destroy the plasmid. Thereafter, long mRNA molecules are selectively recovered by precipitation with lithium chloride. After a wash with 75% ethanol, the mRNA pellet is resuspended in water and quantified by OD260. For a detailed transcription protocol and overview of RNA recovery methods, refer to the manual of commercially available transcription kits such as those from Ambion (mMessagemMachine at www.ambion.com), for example. Messenger RNA resuspended in water can be stored at 4°C for days and at −20°C or −80°C for long-term storage.

2.2 Messenger RNA for Clinical Applications

For good manufacturing practice (GMP) production, the antibiotic used in fermentation of the pDNA should preferably not be of the ampicillin family. This avoids potential clinical problems due to penicillin allergies. The production process is similar for research (as described above) and pharmaceutical grade products. However, for mRNA in GMP quality, the nucleic acids can be purified using a chromatographic method that allows elimination of traces of contaminants from the transcription reaction (proteins, DNA fragments, endotoxins). Eventually the chromatography method can also allow the recovery of the mRNA according to its size. The advantage of this method is that it eliminates abortive (shorter) or aberrant (eventually longer) transcripts produced during the enzymatic reaction (see www.curevac.com for more information). Should the chromatography method use other ions than sodium, a precipitation of the mRNA with NaCl and ethanol will guarantee that the counterion in the RNA batch is sodium.

The final batch should appear as a transparent colorless solution and fulfill the following specifications:

(i) Identity: Sequencing of the plasmid used for *in vitro* transcription should show 100% identity with the expected sequence. At best, reverse transcription and sequencing of the final mRNA could be performed. Agarose gel electrophoresis is used to document the size of the mRNA and prove that only one species of mRNA (one size) is present. Susceptibility to RNase can additionally be used as a proof of molecular identity.

(ii) Content: Quantification should be performed by light absorbance at 260 nm. Osmolarity and pH should also be measured. All these values should be in-between prespecified limits.

(iii) Purity: Residual proteins, chromosomal bacteria DNA, bacteria RNA, and endotoxin must be below specified limits. Sterility must be controlled by standard microbiological assays. Residual pDNA and aberrant mRNA transcripts (smaller or larger byproducts of the transcription) should be checked. The former can be done by using quantitative PCR with primers specific for the plasmid that was used for transcription. The latter can be done by agarose gel electrophoresis. The amount of eventual contaminants should remain below specified limits.

Moreover, counterions (which should be NaCl because of the final precipitation of the nucleic acids with alcohol plus NaCl), residual solvents (if they are used during the production), and potency (functional assay using, for example, transfection of cells and verification of the expression of the protein of interest or testing of the immune response after adequate application in an animal model) can ideally be tested.

Pharmaceutical grade mRNA is offered by two companies: Asuragen in the USA (www.asuragen.com) and CureVac in Europe (www.curevac.com).

2.3 Optimization of mRNA for Vaccination

It can be assumed, although it is not firmly proven, that a high and long-term expression of the protein encoded by the mRNA would favor the efficacy of the mRNA-based vaccine. In order to enhance the transcription rate (high expression) and stability (long-term expression) of the mRNA, several features of the molecule can be optimized.

2.3.1 Optimizing the 5′ Cap Structure

The Cap dinucleotide analogue usually used in the transcription reaction can be incorporated in two directions: either the 3′OH of the pentose carrying the methylated guanine or the 3′OH of the pentose carrying the non-methylated guanine is used for the phosphodiester bridge to the second residue of the mRNA. Only, the second case will lead to a functional mRNA because the initiation elongation factor 4 (eIF4) protein recognizes the methylated base at the 5′ end position only. Thus, using the standard Cap analogue, only half of the 80% mRNA molecules carrying the Cap are functional. As a remedy, a modified Cap can be used. The most common one is called ARCA (anti-reverse Cap) and consists of a Cap analogue with a modification on the 3′OH of the ribose carrying the methylated guanine (Stepinski et al., 2001). Consequently, this side cannot be used for the incorporation of the Cap. Thus, only correctly capped molecules are generated. Moreover, the modification on the sugar may in some unknown ways improve the mRNA since ARCA Cap mRNA molecules are not two-fold but five-fold more efficiently translated than mRNA made with the standard Cap.

Another method to get only correctly capped molecules is to do a transcription reaction without Cap analogue and to perform on the synthesized mRNA a capping reaction. This reaction can be done using the vaccinia virus-encoded capping complex. It consists of two subunits—D1 and D12—and is also known as guanylyltransferase. This enzyme is commercially available as a recombinant molecule (www.ambion.com). In the presence of GTP and S-adenosyl methionine (SAM), the guanylyltransferase can add a natural Cap structure (7-methylguanosine) to the $5'$ triphosphate of a RNA molecule. However, because the efficacy of this reaction cannot be controlled (no simple test allows one to check the level of capping on mRNA molecules), the enzymatic capping is not used routinely. Excess of Cap analogue or, at best, ARCA compared to GTP in the transcription reaction are the standard, reliable methods to produce capped mRNA.

2.3.2 Optimizing the Untranslated Regions

The half-life of mRNA molecules in the cytosole is highly regulated (Ross, 1995). It is in the range of minutes, for example, for messenger-coding cell cycle-controlling proteins or cytokines; up to weeks, for example, for messenger-coding globins in red blood cells. Destabilization and stabilization sequences are usually located at the untranslated (UTR) $3'$ end of the mRNA (between the stop codon and the poly-A tail). The most common destabilization mode is signaled by AU rich sequences called AUREs in the $3'$ UTR. Thus, if they are present in the cDNA of interest, those AUREs sequences should be deleted from the pDNA construct that is used to produce the mRNA. On the opposite side, the most common stabilization mode is signaled by pyrimidine-rich sequences located in the $3'$ UTRs. They are recognized by the ubiquitous "α-complex" (Holcik and Liebhaber, 1997). The most characterized sequences recognized by the alpha complex are the approximately 180-base or approximately 80-base UTRs in the β- or α-globin genes, respectively. They allow the long-term stability of those mRNA in terminally differentiated red blood cells devoid of nuclei. ß- or α-globin UTRs can be added to the end of any cDNA of interest in the pDNA construct that is used to produce the mRNA. Messenger RNA used for therapy usually possess such globin stabilization UTRs (Hoerr et al., 2000; Klencke et al., 2002; Conry et al., 1995; Malone et al., 1989). Together with a poly-A tail of a minimum of 30 residues but of preferably more than 100 residues (Mockey et al., 2006; Holtkamp et al., 2006), the globin UTRs provide stability to the mRNA.

2.3.3 Optimizing the Translated Region

Optimizing the Translation Process

To optimize the production of the desired protein from mRNA molecules, the correct start codon should be the first ATG triplet met by the ribosome after it starts scanning the mRNA from the $5'$ end towards the $3'$ end. This start codon should be in "Kozak" surrounding which is: A/GNNATGG (Kozak, 1978). On this sequence the ribosome will incorporate the N-terminal methionine and move toward the $3'$ end to the next codon. No alternative cryptic start codon should be upstream of the correct start codon since they would induce the production of unwanted upstream protein and reduce the production of the expected antigen.

Most amino acids are encoded by several codons. Some of them are more favorable since they correspond to more abundant tRNA. This feature allows the ribosome to perform translation quickly. Thus, mRNA highly translated, such as, for example, mRNA coding for structure proteins (actin, etc.) contain mostly favorable codons. Unfavorable codons slow down the ribosome and may also induce abortion of the translation process. Because the relative abundance of tRNA is not conserved between species, the codon preference or "codon usage" is also species-specific. For example alanine, which is encoded by four codons, would be optimally coded by GCG in *Escherichia coli*, by GCT in *Saccharomyces cerevisiae*, by GCA in *Bacillus subtilis*, and by GCC in *Homo sapiens*. As a consequence, genes from bacteria or fungi are not well translated by the mammalian cell machinery. As a standard method for optimizing gene therapies, even when the therapeutic gene is of mammalian origin, a codon optimization should be performed to enhance the efficacy of transgene expression in humans. To this end the protein sequence of interest is converted into an optimal mRNA sequence using algorithms that take into account the precise codon usage of human cells. This virtual gene is then created using assembly of chemically synthesized DNA oligonucleotides. Many companies offer this service such as Geneart (www.geneart.com) or Entelechon (www.entelechon.com) or Blueheron (www.blueheronbio.com), for example. The synthetic gene can be cloned in an mRNA production vector as described above. Not only will this allow the generation of mRNA that is optimal for the translation machinery but it will also facilitate the description and full documentation of the genetic starting material for authorities in charge of clinical trials.

Optimizing the Antigen Presentation

Although epitopes presented by MHC class I molecule may mostly come from quickly degraded natural defective translation products ("DRiPs"), it is possible to specifically enhance this antigen presentation pathway thanks to the addition of ubiquitin, calreticulin (Anthony et al., 1999), or herpes simplex virus VP22 (Chhabra et al., 2004) moieties. These additional protein sequences can increase the utilization of the attached antigen for generation of epitopes to be loaded on MHC I molecules. Although these methods were not used for mRNA-based vaccines, they were proven useful to enhance the immunogenicity of antigens delivered by pDNA-vaccination. Thus, mRNA-based vaccinations could be expected to be similarly optimized thanks to the introduction of sequence tags coding for such MHC I optimizing moieties.

The presentation of MCH class II epitopes depends on the availability of the antigen in endosomes of antigen presenting cells (APCs). MHC II antigen processing and loading takes place in these vesicles. For antigens that are normally located in the cytosole, the addition of sequences addressing to the endosomes is a validated method to enhance mRNA-based vaccines at least *in vitro* using transfected APCs. In this context, invariant chain (Momburg et al., 1993) or LAMP (Ruff et al., 1997) moieties that naturally target the attached protein to the endosomes were shown to optimize MHC II presentation of the mRNA-encoded antigen. Another generic method to enhance the presentation of an antigen to the immune system is to address it to the secretory pathway resulting from a signal sequence introduced in front of the antigen (a leader sequence), and at the same time, target it to APCs by adding the sequence of an APC-ligand such as CD40L, Flt-3L, or CTLA4 (Boyle et al., 1997; Hung et al., 2001). These combined modifications allow the secreted antigen to be taken up by APCs and thereby enhance the efficacy of cross-presentation (natural uptake by an APC of an antigen expressed by a somatic cell).

3 Methods of mRNA-Based Vaccination

3.1 Delivery

There are four different formulations of mRNA, which were described in mice to trigger the development of an immune response against the coded antigen. In chronological order of publication, those are:

1. Encapsulation of the mRNA into cationic liposomes (Martinon et al., 1993; Hoerr et al., 2000; Hess et al., 2006). Mice injected with as little as one microgram of mRNA encapsulated in liposomes developed an immune response against the encoded foreign antigen. Intravenous delivery was the most efficient route of vaccination, although intradermal and eventually subcutaneous injections could also induce immunity. Instead of liposomes, the mRNA can be entrapped in cationic polymers such as protamine, with which it spontaneously forms particles (Hoerr et al., 2000; Scheel et al., 2005). Intradermal injections allow these complexes to trigger an immune response specific for the encoded protein (Hoerr et al., 2000).
2. Direct injection of naked mRNA into the dermis (Conry et al., 1995 and Hoerr et al., 2000). Surprisingly, in spite of the presence of ubiquitous RNases on the skin (Probst et al., 2006), naked mRNA when injected in the dermis of mice is spontaneously taken up and translated. The expressed protein is recognized as antigen by the immune system. Formulation of the mRNA in a buffer that contains calcium such as the Ringer solution promotes the spontaneous active uptake of the injected mRNA (Probst et al., Gene Ther. 2007 Aug 14(15):1175–80).
3. Needleless delivery of gold particles coated by mRNA using a gene gun (Qiu et al., 1996; Steitz et al., 2006). The mRNA is precipitated on micrometric gold particles. They are dried inside a tube, which is cut in small pieces used as cartouche in the helium-powered gene gun. By shooting, helium goes through

the cartridge and propels the gold beads, which, thanks to their kinetic energy, penetrate through the *stratum corneum* and directly transfect with the loaded mRNA all type of cells present in the dermis. This mechanical transfection allows the expression of the mRNA-encoded protein. It is followed by the triggering of an immune response against foreign and also against self mRNA-encoded protein (Steitz et al., 2006).

4. Transfection of *in vitro* generated autologous APCs that are re-administered to patients (Boczkowski et al., 1996). APCs, generally monocyte-derived dendritic cells (MoDC), are prepared from the patient's peripheral blood. This requires one week of *in vitro* culture. The cells are then transfected with the mRNA using usually electroporation. After this transfection they are matured by culture one or two days in a medium containing maturation signals and then re-injected into the patients. Mature transfected APCs can efficiently stimulate *in vitro* and *in vivo* naïve or memory CD4- and CD8-positive T cells specific for epitopes from the foreign mRNA-encoded protein.

Although all four technologies were validated in mice, only methods (2), naked mRNA, and (4), transfected MoDC were evaluated in humans through phase I/II trials as presented below in paragraph 4. Probably because of formulation/stability and toxicity issues, the liposome formulation of mRNA was not yet tested in humans. Since the gene gun delivery method was shown to be very efficient and absolutely safe in humans with pDNA vaccines, it was not tested using mRNA.

3.2 Adjuvants

3.2.1 Vaccination by Direct Application of mRNA

When the mRNA is delivered naked, encapsulated, or through a gene gun, mostly somatic cells are transfected. Thus, as opposed to the mRNA-transfection in APCs (see next paragraph), using these three methods, cross-presentation of the antigen may be the primary mechanism for the priming of the immune response. To this end professional APCs need to be present at the site of mRNA delivery. These pick the antigen produced by somatic cells and, being mature, carry it to the draining secondary lymphoid tissues, where stimulation of specific lymphocytes takes place. Thus, enrichment of the mRNA injection site with APCs could be a method to improve the efficacy of vaccination. One well-characterized reagent available at pharmaceutical grade and capable of attracting or inducing APCs is GM-CSF. In mice, several peptide or pDNA-based vaccine formulations were found to be enhanced thanks to concomitant GM-CSF injections. In humans, peptide vaccines are often delivered with recombinant GM-CSF. Accordingly, GM-CSF was tested as an adjuvant for mRNA vaccination in mice using both the naked and liposome formulations. Using naked mRNA injections (Carralot et al., 2004), the application of recombinant GM-CSF either at the site of mRNA injection (dermis: ear pinna) or at a distant site (subcutaneous: flank) was efficient in enhancing the Th1-type of immunity against the mRNA-encoded antigen. However, the recombinant GM-CSF had to be administered one day after the mRNA. Injecting recombinant GM-CSF before or at the same time as the mRNA did not result in any improvement of the immune response. Using liposome-encapsulated mRNA, the co-administration of mRNA coding for a foreign antigen (Ovalbumin) and mRNA coding for GM-CSF could enhance the immunogenicity of the vaccine as well as the development of the primed T cells towards memory lymphocytes (Hess et al., 2006). In this set-up, GM-CSF is actually present some time after the injection since uptake of the liposomes and translation of the mRNA require several hours. Thus, in both reports (Carralot et al., 2004; Hess et al., 2006), the potential of GM-CSF to enhance the efficacy of mRNA-vaccines is evidenced when this chemokine is present after mRNA injection and not, as could be hypothesized from the known capacity of GM-CSF to attract/differentiate DCs, before mRNA application.

3.2.2 Vaccination Using mRNA-Transfected APCs

The optimal status of vaccinating MoDCs is still a mater of debate: Although *in vitro* matured DCs are more efficient than immature DCs for priming T cells, they are eventually too exhausted for migrating to the lymph nodes *in vivo*. This would suggest that DCs on the way to maturation rather than fully matured DCs should be injected. Consequently, the optimal maturation signal to use *in vitro* should induce a slow maturation and induce the capacity to migrate to lymph nodes (through CCR7 expression, for example). Once in the lymph node, the DCs should express adequate cytokines such as IL-12 and co-stimulation signals such as CD80 or CD86. To this end, a cocktail of four molecules is frequently used in order to induce maturation of vaccine DCs: TNF-alpha, IL-6, IL-1 beta, and prostaglandin E2 (Thurner et al., 1999). Two general improvements for the DC-based vaccines have been tested: (i) the pretreatment of the DC-injection site with inflammatory cytokines (Martin-Fontecha et al., 2003), and (ii) the direct intralymphatic injection (Grover et al., 2006). The first method is based on induction of the CCR7 ligand CCL21 in lymphatic endothelial cells by inflammatory cytokines. This creates a lymphatic avenue from the skin to the lymph node. DCs subsequently injected at the same site use this pre-made avenue and migrate efficiently to the draining lymph node. This approach was not yet reported in human clinical trials. The second method consists in the mechanical delivery of the DCs at the site where they prime T cells, which is the lymph node. Such a method can be performed in humans thanks to the monitoring of the injection by ultrasound. Injection is performed while the tip of the needle is in a targeted subcutaneous lymph node such as an inguinal lymph node. Intra-lymphatic injection of peptide pulsed dendritic cells was reported to enhance the efficacy of vaccination. Up to now however, as detailed below, mRNA-transfected dendritic cells were not more potent in inducing an immune response when injected via intralymph node compared to intradermal (Kyte and Gaudernack, 2006).

4 Results of Clinical Trials

Messenger RNA-based vaccines in humans were up to now only tested as immunotherapies to induce or boost anti-tumor immunity in cancer patients.

4.1 Monocyte-Derived Dendritic Cells Transfected with mRNA In Vitro

As mentioned above, the method described by the team of E. Gilboa in 1996 (Gilboa et al., 2003; Boczkowski et al., 1996) was the first to be used as an mRNA-based vaccination regimen in humans. In one of the first trials metastatic prostate cancer patients received several injections of autologous MoDCs transfected with prostate-specific antigen (PSA) coding mRNA (Heiser et al., 2002). After this treatment, specific T cells against PSA could be evidenced in the peripheral blood of all patients (9/9). No severe adverse event was recorded. Thus, mRNA-tranfected MoDCs can safely trigger the desired T cell immunity in human patients. This trial also indicates that the newly induced T cell response may have had a clinical impact (decrease in the log slope of PSA and transient clearance of circulating tumor cells) in some patients. In another trial made by the same team, MoDCs were transfected with the total mRNA from autologous renal tumors (Gilboa et al., 2003; Su et al., 2003). Most treated patients (6/7) responded to the vaccine as shown by monitoring antitumor T cells. Superior results were obtained in a subsequent trial where on top of the mRNA vaccine, patients received ONTAK, which is a IL-2-toxin fusion that kills CD25-expressing T cells such as the CD4+/CD25+Tregs (Dannull et al., 2005). In this case the ablation of Treg could allow a better proliferation and activity of antitumor (antivaccine) T cells. Several other groups have also evaluated this technology. In particular, the team of G. Gaudernack published the results of two trials, in which either allogeneic total tumor mRNA (prepared from three prostate tumor cell lines) or autologous total tumor mRNA (prepared from a surgically removed melanoma metastasis) was transfected by electroporation in autologous MoDCs and injected four times at weekly intervals. Those investigators could record the induction of a T cell response against the tumor in approximately half the vaccinated patients (Kyte et al., 2006) (Mu et al., 2005): 12/19 in the prostate cancer trial; 10/19 in the melanoma trial. In the prostate carcinoma trial, 11 patients had stable disease as judged by PSA levels in the blood. Ten of those eleven patients had a detectable vaccine-induced T cell immune response while only two out of the eight patients with progressive disease (increasing PSA levels) had a detectable vaccine-induced T cell response. Thus, this allogeneic vaccination strategy may have had a positive impact on the tumor disease. In both of these trials, the intradermal injection of transfected MoDCs was compared to the intralymph node injection. However, surprisingly, the vaccine induced T cell response rate was higher in the group of patients receiving intradermal injections (8/9 in the prostate trial) compared to the group of patients receiving intralymph node injections (4/10 in the prostate trial).

Thus, using the MoDC preparation protocol proposed by Gaudernack's team, intradermal injections are sufficient to trigger a potent and clinically relevant antitumor immune response. Follow-up trials designed to further improve this strategy are ongoing. They include the concomitant systemic injection of IL-2 or the application of TLR agonists on the skin at the injection site (Kyte and Gaudernack, 2006).

To conclude, mRNA transfected MoDCs is a safe and efficacious vaccine formulation that can trigger antigen-specific T cells. The forthcoming results of phase II and phase III trials will, it is hoped, firmly demonstrate that this method can induce clinically relevant T cell immune response that can be beneficial for patients' health and survival (for an update, see www.clinicaltrials.gov).

4.2 Direct Injection of mRNA

The direct intradermal injection of mRNA was only recently evaluated in humans although it was described in mice as a vaccination method earlier than the mRNA-transfected MoDC technology. In the first trial, progressive stage III and stage IV melanoma patients were recruited. Total mRNA corresponding to the whole transcriptome of a surgically removed autologous metastasis was produced, formulated, and injected in the dermis. One day after the mRNA injection, recombinant GM-CSF was applied subcutaneously in the same area. Fifteen patients were recruited and altogether 114 mRNA injections were performed. No WHO grade III or grade IV adverse event was recorded. Three of thirteen evaluable patients showed an increased antitumor antibody response during the treatment period (Weide et al., Journal of Immunu therapy, in press). The antivaccine T cell response was eventually induced in 5 of 13 evaluable patients. Although no objective clinical response was observed in this trial, some patients showed an unexpected favorable course of disease. This technology is being further evaluated in melanoma patients and in renal cell carcinoma patients. However, in these subsequent trials defined mRNA species are used (cocktails of 4 to 6 different mRNA coding for defined tumor antigens). Thus, immunomonitoring will be facilitated compared to the autologous whole mRNA approach used in the first trial. These studies should indicate whether the direct injection of mRNA is a method that can efficiently prime an immune response in human.

5 Conclusion

Four methods of mRNA-based vaccinations were validated in animal models and two of them (mRNA transfection *in vitro* in MoDCs and direct injection in the dermis of naked mRNA) were evaluated in clinical trials. The very encouraging results obtained by different academic groups using mRNA-transfected MoDCs may lead to the validation in pivotal phase II or phase III trials of this method. As an alternative, the simpler direct injection of mRNA needs to be further evaluated in phase I/II clinical trials. Meanwhile, our understanding of the immune system and in particular of the suppression mechanisms as well as of the adjuvant effects through TLR signaling allow us to design more efficacious vaccination strategies that will certainly help in turning mRNA-based vaccine strategies into potent therapeutic and prophylactic modalities.

References

Anonymous (2003) Anti-vascular endothelial growth factor therapy for subfoveal choroidal neovascularization secondary to age-related macular degeneration: Phase II study results. Ophthalmol 110: 979–986

Anthony LS, Wu H, Sweet H, Turnnir C, Boux LJ, Mizzen LA (1999) Priming of CD8+ CTL effector cells in mice by immunization with a stress protein-influenza virus nucleoprotein fusion molecule. Vaccine 17: 373–383

Boczkowski D, Nair SK, Snyder D, Gilboa E (1996) Dendritic cells pulsed with RNA are potent antigen-presenting cells *in vitro* and *in vivo*. J Exp. Med. 184: 465–472

Boyle JS, Koniaras C, Lew AM (1997) Influence of cellular location of expressed antigen on the efficacy of DNA vaccination: Cytotoxic T lymphocyte and antibody responses are suboptimal when antigen is cytoplasmic after intramuscular DNA immunization. Int Immunol 9: 1897–1906

Carralot JP, Probst J, Hoerr I, Scheel B, Teufel R, Jung G, Rammensee HG, Pascolo S (2004) Polarization of immunity induced by direct injection of naked sequence-stabilized mRNA vaccines. Cell Mol Life Sci 61: 2418–2424

Chhabra A, Mehrotra S, Chakraborty NG, Mukherji B, Dorsky DI (2004) Cross-presentation of a human tumor antigen delivered to dendritic cells by HSV VP22-mediated protein translocation. Eur J Immunol 34: 2824–2833

Conry RM, LoBuglio AF, Wright M, Sumerel L, Pike MJ, Johanning F, Benjamin R, Lu D, Curiel DT (1995) Characterization of a messenger RNA polynucleotide vaccine vector. Cancer Res 55: 1397–1400

Dannull J, Su Z, Rizzieri D, Yang BK, Coleman D, Yancey D, Zhang A, Dahm P, Chao N, Gilboa E, Vieweg J (2005) Enhancement of vaccine-mediated antitumor immunity in cancer patients after depletion of regulatory T cells. J Clin Invest 115: 3623–3633

Grover A, Kim GJ, Lizee G, Tschoi M, Wang G, Wunderlich JR, Rosenberg SA, Hwang ST, Hwu P (2006) Intralymphatic dendritic cell vaccination induces tumor antigen-specific, skin-homing T lymphocytes. Clin Cancer Res 12: 5801–5808

Heiser A, Coleman D, Dannull J, Yancey D, Maurice MA, Lallas CD, Dahm P, Niedzwiecki D, Gilboa E, Vieweg J (2002) Autologous dendritic cells transfected with prostate-specific antigen RNA stimulate CTL responses against metastatic prostate tumors. J Clin Invest 109: 409–417

Hess PR, Boczkowski D, Nair SK, Snyder D, Gilboa E (2006) Vaccination with mRNAs encoding tumor-associated antigens and granulocyte-macrophage colony-stimulating factor efficiently primes CTL responses, but is insufficient to overcome tolerance to a model tumor/self antigen. Cancer Immunol Immunother 55: 672–683

Hoerr I, Obst R, Rammensee HG, Jung G (2000) *In vivo* application of RNA leads to induction of specific cytotoxic T lymphocytes and antibodies. Eur J Immunol 30: 1–7

Holcik M, Liebhaber SA (1997) Four highly stable eukaryotic mRNAs assemble 3′ untranslated region RNA-protein complexes sharing cis and trans components. Proc Natl Acad Sci USA 94: 2410–2414

Holtkamp S, Kreiter S, Selmi A, Simon P, Koslowski M, Huber C, Tureci O, Sahin U (2006) Modification of antigen-encoding RNA increases stability, translational efficacy, and T cell stimulatory capacity of dendritic cells. Blood 108: 4009–4017

Hung CF, Hsu KF, Cheng WF, Chai CY, He L, Ling M, Wu TC (2001) Enhancement of DNA vaccine potency by linkage of antigen gene to a gene encoding the extracellular domain of Fms-like tyrosine kinase 3-ligand. Cancer Res 61: 1080–1088

Klencke B, Matijevic M, Urban RG, Lathey JL, Hedley ML, Berry M, Thatcher J, Weinberg V, Wilson J, Darragh T, Jay N, Da Costa M, Palefsky JM (2002) Encapsulated plasmid DNA treatment for human papillomavirus 16-associated anal dysplasia: A Phase I study of ZYC101. Clin Cancer Res 8: 1028–1037

Kozak M (1978) How do eukaryotic ribosomes select initiation regions in messenger RNA? Cell 15: 1109–1123

Kyte JA, Gaudernack G (2006) Immuno-gene therapy of cancer with tumour-mRNA transfected dendritic cells. Cancer Immunol Immunother 55: 1432–1442

Kyte JA, Mu L, Aamdal S, Kvalheim G, Dueland S, Hauser M, Gullestad HP, Ryder T, Lislerud K, Hammerstad H, Gaudernack G (2006) Phase I/II trial of melanoma therapy with dendritic cells transfected with autologous tumor-mRNA Cancer Gene Ther 13: 905–918

Malone RW, Felgner PL, Verma IM (1989) Cationic liposome-mediated RNA transfection. Proc Natl Acad Sci USA 86: 6077–6081

Martin-Fontecha A, Sebastiani S, Hopken UE, Uguccioni M, Lipp M, Lanzavecchia A, Sallusto F (2003) Regulation of dendritic cell migration to the draining lymph node: Impact on T lymphocyte traffic and priming. J Exp Med 198: 615–621

Martinon F, Krishnan S, Lenzen G, Magne R, Gomard E, Guillet JG, Levy JP, Meulien P (1993) Induction of virus-specific cytotoxic T lymphocytes *in vivo* by liposome-entrapped mRNA. Eur J Immunol 23: 1719–1722

Mockey M, Goncalves C, Dupuy FP, Lemoine FM, Pichon C, Midoux P (2006) mRNA transfection of dendritic cells: Synergistic effect of ARCA mRNA capping with Poly(A) chains in cis and in trans for a high protein expression level. Biochem Biophys Res Commun 340: 1062–1068

Momburg F, Fuchs S, Drexler J, Busch R, Post M, Hammerling GJ, Adorini L (1993) Epitope-specific enhancement of antigen presentation by invariant chain. J Exp Med. 178: 1453–1458

Mu LJ, Kyte JA, Kvalheim G, Aamdal S, Dueland S, Hauser M, Hammerstad H, Waehre H, Raabe N, Gaudernack G (2005) Immunotherapy with allotumour mRNA-transfected dendritic cells in androgen-resistant prostate cancer patients. Br J Cancer 93: 749–756

Nishikawa M, Hashida M (2002) Nonviral approaches satisfying various requirements for effective *in vivo* gene therapy. Biol Pharm Bull 25: 275–283

Probst J, Brechtel S, Scheel B, Hoerr I, Jung G, Rammensee HG, Pascolo S (2006) Characterization of the ribonuclease activity on the skin surface. Genet Vaccines Ther 4: 4

Probst J, Weide B, Scheel B, Pichler BJ, Hoerr I, Rammensee HG, Pascolo S (2007) Spontaneous cellular uptake of exogenous messenger RNA in vivo is nucleic acid-specific, saturable and ion dependent. Gene Ther. 2007 Aug; 14(15):1175–80. Epub 2007 May 3

Qiu P, Ziegelhoffer P, Sun J, Yang NS (1996) Gene gun delivery of mRNA *in situ* results in efficient transgene expression and genetic immunization. Gene Ther 3: 262–268

Ross J (1995) mRNA stability in mammalian cells. Microbiol Rev 59: 423–450

Ruff AL, Guarnieri FG, Staveley-O'Carroll K, Siliciano RF, August JT (1997) The enhanced immune response to the HIV gp160/LAMP chimeric gene product targeted to the lysosome membrane protein trafficking pathway. J Biol Chem 272: 8671–8678

Steitz J, Britten CM, Wolfel T, Tuting T (2006) Effective induction of anti-melanoma immunity following genetic vaccination with synthetic mRNA coding for the fusion protein EGFPTRP2. Cancer Immunol Immunother 55: 246–253

Stepinski J, Waddell C, Stolarski R, Darzynkiewicz E, Rhoads RE (2001) Synthesis and properties of mRNAs containing the novel "anti-reverse" Cap analogs 7-methyl(3'-O-methyl)GpppG and 7-methyl (3'-deoxy)GpppG RNA 7: 1486–1495

Su Z, Dannull J, Heiser A, Yancey D, Pruitt S, Madden J, Coleman D, Niedzwiecki D, Gilboa E, Vieweg J (2003) Immunological and clinical responses in metastatic renal cancer patients vaccinated with tumor RNA-transfected dendritic cells. Cancer Res 63: 2127–2133

Thurner B, Roder C, Dieckmann D, Heuer M, Kruse M, Glaser A, Keikavoussi P, Kampgen E, Bender A, Schuler G (1999) Generation of large numbers of fully mature and stable dendritic cells from leukapheresis products for clinical application. J Immunol Meth 223: 1–15

Ulmer JB, Donnelly JJ, Parker SE, Rhodes GH, Felgner PL, Dwarki VJ, Gromkowski SH, Deck RR, DeWitt CM, Friedman A and (1993) Heterologous protection against influenza by injection of DNA encoding a viral protein. Science 259: 1745–1749

Wolff JA, Budker V (2005) The mechanism of naked DNA uptake and expression. Adv Genet 54: 3–20

Wolff JA, Malone RW, Williams P, Chong W, Acsadi G, Jani A, Felgner PL (1990) Direct gene transfer into mouse muscle *in vivo*. Science 247: 1465–1468

Index